Genius of Homeopathy

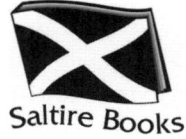
Saltire Books Limited, Glasgow, Scotland

Genius of Homeopathy

by

Francis Treuherz MA, RSHom, FSHom

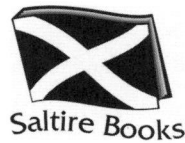

Saltire Books Limited, Glasgow, Scotland

Published by Saltire Books Ltd

18–20 Main Street, Busby, Glasgow G76 8DU, Scotland
books@saltirebooks.com   www.saltirebooks.com

Cover, Design, Layout and Text © Saltire Books Ltd 2010

 is a registered trademark

First published 2010

Typeset by Type Study, Scarborough, UK in 11 on 13½ Dyadis
Printed by Information Press Ltd, Eynsham, Oxford, UK

ISBN-978 0 95 590652 7

All rights reserved. Except for the purpose of private study, research, criticism or review, as permitted under the UK Copyright, Designs and Patent Act 1988, no part of this publication may be reproduced, stored or transmitted in any form or by any means, without prior written permission from the copyright holder.

The publisher makes no representation, express or implied, with regard to the accuracy of the information contained in this book and cannot accept any legal responsibility or liability for any errors or omissions that may be made.

The right of Francis Treuherz to be identified as the author of this work has been asserted in accordance with the UK Copyright, Designs and Patent Act 1988.

A catalogue record for this book is available from the British library

For Saltire
Project Development: Lee Kayne
Editorial: Steven Kayne
Design: Phil Barker

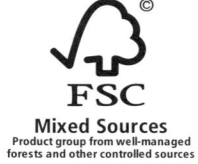

Forest Stewardship Council is a non-profit international organisation established to promote the responsible management of the world's forests. Products carrying the FSC label are independently certified to assure consumers that they are sourced from forests managed to meet the social, economic and ecological needs of present and future generations.

CONTENTS

	Foreword	vii
	Preface	ix
	About the Author	xi
	Acknowledgements	xiii
	Notes on the Text	xv
1	Introduction	1
2	Examples of Hahnemann's Communications	13
3	The Life Force, Hahnemann's Method	39
4	Hering's Preface to Hahnemann's *Chronic Diseases*	55
5	Prefaces to the British and American Editions of the *Organon*	67
6	Homeopathic Reminiscences	79
7	Memorial	87
8	*Ecce Medicus*	99
9	Hahnemann as a Medical Philosopher	139
10	Hahnemann as a Scientist by his Chief Translator	165
11	Hahnemann's Work and Results	197
12	Clarke on Revolution	221
13	More Commentary from Dudgeon	241
14	The Sycosis of Hahnemann	259
15	The Clarke Memorial Meeting	273
16	The Porcelain Painter's Son	297
	Index	329

FOREWORD

Walking into Francis Treuherz's home in North London is like walking into the long history of homeopathy. Over his lifetime Francis has respectfully collected thousands of homeopathic texts and items that reflect homeopathy's rich history and profound information. And then to sit down with him and hear him eloquently speak about Hahnemann's life and each contributing homeopath over time is quite an experience too. I have had the fortune to both listen and see his extensive library. Without a doubt he is one of the most knowledgeable and able curators of our history and knowledge. As well, he brings such a deep passion and love for homeopathy to his skills as both a homeopath and an editor. This book reflects that.

The question for someone not so acquainted with the history of homeopathy is where to start and where to finish, in appropriately selecting reading materials from classical authors and biographers. Not to worry, Francis has done so in this book and it is a profound yet delightful read.

Francis has chosen to highlight many writings that are most relevant to the current conflict in which homeopathy is embroiled. He highlights the early period when Hahnemann attempted to turn the tide of hundreds of years of medicine using treatments via opposites and material perspective, changing that to the use of similars and a vitalist approach. This book emphasises the process by which Hahnemann and followers introduced the core principals of energetic medicine.

Hahnemann's little known article on "The Life Force" is one such superlative piece of writing explaining his position on homeopathy versus mechanical science. As if to foretell the skeptics, he succinctly laid out his belief, which we reiterate today.

The life of man, as well as his twofold condition (health and sickness), can never be demonstrated in a manner usual in demonstrating other objects according to definite principles; it cannot be compared with anything else in this world but with itself; it cannot be compared with a wheelwork, with a hydraulic machine, with chemical processes, with decomposition or formation of gases, with a galvanic battery, nor with anything inorganic. Life is in *no respect* controlled by any physical laws, which govern only inorganic substances. (p. 42)

As you can see, this is an important book for our times. I am so happy to see Francis Treuherz actively realise his superb editorial and writing talent in this book.

Louis Klein FSHom
Bowen Island, British Columbia
May 2010

With over 30 years of continuous practice and teaching, Louis Klein is acknowledged as a leader in the homeopathic profession and as an exceptional practitioner. He was awarded a Fellowship of the Society of Homeopaths in recognition of an outstanding contribution and service to homeopathy.

PREFACE

It is tempting to leave Samuel Hahnemann on a pedestal, to present hagiography, to do as some Indian writers do and create a 'guru' figurehead. He has indeed inspired so many. It is hoped that this book will show him in perspective.

As the reader works through the varied biographies a dramatic picture builds up of Hahnemann's life where we know the outcome but are shown the different roads along which he travelled. It is like the story of the blind men and the elephant.[1] Each writer interprets Hahnemann in his own way, but each with such delight and personal and professional fulfillment, and we may learn from them all.

This volume is published to coincide with the 200th anniversary of the first edition of Samuel Hahnemann's *Organon of the Rational Art of Healing* in 1810[2] which was translated into English in 1913.[3] Rather than attempt a new history of homeopathy or a biography of Hahnemann, here is an exhibition of some gems from the forgotten literature of homeopathy. The essays are by or about Hahnemann, his life and work, his philosophy and his *Organon*. These are valuable examples of the early literature of homeopathy, mainly from Britain, enhanced by descriptions of the writers, and exchanges of correspondence between them.

References

1 Saxe, GJ. *Blind Men and the Elephant*: www.wordinfo.info/words/index/info/view_unit/1/?letter=B&spage=3 [accessed 21:28 30.06.2009].
2 Hahnemann, S. *Organon der rationelle Heilkunde*, Leipzig: Arnold, 1810.
3 Hahnemann, S. Wheeler, C. trans., *Organon of the Rational Art of Healing*, London, JM Dent, 1913.

ABOUT THE AUTHOR

Francis Treuherz's initial career was in the youth and social care services of the Jewish community, and as a university teacher of social sciences. On becoming a successful patient of homeopathy, he retrained and, in his own words, "started my life again".

Francis has been in private practice since 1984, and part time in NHS primary care from 1990-2003. He is a Fellow of the Society of Homeopaths, former editor of the journal *The Homeopath* for 10 years, and is currently Board member and Hon Secretary of the Society. He also teaches worldwide and has written many articles, a research report and a book, and helped create specialist software for homeopaths. Francis describes his 'incurable disease' as collecting books on homeopathy, with a library comprising about 8500 volumes.

ACKNOWLEDGEMENTS

Many thanks to Catherine Boyd of Perth, Western Australia, whose invaluable secretarial help continued via the internet after she left NW London.

Thanks to homeopathic colleagues Annette Gamblin, Suse Moebius and Sue Young for their helpful observations and information.

Thanks to Steven Kayne for his extraordinary and conscientious editorial advice.

Thanks to my family for giving me the love, security and strength to continue working.

NOTES ON THE TEXT

Contents
The contents show the date when an article was written with the title, when this differed from the date of first publication or translation into English.

The contributors
Information about each author is given at the beginning of each chapter in the form of obituary notices or excerpts from contemporary or modern biographical sources.

Spelling
The modern spelling of homeopathy has been adopted in the introduction and the titles of this book. The traditional usage of 'homoeopathy' has been retained in the old texts and in proper names. The older form of the diagraph 'œ' has not been used.

Footnotes
Most footnotes to articles reprinted from older journals are reproduced as they appeared.

Photographs
Photographs are of the best quality available.

1

INTRODUCTION

Even without the trappings of modern electronic technology, homeopaths were able to create dozens of journals dealing with homeopathy[1] and thousands of books in many languages.[2] All the homeopathic literature crossed continents and oceans and much was translated.[3] So here are some excerpts. Here also is a selection of contemporary obituaries and appreciations to describe the authors, even if some of these are hagiography in addition to biography.

1755	Hahnemann born
1800	Hering b
1812	Lippe b
1820	Dudgeon b
1828	Dunham b
1830	Pope b
1834	Jones b
1836	Hughes b
1840	Burnett b
1843	Hahnemann died
1853	Clarke b
1877	Dunham d
1880	Hering d
1886	Lippe d
1901	Burnett d
1902	Hughes d
1904	Dudgeon d
1908	Pope d
1912	Jones d
1931	Clarke d

Dates for Stratten, Devrient and Cleave not known.

Figure 1.1 Samuel Hahnemann and his followers

1779	Hahnemann qualified in medicine at Erlangen
1790	First *China* experiment performed (published in 1796)
1805	Publication of *The Medicine of Experience* in German
1805	Publication of *Fragmenta de viribus medicamentorum positivis* in Latin
1805	1793-1805 *Letters to a patient* (translated 1887)
1810	First publication of the *Organon* in German
1821	Hahnemann moved to Köthen
1833	Third edition of the *Organon* in German
1833	Hahnemann: *The genius of the homoeopathic healing art* (translated 1895)
1833	Stratten: Preface to the 4th edition of the *Organon* 1828
1835	Hahnemann arrived in Paris (medal struck)
1836	Hering: Preface to the 4th edition of the *Organon* 1828
1836	Hahnemann: *Homoeopathic Reminiscences* (published 1905)
1839	Jubilee of Hahnemann's medical qualification (medal struck)
1845	Hering: *Preface to Hahnemann's Chronic Diseases* 1828
1865	Lutze's spurious 6th edition of *The Organon*
1865	Dunham: *Memorial*
1880	Burnett: *Ecce Medicus*
1881	Hughes: *Hahnemann as a medical philosopher*
1882	Dudgeon: *Hahnemann, the founder of scientific therapeutics*
1883	Pope: *Hahnemann, his work and his results*
1886	Clarke: *The revolution in medicine*
1887	Dudgeon: *The Hahnemann Oration*
1889	Burnett: *On gonorrhoea in its constitutional aspects*
1890	Clarke: *The two paths in homoeopathy*
1898	Jones: *The porcelain painter's son: a fantasy*

Figure 1.2 Some historical events of homeopathic literary importance

As the following essays make clear, there was no unanimity about how to interpret Hahnemann's life and writings. All the British and other homeopaths whose work is presented here differed markedly in their approaches. We can learn from all of them, even as we can enjoy the controversies, which are also presented. We can better understand their approach to Hahnemann through understanding their life stories. They were closer to Hahnemann than modern historians, they knew Hahnemann or knew someone who knew him.

The essays are presented in chronological order of their original publication, with a further introductory commentary at the start of each chapter. Figures 1.1 and 1.2 show time-lines for each of the authors and their contributions.

The contributions are varied in style and content and chosen for various reasons. Some are by well-known authors most of whose works have been reprinted and are still consulted, and these valuable insights were overlooked. Burnett on sycosis and gonorrhoea is an example. Some are my personal favourites like the last essay by Jones. Other parts illustrate the complex relationships between some of the authors, who are often studied out of context with the modern reader not aware even that they knew each other. I have discovered some from extensive reading, especially the Hahnemann lecture series, which I recently found, and which impelled me to create this collection.

A short biography of Hahnemann follows taken from the *Biographical Cyclopaedia of Homoeopathic Physicians and Surgeons*, published in 1873.[4] The book, originally sold by subscription, was by American author Egbert Cleave[5] and contained 705 short biographies and 65 steel-engraving portraits.

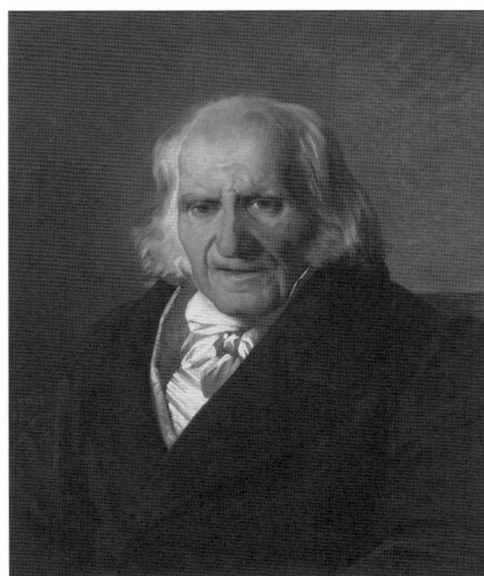

Figure 1.3 Portrait of Christian Friedrich Samuel Hahnemann (1755-1843) by Alexandre Jean-Baptiste Hesse (1806-1879).

Reproduced with the permission of Institut für Geschichte der Medizin, Stuttgart.

About Samuel Hahnemann

Christian Friedrich Samuel Hahnemann was born on the 10th of April, 1755, at Meissen, in Cur-Saxony, one of the most beautiful regions of Germany. Among the papers left behind him is one, dated August, 1791, which gives some interesting particulars respecting his family and early youth.

> *My father, Christian Gottfried Hahnemann, who died four years ago, was a painter in the porcelain manufacture, and had written a little work on that art. He had the soundest ideas on what was to be reckoned good and worthy in man, and had arrived at them by his own independent thought. He sought to*

implant them in me, and impressed on me, more by action than by words, the great lesson of life, 'to act and to be, not merely to seem.' When a good work was going forward, there, often unobserved, he was sure to be helping hand and heart. Shall I not do likewise?

His mother's name was Johanna Christian, née Spiess. His parents taught him to read, and perhaps some other rudimentary education, while he was at play.

He passed several years at the Stadtschule (Town school), and, at the age of sixteen, began to attend the Fürstenschule (Prince's school), of Meissen. He states that he was beloved by his rector, Magister Miller, as if he had been his own son; that he was permitted by him – on account of the delicacy of his health, induced by over study – to omit some of the regular tasks of the school, and to spend the hours they would have occupied in general reading. He had access to him at all hours of the day, and, strange as it may appear, though thus eminently favoured, he was nevertheless a general favourite with the other scholars. His father, he tells us, was opposed to his studies; he wished him to pursue a calling more in accordance with his own income, and frequently withdrew him from school. He was, however, permitted to remain for eight years at the request of his teachers, who allowed him to attend without requiring the usual fees paid by scholars.

Anecdotes of the youth of most great men are on record, which would have but little interest did we not know that 'the boy is father of the man,' and that the bias of mind displayed in youth is usually carried out in after years. Washington had his cherry-tree; Napoleon had his snow-ball matches, and, as the following clearly shows the inherent thirst for knowledge which prevailed in the mind of Hahnemann, we record it.

His parents were very poor, and his father, objecting to the extravagant quantity of oil consumed by his son's nocturnal studies, deprived him of the family lamp, except at stated hours. The youth, however, by exercising his ingenuity, contrived to make a lamp out of clay; and then persuaded his indulgent mother to supply him with oil out of her stores. This determination to overcome difficulties remained as a characteristic trait during his subsequent career.

The time had now arrived for him to enter upon a university course, and, having obtained the permission of his father, he set out for Leipzig, at Easter, in 1775, with twenty crowns in his pocket; the last money he ever received from his parent. This little capital would have lasted for a considerable time; but, like another Gil Blas, he was unfortunately robbed of the greater portion of it.

Thus deprived of the means of existence, he was compelled to support himself at the university by giving lessons and making translations into the German. During the two years of his residence at Leipzig, besides attending lectures the greater part of the day, and giving instruction in the evenings, he translated the following works: Steadman's *Physiological Essays*, Nugent's *Essay on Hydrophobia*, Falconer on the *Waters of Bath*, in two volumes, and Ball's *Modern Practice of Physic*, in two volumes. The only time he could devote to these labours was the night, and he was in the habit of sitting up altogether every alternate night. Such indefatigable industry is astonishing and almost unparalleled. Notwithstanding the difficulties in his path, he contrived by his abstemious habits and incredible exertions to save sufficient money to carry him to Vienna, where he studied under Dr Quarin and practised in the hospitals for two years, when his necessities compelled him to accept the offer of Baron von Bruckenthal, Governor of Transylvania, to accompany him to Hermanstadt, as his private physician, librarian, and superintendent of a museum of coins. From Hermanstadt he went to Erlangen, where he took his degree of Doctor of Medicine, on the 10th of August 1779.

The real history of his life may now be said to commence, as, after leaving Erlangen, he first began the practice of medicine at Hetstadt, a little town among the mountains; but, that place proving much too circumscribed a sphere of action, he removed to Dessau, where he remained but a short time, being tempted by the offer of a governmental appointment of District Physician, at Gommern. The position was almost a nominal one, and of little importance in his life; save that in this place he fell in love with Henrietta Bücklerin, whom he married. In 1784, he went to Dresden, where he resided for four years, maintaining himself chiefly by his pen. Here he wrote eighteen treatises, the most remarkable one being on a new salt of mercury, which he called *Mercurius solubilis*; a name it still retains. We next find him in Leipzig, in 1789, ten years after taking his degree. Here he applied himself with his accustomed energy and industry to the study of medicine, chemistry, mineralogy, and other kindred sciences – besides continuing to make translations from foreign languages – making many important discoveries, which gained for him a high and widely spread reputation among the *savants* of Europe, and also a membership, of the Leipzig Society of Economical Science, and some others.

In spite of all this, he seems at this time to have been inspired by some innate conception of the future. He was dissatisfied with the existing state of medical science, which he considered as imperfect and more the result of guesswork than of positive knowledge. At length, the truth dawned upon him, and an inkling of the theory, which he subsequently elaborated with so much care, toil, and personal suffering, was revealed to him.

His attention was drawn to the fact that cinchona, or Peruvian bark – a well known remedy in cases of intermittent fever- when taken by persons in sound health, produced a disorder very similar to that disease; but, as the district where this occurred was malarious, he was not certain that these effects might not have been produced by natural causes. In order to be assured on this point, he tools a quantity of the drug, and was inexpressibly gratified to find himself severely attacked by the disorder. He was now in possession of a tangible fact; a remedy that would cure a certain disease, would also produce it in a healthy person, and it was certain that the converse was equally true, i.e. that a drug, which produced a certain disease in a healthy body, would cure it in a sick one. But this was only one instance and might be an exception. He therefore set himself to the task of testing a great number of drugs, and with heroic self-sacrifice took them himself, carefully noting the minutest effects produced, and comparing them with the symptoms of well-known diseases. By this means a species of code was established. He likewise induced some of his friends to join him in these tests or *provings*, and by mutually comparing notes certain positive facts were established. This was the origin of the famous axiom that *similia similibus curantur*, which, with his theory of infinitesimal doses, was destined to subvert the existing order of things, and so embittered the medical world, as to draw upon its author ridicule, abuse, and even persecution. In this he merely suffered the fate of most discoverers and inventors. Galileo was forced by the inquisition to recant the heresy of his theory, that the earth revolved around the sun; but on leaving its halls, he muttered, "nevertheless it moves;" Columbus was ridiculed for believing in the existence of a new world, and the man who first proposed to cross the Atlantic by means of steam was laughed at. There is scarcely less folly in denying the motion of the earth, the existence of a new world, or the passage of the Atlantic by steam, than in refusing to give credence to the manifest truths of the Hahnemannian theory.

To this new system of cure Hahnemann gave the name of Homoeopathia, derived from two Greek words, *homoios*, similar, and *pathos*, feeling, or suffering.

Seven years afterwards he published his first trial of the application of the new system in Hufeland's *Journal*. The case was one of colicodynia in its severest form, and after trying in vain all the usual remedies, he cured his patient by administering *Veratrum album*, a drug which produces similar symptoms. The next case noticed, also a very remarkable one, was in 1799. The patient was attacked by scarlet fever, and Hahnemann, having observed that children who ate the berries of the *Belladonna*, suffered from eruptions similar to those incident to the disease itself, administered the extract as a remedy with perfect success, and, furthermore, he found that by giving it in proper doses to persons in infected districts, it prevented them from being seized with the disorder. Notwithstanding much opposition, many German physicians tried this preventive; the result being that out of 3747 persons exposed to the infection only 91 took the disease. If *Belladonna* be fairly tried, it may perhaps prove as successful against scarlet fever, as vaccination has shown itself against smallpox. It was Hahnemann who first recommended *Aconite* in cases of pure inflammatory fevers, with or without eruption; "and," says a recent writer, "even were we under no other obligation to him, he would, like Jenner, deserve to be ranked among the greatest benefactors of suffering humanity." He spent his whole life, after the age of forty-five, in the utmost self-abnegation, giving up everything, denying himself everything, suffering everything, in the cause of humanity. Mathiolus, of old, poisoned criminals, given up to him by the state; the modern Magendie poisoned dogs and cut up horses by vivisection; and some physicians poison their patients by experiments in the interest of science; but Hahnemann poisoned himself to perfect the system he was promulgating. He has left us a record of no less than *one hundred and six* medicinal substances with which he had experimented on his own person. And yet, this man has been called an immoral scoundrel. He has, however, left ten volumes of the *Materia Medica Pura* to disprove so odious a falsehood.

In a letter to Dr Stapf, not intended for publication, he says: "The man who undertakes and carries through with steadfast resolution to benefit humanity – for, in my case, there could be no other motive, since beyond the miserable sum given me by the booksellers, which was no compensation for a life of such self-sacrifice, I met only with persecution – a man that so lives and works must be good at bottom."

Jean Paul Richter says: *"His detractors are more given to detest the man than to read his works."*

Such accusations are mere blinds to cover the real causes of animosity against him, which were that, while at Leipzig, he had performed some remarkable cures on persons of eminence, and his promulgation of the theory of minimum doses, which – impressed with his great responsibility – he would only administer when prepared by himself; the former exciting the jealousy of the medical profession, and the latter touching the pockets of the apothecaries. Amongst them they discovered an obsolete law, forbidding physicians to dispense medicines; thus obliging Hahnemann, whose conscience would not allow him to entrust the preparation of his remedies to other hands, to relinquish a profitable practice in Leipzig, and repair to Köthen. The Duke of Anhalt-Köthen became his friend, giving him full permission to practise as he pleased.

It is not possible in this place to enter into details respecting his great work, which he called the *Organon of Rational Medicine*, and with which the profession is already so familiar; suffice it to say that he incurred much blame for his supposed presumption in endeavouring to assume to himself the position of the Bacon of Medicine. But on reflection this idea will be seen to be erroneous. Bacon introduced a new organ, or instrument, called the *Novum Organum*, for the advancement of science, and Hahnemann justly conceived that he had found a new organ for the discovery of specifics, and the results have fully supported his belief. The *Organon*, with its four propositions, has ever been, and, doubtless, will continue to be the text-book of the homoeopathic profession.

We must also summarily dismiss the *Materia Medica Pura*, the value of which is so perfectly appreciated by every homoeopathist that, without its aid, all would be at a loss in finding the remedies needed. With its ten volumes it is almost a life study in itself. The *Fragmenta* is a work of less importance, though replete, as is every thing from Hahnemann's pen, with useful information.

In 1805, he published a little work on *The Positive Effects of Medicine*, i.e. the effects produced by drugs on a healthy body. This was written in Torgau; but to make the experiments more perfect, he was compelled to return to Leipzig.

In 1831, the cholera raged with fearful violence in Eastern Europe. Hahnemann suggested the use of *Camphor* as a remedy, which led the way to the trial of the homoeopathic system in some of the hospitals of Russia with the most gratifying results. Again, in 1836, when a similar epidemic prevailed in Vienna, Dr Fleischmann adopted that mode of treatment in the hospital of the Sisters of Charity with even greater success. Mr. Wilde remarks, in connection with this fact, that "on comparing the report made of the treatment of cholera in that hospital, with that of the same epidemic in other hospitals in Vienna, at the same time, it appeared that while two-thirds of those treated by Dr Fleischmann recovered, two-thirds of those treated by the ordinary methods died."

Hahnemann resided fifteen years at Köthen, under the protection of the Duke, pursuing one of the most brilliant careers on record. He was constantly perfecting his system by experiments upon himself and his friends, many of them accompanied with extreme suffering. Not only did he enjoy the highest reputation at home, but the fame of his marvellous cures had spread itself throughout the whole of Europe, so that thousands of strangers of the highest rank flocked from abroad to profit by the advice of the illustrious founder of the new school of medicine. Here one of the most romantic marriages we have heard of took place.

Mademoiselle Marie Melanie D'Hervilly-Gohier, a member of one of the most distinguished families in France, was amongst the number of his patients. She was suffering from an apparently incurable pulmonary complaint and disease of the heart; had consulted almost every physician of eminence in Europe, had tried the climate of Italy, and employed all the ordinary methods of cure without avail, being pronounced by her physicians to be beyond medical aid. Hahnemann effectively mastered the disease in an incredibly short space of time, and, upon her recovery, they were married, when he was in his eightieth year, his wife being some forty-five years his junior. She was charmed with his genius, his manners, and his noble character, and positively adored him till the day of his death. He, on his side, cherished and almost reverenced her; was never tired of speaking of her devotion and her brilliant talents, and regarded her as his ministering angel, as well he might. Shortly after their marriage, he was persuaded by his wife to remove to Paris; not to increase his already oppressive popularity; but, on the contrary, to enjoy that ease and repose his declining years required. They travelled *incognito*, even his immediate friends and pupils being left in ignorance of their destination. His retreat, however, did not long remain undiscovered, and, thenceforward, his doors were daily besieged by throngs of sufferers, anxious to benefit by the skill of the great innovator. Indeed, such was the pressure upon him that, without the aid of his wife, he could not have borne it. We are indebted to the pen of an American lady, Helen Berkley, for a delightful and graphic picture of their joint lives in Paris. She saw them frequently both in private and during their hours of business.

Madame Hahnemann was a woman in every way worthy of her husband, and possessed of most extraordinary talents. Wealthy in her own right, she refused to participate in her husband's fortune; a poetess of no mean order, and an artist, whose paintings had been admitted into the galleries of the Louvre. She spoke and wrote fluently five or six languages, and had studied the homoeopathic system under her husband to such advantage, that she

> took almost the entire burden of consultation from his shoulders. She was always present at his receptions, putting questions, receiving replies, and noting minutely the symptoms of every case, merely appealing to Hahnemann in cases of difficulty, when he would reply, "yes, my child," or, "good, my child," and the consultation proceeded; she was tenderly beloved by her step children, and in short a family so united is rarely to be met with.
>
> At this period he was eighty-four years of age, of a slender and diminutive form. His head was large and beautifully proportioned; his forehead broad and massive, set off by a few silvery locks; his eyes deep set, dark, piercing and animated, and his whole appearance indicative of the highest order of genius. He constantly smoked a long pipe with a painted bowl, even during his hours of reception. He read and wrote without the use of spectacles; his handwriting was firm and delicate – almost equal to copperplate – and his activity and animation still exhibited some of the traces of youth.
>
> Hahnemann continued to reside in Paris till his death, that occurred on 2nd July 1843. In his last illness, he was waited on by his devoted wife, with that loving care, which tended so much to alleviate his sufferings. Shortly before his death, his wife, by way of imparting some comfort to the invalid, whispered: "Surely some mitigation of suffering is due to you who have alleviated the sufferings of so many." To this he replied with his latest breath "Every man on earth works as God gives him strength, and meets from man with a corresponding reward; but no man has a claim at the judgment Seat of God. God owes me nothing. I owe him much – yea all."
>
> With these beautiful sentiments on his lips he departed, and the world was deprived of one of the noblest, purest, and grandest characters that have ever ministered to the good of humanity.

There were statues and commemorations to Samuel Hahnemann around the world.[10] In 1855, on the 100th anniversary of his birth, crowds gathered in Meissen in celebration (see figure 1.4 below). In 1900 the only statue of a doctor on Capitol Hill in Washington DC was erected at Scott Circle by the American Institute of Homeopathy. It was restored and rededicated in the year 2000.

Introduction 11

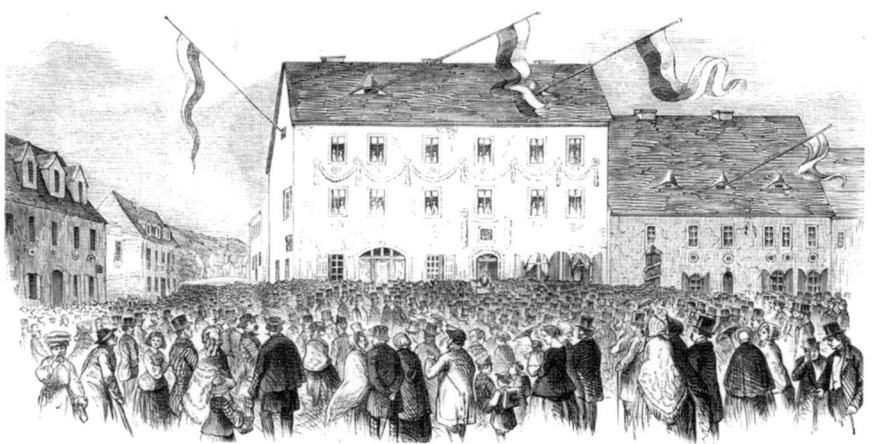

Figure 1.4 Celebration in Meissen of the 100th anniversary of the Birth of Hahnemann.[11] (From the author's personal collection).

References

1. Baur, J. Gypser, K-H. von Keller, G. & Thomas, PW. *Bibliotheca Homoeopathica, International Bibliography of Homoeopathic Literature, volume 1*: Journals, Lyon, Aude Sapere, 1984.
2. Bradford, TL. *Homoeopathic Bibliography of the United States for the year 1825 to the year 1891 inclusive*, Philadelphia, Boericke & Tafel, 1892.
3. Haehl, R, *Homöopathische Bibliothek Richard Haehl*, Marburg, Elwert & Stargardt, 1955.
4. Rozet, C. *Bibliographie de l'homeopathie, Publications en Langue Française de 1824 a 1984*, Lyon, Boiron, 1984.
5. Rabanes, O. & Sarembaud, A. *Dictionnaire des auteurs d'ouvrages d'homeopathie en langue francaise*, Lyon, Boiron, 2003.
6. Schroers, FD. *Lexikon deutschsprachiger Homöopathen. Herausgegeben vom Institut für Geschichte der Medizin der Robert Bosch Stiftung*, Heidelberg, Haug, 2006.
7. Baur, J. *Un Livre Sans Frontières, Histoire et Metamorphoses de l'Organon de Hahnemann*, Lyon, Boiron, 1991.
8. Cleave, E. *Biographical Cyclopædia of Homoeopathic Physicians and Surgeons*, Philadelphia, Galaxy Publishing, 1873.
9. Kirk, JF. *Allibone's Critical Dictionary of English Literature: A Supplement. British and American authors*. Two volumes. Philadelphia: J.B. Lippincott, 1891.
10. Schweitzer, W. *Ikonographie Sammlung, Dolumentation, Historie und Legenden der Bilder des Hofrates Dr.med habil. Christian Friedrich Samuel Hahnemann*, Haug, Heidelberg 1991.
11. *Illustrirte Zeitung*, Meissen, Mai 1855, p 300.

2

EXAMPLES OF HAHNEMANN'S COMMUNICATIONS

Introduction

Samuel Hahnemann was a good communicator and wrote widely. In this chapter there are examples of his letters to a patient, some notes from the patient concerned and an example of an open letter.

Communications with a patient[1]
(See also Chapter 13)

A book by Thomas Lindsley Bradford and published at Tübingen by Dr Bernhard Schuchardt in around 1887, contains a series of letters written by Hahnemann between the years 1793 and 1805, to a patient ('Mr X') who seems to have been a tailor in Gotha. The patient died in 1851, at the age of 92, and he probably profited by the good advice and treatment of his physician.

The letters, of which a selection is presented here, were written at an interesting period of Hahnemann's career. In 1790 he took the *Cinchona* and in 1796 he published the results of his experiment. In 1805 he began to publish work about similars in *The Medicine of Experience*.[2] The *Organon* appeared in 1810.

Hahnemann appears to care deeply what happens to his patient, and gradually changes therapy, already naturopathic in his approach with his use of cold water and dietary advice, as he begins to use the homeopathic medicines, *Hyoscyamus* and *Opium*. We can share in the demonstration of his concern and care for his patients.

The letters are signed in different ways by Hahnemann; some are dated and have the location at which they were written – others do not.

Georgenthal, 22nd April 1793.

My dear Mr X

You do well to write me full particulars; though you may consider some of the details of a trifling character, they are useful to me. No doubt worry has had a bad effect on you.

Henceforward we shall arrange the treatment in this way, that you will get the powders[3] again made up, but you will only take one every other morning. On the alternate days, take at the same hour in the morning 20 drops of the medicine here prescribed[4] in a teaspoonful of water, increasing the dose each time by two drops. On the evening of the day you take the prescribed pills[5] with a mouthful of water.

Keep up your spirits, and take as much exercise as you can without fatigue.

If you are in the habit of reading in the evening, cease to do so at present. It is not good for you, and it excites your nervous system. I do not approve of your reading even by day. I trust you may soon be better. Write as often as you please: I will answer when I think it necessary. You do not need to pay the messenger; I have made an arrangement with him.

Dr Hahnemann.

Georgenthal, 6th May 1793.

My dear Mr X

You see from your own experience what a bad effect reading, and indeed any mental exertion, has on your nervous system. Avoid it, please, until you are better, which you will be soon. The blood you spat only came from the mouth or the back of the nose, if it was not brought up by coughing; it is only by coughing that anything can come from the lungs, not otherwise.

Be always moderate in eating, but I advise you not to be afraid of any kind of food. Variety in diet is very good for you.

Take a walk between 5 and 6 p.m. before eating a little bread. An important point of diet, I may remind you, is rather to eat a full meal at mid-day, but not in evening. You should bear in mind that it is best to eat chiefly dry bread or a dry roll.

If you have a feeling of tension in the chest, that is usually caused by flatulence in the stomach, nothing more! But in order to get on further with our treatment and so advance towards health, I will add the following directions to the remedies hitherto employed, and which should still be continued.

Every morning just before you take your walk, strip yourself naked, put on a pair of woollen gloves, put on the table before you a basin of fresh spring water, put your gloved hands in it and standing up rub your whole body over with the wet gloves. The first day dip your hands twice in the water, after three days dip them three times, and afterwards more frequently. This rubbing or washing should only be done on the first days for minute or while you can say a pater noster. Then dry yourself quickly, so that no moisture remains on the body, dress rapidly and go out without loss of time.

I would advise you to dress yourself in the lightest clothes you have for your walk. Let the weather be what it will. After the cold washing you will find that the best and most comfortable for walking in. Do this exactly as I have said; you will not regret it.

Eight days after the first washing you may commence to rub yourself for two minutes, not sooner.

Increase the number of drops until it tastes a little too acid, then keep to that quantity.

I cannot allow you to visit me until I have changed my residence, which I shall do in ten or twelve days. I am coming nearer to Gotha. I will let you know where.[6]

Farewell, and rely on being cured.

Yours,

Dr Hahnemann.

My dear Mr X

It will now be much better that you take your bath quite early, before the sun is powerful, and at once to for your walk after drinking a cup of coffee. You may eat a couple of rolls after your walk. Your strength seems still insufficient, so you had better discontinue sawing wood for the present.

I have no objection to your taking a pill every other night, but I believe that your sleeplessness is more owing to over-exertion and the heat of the weather, than to the pills. But we continue them now only every other day.

Tell me if a single glass of wine makes you hot. If it does then I would like you always to take one at dinner time.

As the itching has ceased do not take a hip bath at present.

Does your morning cup of coffee cause no commotion in your blood – no heat? Drink once or twice three cups and see what effect they have.

Don't forget to open the windows of your bedroom during the day, and of your working room at night.

Yours very truly,

Dr Hahnemann.

My dear Mr X

It is evident from your last letter, as I suspected, that coffee does not agree with you, and that you would do well to diminish your morning allowance to one cup. After doing so for fourteen days, you may for the same length of time drink a cup every other day, and after that if possible leave it off altogether. Instead of it you may drink what you will – a couple of cups of boiled milk, or nothing at all, or a mouthful of water. But you ought not to discontinue the use of coffee more rapidly than I have said.

As regards wine, I see very well that you must be very moderate. But I do not wish you to leave it off altogether. As you no longer take the powders with their accompanying glass of wine, you may try every day at dinner a wine-glassful of half wine half water, and go on thus till I see you again.

If you can come here some day soon, and let me know the day before, I shall be much pleased. Continue to take the drops and pills.

You may now increase the drops, and that as rapidly as possible, so as to attain the largest portion the taste will permit. Then remain at that, and continue without change for several days, but get a fresh supply from the Chemist's, and keep it for future use.

As regards bed clothes at night, you should adapt the quantity to your feelings, but you should rather lie cool than hot. If you can avoid perspiring without much trouble, that would be advantageous.

You do well to take the pills only every other night; should you be restless the nights you don't take a pill, then you might take one at night and see what effect it has.

As regards exercise, you may increase or diminish that according to your feelings, always bearing in mind that exercise is necessary for your health.

Do not make use of electricity at present, your system is too irritable for that.

Tell me exactly how the morning washing agrees with you; I think you might now use it more vigorously.

Above all be of good courage, it will all come right.

Yours,

Dr Hahnemann.

My dear Mr X

I would like you to drink pure milk; you will by-and-by find benefit from it.

Continue to take the drops as before. You do not need to drink more than your thirst requires.

Observe if the toothache comes on from a chill after the bath. Get through with it quickly and energetically, use a good deal of force in rubbing with your hands, even when you have washed yourself all over. Dry yourself quickly and strongly; dress yourself rapidly and go for your walk. Do not be sparing of the cold water. I would prefer that you should pour the water all over your body.

I send herewith a fresh supply of pills for you to go on with as before, and remain

Yours,

Dr Hahnemann.

The following directions of the doctor given on the 7th July 1793 were written by the patient

After having washed myself over with my hands in the morning, I should on the first three days pour three handfuls of water over me, and after three days an additional handful every day; after five days two additional handfuls up to ten handfuls, thereafter I should do the same with a jugful of water, and go on increasing the quantity up to 20 jugfuls. I should also wash my face and neck, and dip my face several times in water.

Any morning, if my appetite is good, I may eat an additional roll, and at 3 p.m., if I have appetite, I may eat half a meal.

> I should not drink my wine and water at dinner, but half and three-quarters of an hour thereafter. I should increase the drops every day by three until I come to 100, then go on with that amount, measuring that quantity, or thereabouts, in a spoon. I am to take one day two pills, then wait two days, and the third day again two, and observe the effect.

This letter, which is undated, seems to belong to this period, though in Schuchardt's book it is placed much further on.

> My dear Mr X
>
> I send you six pills, of which you will take one every morning if they do not cause you any great discomfort, and let me know how they act before you have taken them all.
>
> Let me know if you have your electric machine in the house. I would very much like Secretary Kayser[7] to make a trial of electricity. Be so good as to help him to it. He is rather clumsy but deserves compassion. I would charge him with electricity and draw simple sparks from the renal and cardiac regions. You should get him to come to you.
>
> Yours,
>
> Dr H.

> My dear Mr X
>
> I am very glad that you have seen Mr Secretary Schröder. He is an intelligent man. Get him to lend you a spark-drawer, the blunt end of which is cased in wood, and when you are charged with electricity let it be passed over all the weak parts through the clothes. This will cause conduction without your feeling it; he will tell you how to do it. But the machine must be very powerful in order to do you good. This drawing out of sparks must be done with the hand of another person. Let Mr Schröder give you slight sparks with the Leyden jar, in order that you may learn how it is done. For when simple drawing out of sparks ceases to have any effect you must proceed to slight shocks.

You can apply to the chilblains in your fingers some petroleum, which you can get from the druggist.

Come soon to see me. For the enclosed thaler we will feel obliged to you to get for us some butter and six good sausages, and six groschen worth of the dark gray wool for the purpose of darning the women's stockings you sent us, and six groschen worth of the pale gray wool similar to that of the two pairs of children's socks.

Dr Hahnemann.

My dear Mr X

You have done right to take only three pills; we cannot go further with them. Your strength should now be restored; but as long as you have uneasy dreams you should continue to take the night pills; you may now take two if necessary.

But I should like to know how it is with your gouty symptoms, whether the morning pills have had any effect on them. If possible increase your cold bath and douche yourself with a jugful.

If the machine is in order electrify yourself as directed.

Yours truly,

Dr Hahnemann.

In the final paragraph of the following letter Hahnemann refers to some plants that he evidently desired for his garden in Molschleben, a small village not far from Gotha, where lived at this time

---

My dear Mr X

When you were electrified did you stand on an insulator under which there was glass or rosin? That is essential. You ought not to feel shocks; the sparks may be drawn from you with the finger if you find that the ball makes too large sparks. And if this should cause heat, then let yourself be charged with electricity for a quarter of an hour only, whilst you stand on the insulator protected by glass or pitch, without having sparks taken from you. I have sent you a prescription for a powder, of which you will take every morning a heaped teaspoonful.

We beg you to send us 45 plants of curly kale, 15 of kohlrabi, and 20 of blue cabbage – all with the roots. Enclosed are 16 groschen to pay for them, with thanks for the trouble.

Yours truly,

Dr Hahnemann.

My dear Mr X

The reason why sparks cannot be drawn from you, is probably the weakness of the machine, or the stative on which you stand and on which you should be isolated has some dust or moisture upon it, or if it is a cake of rosin it has perhaps some cracks in it; or if the stative has glass feet these are either cracked, or dusty, or moist. It must depend on one of these things, or maybe you have some pointed piece of metal about you, whereby the electricity escapes. If you cannot find where the fault is yourself, you must get an expert to examine it. Sparks can be drawn from a lifeless body, why not from you?

You can now discontinue the afternoon drops, and instead take daily at the usual time a heaped teaspoonful of the powder in the accompanying prescription in anything you please; it will act as a tonic. Only keep up your courage.

Yours truly,

Dr Hahnemann.

My dear Mr X

As merely charging yourself with electricity has no effect, you may now try drawing sparks from your body. Commence with a few, and go on increasing them. Do you still continue to take your bath and walk?

Yours truly,

Dr Hahnemann.

My dear Mr X

Although you have experienced no improvement as yet, from this time you must make progress. I do not give up. I hope too that you will do exactly as I tell you.

Go on with the powders and pills. But as regards your diet, that must be attended to henceforth. For the next eight days take only half as much meat and meat soup as you have been accustomed to take. When these eight days have elapsed tell me exactly how much of each you have consumed during the week, I well then send you further instructions.

Eat the rolls you have for breakfast henceforth without butter. For supper you should have only plain bread with a little salt, as much as you have appetite for.

Continue your exercise in the open air, but do not increase it. I should like you to try and get some genuine Hungarian wine. You may take daily a tablespoonful of it, at the time when you feel a particular want of strength.

I expect your answer at the time fixed. Put your trust only in God and me, and I rely on your sense and obedience, which has hitherto been exemplary. You will soon be better.

Yours truly,

Dr Hahnemann.

My dear Mr X

I advise you to continue your morning drops, your evening pill and your bath; leave off all the rest. But I would like you to try the electricity occasionally, in the same way as you lately used it, that is, merely charging yourself with electricity, but without drawing sparks. Do it one or twice a week. If it makes you worse you may leave it off, but if it does not do when used in that way, I advise you to try little shocks, they must not be bigger than the thickness of a straw.

Keep up your courage, all will come right. If this does not do, I am not at the end of my resources.

Yours, &c.,

Dr Hahnemann.

My dear Mr X

Probably your toothache and other pains come from a chill. If they should persist or return, go to bed and take every quarter of an hour a cupful of elderflower tea, pretty strong, about two ounces of the flowers to a quart of boiling water. As soon as you experience relief to the pain or get into a gentle perspiration, leave off the tea.

As regards bedclothes you must arrange that according to the weather, but you should always be covered in such a manner that you should not feel hot under the bedclothes, but on the other hand you should never feel cold. That would not be good.

In place of the drops, which you may now leave off, every morning, at a convenient time, take of the enclosed powder as much as will lie on the tip of a penknife, rubbed on a piece of bread, or in water. If after some days it would cause constipation, leave it off for a day or two and take instead the acid drops. But if your bowels continue to act, even though scantily, continue the powder.

As regards the night pills you must increase the number till you find that you get tranquil nights, then stick to that number.

Continue the bath and do not alter its strength. Let me hear from you again. Keep up your courage and listen occasionally for quarter of an hour to good music, or entertain yourself in conversation with your friends. Eat any nourishing food.

Dr Samuel Hahnemann.

My dear Mr X

If the salt is not dissolved then add some more water until it dissolves, you should not throw any of it away.

You may now diminish the quantity of the drops, taking 10 drops fewer every day until you come to 60 drops, then continue to take that quantity.

What I told you about Reinicke is the truth. Nessler,[8] too, keeps this medicine.

Go on with the electricity and keep up your courage.

I remain, yours truly,

Dr Hahnemann.

The following directions on the 22nd September 1794 were written in the patient's handwriting.

> I must for a week have small sparks and then gradually larger ones drawn from me, especially from the jaw.
>
> I may take a douche-bath and a walk at noon again.
>
> As I have in the morning a bad taste and a white tongue, I must continue to eat less at supper till they are gone.
>
> I should dress myself according to the weather.
>
> If the tearing pains in the jaw return, I may apply leeches to the edge near the ear.

> My dear Mr X
>
> Do not think that I have forgotten you. I can understand that your old ailment has not yet gone, although you have undoubtedly not neglected to take the strengthening remedies. In order to afford you complete relief, I enclose a medicine I have carefully prepared for your case, which you are to use along with the cold washing and the acid drops. You will take of this black powder on the point of a knife about as much as a vetch in size, put it on your tongue and drink a mouthful of water to send it down. Do this for eight days every other evening. Then for fourteen days take it every third evening, and then for four weeks every fourth evening. At the same time continue the strengthening remedies, the walking exercise, etc., and at the end of seven weeks tell me how you feel. I hope with all my heart that you will be in the best of health.
>
> Dr Sam. Hahnemann.
>
> Now in Pyrmont (where I think I shall remain).

> *19th October 1794.*
>
> My dear Mr X
>
> I am sorry that you have not quite satisfactorily recovered. It will all come right. I send herewith the prescription for the night pills. Reinicke will make them up for you very well. Get a small pair of scales with little weights from

one grain to 20. I will then send you a powder, and you can weigh out the proper quantity. Your bath should not now be so strong, since your strength is diminished.

I wish you everything that is good.

Dr Hahnemann.

My dear Mr X

Before sending you the powder, you must first take the accompanying drops. About 4 p.m., take 50 drops stirred up in a cupful of water, and continue to take this medicine daily, increasing the dose by 10 drops every day, until the taste ceases to be pleasant, then stick to this quantity.

Take of the pills as many as are required to act satisfactorily. Keep up your spirits.

Yours truly,

Dr Hahnemann.

My dear Mr X

I am pleased to think that you remember me. God will again help you.

In order to go rightly to work, you should just take one of the No. 1 powders in the morning. The following morning take a second powder, then wait a day and observe carefully if immediately after the powder the cough is aggravated, but becomes better than usual in the afternoon, or if on the first day the cough is less frequent, or milder, or more severe, &c.; if your breathing becomes tighter, also if you have any new symptoms. After the day when you take no medicine, take 5 drops of the medicine marked No. 2 in the morning, when the cough commences, and then 5 more every two hours, until the cough evidently increases or evidently diminishes, in either case stop taking them. The following day do the same, but the day after that omit them entirely; next day take one of the No. 3 powders, one in the morning another in the afternoon, next day again two, the day after that omit the medicine and observe all the alternations in your health. You may continue to take two *Hyoscyamus* pills at night. You may leave off the both at present, but keep up your spirits.

Next time you write send me back the prescription, or a copy of it, so that I may remember it.

Yours truly,

Dr Hahnemann.
Königslutter, near Brunswick, 6th October 1796.

K'lutter, 3rd November 1796.

My dear Mr X

I have missed the last post. I write today to tell you not to go on with Nos. 1 and 2. I would rather advise you to resume the use of No. 3, but if you do not find any benefit after taking it for four days, stop it and take of the powders for which I enclose a prescription[9] one about 9 a.m. and another about 3 p.m. in beer. After taking them for eight days write me again. You will be able to judge if the acid drops do your cough any good, I doubt if they will.

Wishing the best result.

Dr Hahnemann.

My dear Mr X

If only you had not left off the *Arnica* powders. That is the best tonic for you. I do not know if you have taken a whole powder at once daily, or how you have done; but that does not matter. Thenceforward take the powders as I directed, but one hour before bedtime take one-third of the daily portion (in addition to the usual daily portion), and if after three or four days you find it agree you may then take half of the daily portion once in the morning. If you require the *Hyoscyamus* pills you may still take them, but somewhat later. You will soon feel if you require them. Write soon.

Yours, &c.,

Dr Hahnemann.

Königslutter, 5th May 1797.

My dear Mr X

Go on with the *Arnica* powders, and take the *Hyoscyamus* pills when you need them to procure sleep.

In order to try something to allay your cough when it is worse than usual, I send you herewith a powder, of which you will take one grain at a time (you have got scales and weights?) once, twice, or thrice daily. While you do this you will leave off the *Arnica* powders. Perhaps this will make you sleep better, but you must not take acids at the same time. Tell me how you are in about three weeks.

Poor Kayser is much to be pitied. Please remember me and mine kindly to M. Zeyss, also to Mr Becker.[10] Farewell.

Dr Hahnemann.

P.S. – Keep this powder in a corked bottle. If the powder does you good you may take less of it; you may even leave it off entirely, and remain for some time without medicine (except, perhaps, the *Hyoscyamus* pills). When necessary go back to the *Arnica* or to the white powder, &c.

My dear Mr X

I send you more of the same powder; use it with judgment. Perhaps it will do your cough good. If it does not seem to answer go back to the *Arnica*.

Poor Kayser seems to be in sad state. God help him!

Farewell, and write soon to yours truly,

Dr Hahnemann.
Königslutter, 28th June 798.

My dear Mr X

As you are so very cautious in your use of medicine, I may safely leave it to yourself to make one more trial of the white powder. It will not weaken you, that you may depend upon. But if it does not agree with you, try what taking half a dose more of *Arnica* will do for you. I think the full dose was 7 grains, so the half dose will be between 3 and 4 grains. Perhaps that will do more for you.

I have had no more news of Mr Kayser; is he dead*?
I heartily wish you the best results.

Your most devoted servant,

Dr Hahnemann.
Königslutter, 29th July 1798.

*Note by Mr X.
Mr Kayser was buried on the 6th August.

Königslutter, 1st Sept.

My dear Mr X

The improvement in your health gives me great pleasure, and I thank you very much for what you have sent me. Go on with the *Arnica* powder. But if the cough does not improve, or even seems to be aggravated, take the *Arnica* powder only every other day, and on the intermediate days take the medicine for which I enclose the prescription. Should you like to take the cough powder for several successive days, you may do so, you will then be able to observe better what it does for you. At first take half a powder in the early morning and the other half at 2 p.m. If it does not suffice in two days then you may take half a powder in water at 10 a.m., and if this is not enough you may take another half at 5 p.m. This will certainly allay your cough. At the same time notice if this makes you wakeful at night or causes any other symptoms. It will assuredly, in any case, do you good.

With every good wish,

Dr H.

Königslutter, 10th Sept. 1798.

My dear Mr X

I much obliged to you for the 10 thalers sent. Even though the increased quantity of *Arnica* powder may have increased your cough somewhat, I advise you continue it for the present. In course of time it will allay your cough all the more. If after a few weeks my prophecy should not prove correct, write me again, so that I may give you further advice. As far as I can judge from your description, your cough is tolerably moderate, and you have nothing to fear from it. Tell me at the same time how it is with your dry chills and heats. If you have had any return of them let me know if they were benefited by the white powder, also if you have regained your strength. In the meantime, I remain, with esteem.

Your friend,

Dr Sam. Hahnemann.

My dear Mr X

You have not acted well to consult another doctor, I don't care who he may be. You have such an irritable system that the slightest improper treatment, even though it be only external, will affect you as much as, or more, than a two years' old child; and without boasting I may say that you would long ago have been in your grave if I had not studied your really uncommon and ticklish constitution.

If you are again in the enjoyment of a tolerable sate of healthy, you may be pleased; you cannot expect ever to possess perfectly unchangeable health, which few indeed enjoy. The clay of which you are made is infinitely more delicate than that of other men.

Now, as regards your knee, I will not enumerate all the errors that have been committed in the treatment of it. Leave off all the remedies instantly; cover the naked skin with some blue taffety made like a wide little boot or boot-leg, which should envelope the joint all round and cover it loosely, and some inches above and below it. All the other covering of the trousers must be very loose and comfortably warm. Thus it must remain until it has got into the state it was before you used the remedies. Try if you can at the same take the arnica powders. Take some *very slight* exercise; as much as you can bear without particular distress. You must not kneel any more, though I will not assert that the malady has been brought on by doing so. As soon as it is better write me again; also if it does not improve write me. Keep up your courage, it will assuredly come all right.

Be so kind as to beg Mr Ettinger[11] to insert this report[12] in his paper as soon as possible. Give my kind regards to Mr Becker and beg him to send me a copy of the *Reichsanzeiger* in which the notice appears.[13]

(Unsigned)

Note by Mr X
Received on the 4th October 1789

My dear Mr X

It is well that you have confessed. That is the first step towards amendment. Henceforth, and, if possible, for the remainder of your life, take a walk every day if you can, if not every other day, and never neglect doing so.

Continue to treat your knee as directed; cover it with silk, but not tightly. You must see that the whalebone bandage you mention does not press in the hollow behind the knee, and helps the swelling; but I will not answer for it. Don't be anxious about it, avoid kneeling, take the needful exercise in the open air and think no more about it. If, after the lapse of some time, the swelling does not yield to the silk dressing you should electrify the naked swelling in such a way that *small* shocks are sent from one end of the swelling to the other, consequently, only a few inches through the swelling in all directions, but not beyond it. As regards medicine, stick to the arnica if nothing prevents you.

Let me hear soon how you feel. You will soon be better, only keep up your courage!

Many thanks for your enclosure, and believe me to be your good friend,

Dr Hahnemann.

Königslutter, December 15, 1798.

I am glad to hear that you children are well, and they will remain so if you bring them up in a robust manner, letting them work more with their hands than with their head. Give them my kind regards and your dear wife especially.

My dear Mr X

I can give you no better advice than to go on in the manner I have told you, and which you inform me you are doing. Avoid all pressure and all tight bandages. Continue the same diet and regimen, and mind you *take your walks in the open air*. All will go on as well as possible, that is to say, you will constantly improve. It is all a work of time and keeping up your courage.

When I see that it is time to do so, I will allow you to employ electricity, not sooner.

I beg you to believe me your faithful friend.

Dr Hahnemann.
KL, 22nd January 1799.[14]

My dear Mr X

Today I make you my confidant. Kindly give the enclosed letter as soon as you can to the Minister von Frankenberg, if he is still alive, but if Zigesar is in his place, give it to him, but before doing so have the goodness to write the name of the present First Minister in Latin characters on the envelope in the blank space. I was not quite sure if Frankenberg is still living, otherwise I would have written his name myself. I am applying in this letter for Dr Buchner's[15] post with the Duke, and would like to return to Gotha in that capacity, for I have always preferred Gotha to Brunswick. But it is impossible for me to have an excuse for changing my abode unless I get an appointment of this sort. But do not let anyone know a world about all this, in order that no intrigues may be set on foot, as would certainly happen. But how will you manage to get this letter at once and with certainty into Frankenberg's hands? As it is, the news of Buchner's death reached me a week later than it ought, so I must now lose no time. Forgive me for the trouble I am putting you to, and with best wishes I remain,

Your most devoted servant,

Dr Hahnemann.

14th March 1799.

My dear X

It is true that I am going to Hamburg, but that need not trouble you. If you do not grudge the few groschen a letter will cost, you can still have my advice when I am there. Merely write my name and Hamburg beneath it, and your letters so addressed will find me.

For the present I must say that you are on the fair road to health, and the chief sources of your malady cut off. One source still remains, and it is the cause of your last relapse. Man (the delicate human machine) is not constituted for overwork, he cannot over-work his powers or faculties with impunity. If he does so from ambition, love of gain or other praiseworthy or blameworthy motive, he sets himself in opposition to the order of nature, and his body suffers injury or destruction. All the more if his body is already in a weakened condition; what you cannot accomplish in a week, you can do in two weeks. If your customers will not wait they cannot fairly expect that you will for their sakes make yourself ill and work yourself to the grave, leaving your wife a widow and your children orphans. It is not only the greater bodily exertion that injures you, it is even more the attendant strain on the mind, and the over-wrought mind in its turn affects the body injuriously. If you do not assume an attitude of cool indifference, adopting the principle of living first for yourself and only secondly for others, then there is small chance of your recovery. When you are in your grave, men will still be clothed, perhaps not as tastefully, but still tolerably well.

If you are a philosopher you may become healthy – you may attain to old age. If anything annoys you, give no heed to it; if anything is too much for you, have nothing to do with it; if any one seeks to drive you, go slowly and laugh at the fools who wish to make you unhappy. What you can do comfortably then do; what you cannot do, don't bother yourself about.

Our temporal circumstances are not improved by over-pressure at work. You must spend proportionately more in your domestic affairs, and so nothing is gained. Economy, limitation of superfluities (of which the hard worker has often very few) place us in a position to live with greater comfort – that is to say, more rationally, more intelligently, more in accordance with nature, more cheerfully, more quietly, more healthily. Thus we shall act more commendably, more wisely, more prudently, than by working in breathless hurry, with our nerves constantly overstrung, to the destruction of the most precious treasure, calmly happy spirits and good health.

Be you more prudent, consider yourself first, let everything else be of only secondary importance for you. And should they venture to assert that you are in honour bound to do more than is good for your mental and physical powers, even then do not, for God's sake, allow yourself to be driven to do what is contrary to your own welfare. Remain deaf to the bribery of praise, remain cold and pursue your own course slowly and quietly like a wise and sensible man. To enjoy with tranquil mind and body, that is what man is in the world for, and only to do as much work as will procure him the means of enjoyment – certainly not to excoriate and wear himself out with work.

The everlasting pushing and striving of blinded mortals in order to gain so and so much, to secure some honour or other, to do a service to this or that great personage – this is generally fatal to our welfare, this is a common cause of young people ageing and dying before their time.

The calm, cold-blooded man, who lets things softly glide, attains his object also, lives more tranquilly and healthily, and attains a good old age. And this leisurely man sometimes lights upon a lucky idea, the fruit of serious original thought, which shall give a much more profitable impetus to his temporal affairs than can ever be gained by the overwrought man who can never find time to collect his thoughts.

In order to win the race, quickness is not all that is required. Strive to obtain a little indifference, coolness and calmness, then you will be what I wish you to be. Then you will see marvellous things; you will see how healthy you will become by following my advice. Then shall your blood course through your blood-vessels calmly and sedately, without effort and without heat. No horrible dreams disturb the sleep of him who lies down to rest without highly strung nerves. The man who is free from care wakes in the morning without anxiety about the multifarious occupations of the day. What does he care? The happiness of life concerns him more than anything else. With fresh vigour he asks about his moderate work, and at his meals nothing – no ebullitions of blood, no cares, no solicitude of mind – hinders him from relishing what the beneficent Preserver of life sets before him. And so one day follows another in quiet succession, until the final day of advanced age brings him to the termination of a well spent life, and he serenely reposes in another world as he has calmly lived in this one.

Is not that more rational, more sensible? Let restless, self-destroying men act as irrationally, as injuriously, towards themselves as they please; let them be fools. But be you wiser! Do not let me preach this wisdom of life in vain. I mean well to you.

Farewell, follow my advice, and when all goes well with you, remember

Dr S. Hahnemann.

P.S. – Should you be reduced to your last sixpence, be still cheerful and happy. Providence watches over us, and a lucky chance makes all right again. How much do we need in order to live, to restore our powers by food and drink, to shield ourselves from cold and heat? Little more than good courage; when we have that the minor essentials we can find without much trouble. The wise man needs but little. *Strength that is husbanded needs not to be renovated by medicine.*

Hamburg, 27th July 1800.

Dear Mr X

This moment I have received yours of July 21st, and I see that at the time you had not yet got my letter of July 11th or the medicine. That is the fault of the slow post. Another time I will try to enclose the medicine in a letter, so that you may be able to get them by the post in five days.

Good heavens! What a fierce onslaught Stickler[16] makes with *Opium* on our weak man – and yet he gives *Epsom salts* at the same time! I read your report with horror. What infinite mischief can be wrought by the *continued* and *excessive* use of *Opium* in chronic diseases, I alone am in a position to know; the good young man knows nothing about it. I cannot tell if I can repair the mischief quickly. Excuse haste for the post is just going out.

Do not allow Stickler to interfere any more with our treatment, whether the patient lives or dies.

Mr Wander must have patience with me, for my conscience will not allow me to use such palliatives (in their after consequences injurious) as anodyne and narcotic remedies. If under my treatment the disease seems to get worse, I go the most direct way to work and softly seize hold on the disease by the roots. Adieu, my folk greet yours,

Dr Hahnemann.

Should the bowels not be opened after taking my medicine several days, he must not take any Epsom salts; at the very most he may have a clyster of lukewarm or cool water.

Hamburg, 3rd Aug. 1800.

Dear Mr X

That dear *Opium* and his previous disease have irritated our patient in the highest degree and weakened him almost to death. The very smallest dose of medicine is too strong for him. This is a very serious state of things. Before I can look about me I may at any moment receive the intelligence that he has died suddenly. I write this for your information and in my own defence.

Your friend and servant

S. Hahnemann.

Dear Mr X

You have done well to resume your walks. Persevere with them. The tonic influence of the open air cannot be replaced by diet or medicine. It is for us an indispensable instrument.

For the first four weeks you should eat rather sparely, hardly enough, so that your stomach may recover its proper power. Otherwise I do not wish you to be particular about your food, except that you should avoid those things which never agree with you and which you can easily give up, as for example, sugar. I send you herewith three bottles. For several years past I prepare the medicines so that they have neither taste nor smell. Do not let their tastelessness prejudice you against them. The medicines are very powerful. Take the first morning a drop of No. 1; drop it in a teaspoon and lick it up, just as it is. Next morning take nothing and observe what alteration has taken place in your cough these two days. The third morning (having taken no medicine the previous day) take another drop of No. 1. You will probably have observed the day before rather an aggravation than an amelioration, or some other new symptom which you have not before experienced. In that case, instead of taking the second drop of No. 1, take instead a drop of No. 2. But if you have not noticed any new symptom from the first drop of No. 1, on either the first or second days, and no aggravation of the cough, then take on the third day another drop (the second drop) of No. 1. Then, if you have felt nothing the first two days, this and the following day will assuredly show you whether you have good reason to expect improvement from it. Then you can judge, if it has done good, that you cannot do better than continue to take a drop of No. 1 every other morning until you write to me.

But if, after taking it in the way I have indicated, no improvement has ensured, then you can take No. 2 as directed and continue it in the same manner. If after two doses (one drop every other day) no improvement is observable, you may then take No. 3 in the same way. Whatever does you good, that you should stick to as long as it is useful – not longer. If none of the three does you good, then write me again, if one has proved successful and you have take it all, then write me.

I should like you also to tell me what alteration or what symptoms you have observed from taking the Iceland moss – whether it causes pressure on the chest, or dysponoea, or anything else.

It is possible that you have some acidity of stomach and in that case you would do well to take every evening one of the powders ordered in the accompanying prescription, whatever drops you may be taking at the time. The powders will not interfere with the drops.

I heartily wish and hope to hear of your improvement as your old friend and servant,

Dr Hahnemann.
Torgau, 21st June 1805.

Dear X

You can now resume your usual meals, only not too much at supper-time. Continue your walking exercise. All this you will be able to do now that your health is so much improved. If the cough is allayed, you can take No. 1 twice a week, and after two weeks only once. You will not require the powders any longer. Your strength will soon be completely restored, as I am convinced you will tell me when you write me again in a few weeks.

Your most devoted friend,

Dr Hahnemann.
Torgau, 4th Aug. 1805.

This concludes the correspondence with the patient.

Public communication

Dr Schuchardt gives a letter in his book, which Hahnemann caused to be inserted twice in the newspaper *Reichsanzeiger*.

He commissioned his patient, Mr X, to pay for it, and a memorandum of the payment was found among X's papers, from which we find that Hahnemann had to pay 1 thaler, 8 groschen for the two insertions.

(The thaler was a silver coin used throughout Europe for almost four hundred years and minted in Saxony until 1872. It comprised 30 groschen)

The letter, which is reproduced below is interesting because it shows that Hahnemann was exposed, like many other doctors, to have advice stolen from him without remuneration, and that he adopted very effectual means for putting a stop to such fraudulent conduct.

Complaint and Resolve

Dear Public!

It will scarcely be credited that there are people who seem to think that I am merely a private gentleman with plenty of time on my hands, whom they may pester with letters, many of which have not the postage paid, and are consequently a tax on my purse, containing requests for professional advice, to comply with which would demand much mental labour and occupy precious time, while it never occurs to these inconsiderate correspondents to send any remuneration for the time and trouble I would have to expend on answers by which they would benefit. In consequence of the ever-increasing importunity of these persons I am compelled to announce:

1. That henceforward I shall refuse to take in any letters which are not post paid, let them come from whom they may.
2. That after reading through even paid letters from distant patients and other seeking advice, I will send them back unless they are accompanied by a sufficient fee (at least a Friedrich's d'Or) in a cheque or in actual money, unless the poverty of the writer is so great that I could not withhold my advice without sinning against humanity.
3. If lottery tickets are sent to me, I shall return them all without exception; but I shall make the post office pay for all the expense of the remission, and the senders will get them back charged with this payment.

Samuel Hahnemann, Doctor of Medicine.
Altona, by Hamburg, 9th Nov. 1799.

References and notes

1 Published in the *Monthly Homoeopathic Review*, 1887; 31: 543-557 & 615-623. Discussed by RE Dudgeon in his *Hahnemann Oration* of 1887 in Chapter 13 of this book.
2 Hahnemann, S, *The Medicine of Experience 1805* in *The Lesser Writings of Samuel Hahnemann*, trans Dudgeon RE. London, W. Headland, 1852.
3 R. Pulv. *Cortic. Peruvian. optim.* 3j, divide in 16 part. æqual. D. S., one to be taken between 9 and 10 a.m., mixed in a glass of wine.
4 Elixir *acidi Halleri* 3j.
5 Of Extract. *Hyoscyami*.
6 He removed to Molschleben, a village near Gotha.
7 A Secretary of State in Gotha, in whom Hahnemann seems to have been much interested.
8 Two druggists in Gotha.
9 R. *Recentis pulveris radicis Arnicæ* gr. vij.; *denture tales doses*, xvij. Dr Hahnemann. But they must be freshly triturated from the fresh root.
10 The publisher of the *Reichsanzeiger*, a widely circulated paper, in which many of Hahnemann's essays appeared.
11 Publisher of a scientific journal in Gotha.
12 The report was that Hahnemann had received a call to become a professor in the University of Mietan, which was not the case.
13 No report of the sort is to be found in the *Reichsanzeiger*, of which Becker was the publisher.
14 On the back of this letter the following prescriptions are attached. 1. R. *Pulv. rad. valerianæ sylv.* 3ij d. D. H. 2. R. *Salis volatilis salis ammoniaci* 3ss. Solve in *aquæ calideæ* 3iss. d. Dr H.
15 The former physician in ordinary to the Duke, who had died a month previously. Hahnemann did not obtain this appointment.
16 A young doctor practising in Gotha.

3

THE LIFE FORCE, HAHEMANN'S METHOD

Introduction

This chapter presents a forgotten essay by Hahnemann from 1813 together with lengthy footnotes, which did not appear until 1833, translated by Adolph Lippe. It then seems to have vanished from the modern canon of Hahnemann's writings.

Hahnemann has progressed in his ideas and in his confidence and in his ethics. If Hippocrates is known to promulgate a negative ethic 'at least do no harm', Hahnemann is at once more positive and more assertive. He says in the essay:

> I will now show what we discern as indubitably curable in diseases; how the curative virtues of medicines can become clearly perceivable, and how then they can be applied for the cure of the sick.

Hahnemann relies on discerning a life force which medicine has to cultivate. Illness and healing are dynamic and dynamic medicines are to be employed. He is confident that his method is the right one and the only one:

> The sick person can by no other possible means of cure be more easily, more quickly, more certainly, in a more reliable and permanent manner, liberated from disease, than through homeopathic medicines in small doses.

A short biography of Lippe, the translator of the essay follows, showing a typical career of that time, of a dedicated German immigrant homeopathic physician. His single-minded support of Hahnemann and his philosophy, and to creating his own lasting works was outstanding, and his legacy lies in the surviving philosophy and journals of the International Hahnemannian Association. The original spelling is preserved.

> **About Adolphus Lippe, the translator**[1]
> Adolphus Lippe MD, 1812–1888, of Philadelphia, one of the most celebrated homoeopathists in this country, is a native of Germany, and was born at the family estate of See, 11th May 1812. He is the oldest son of the late Count Ludwig and Countess Augusta zur Lippe, and was destined by them for the

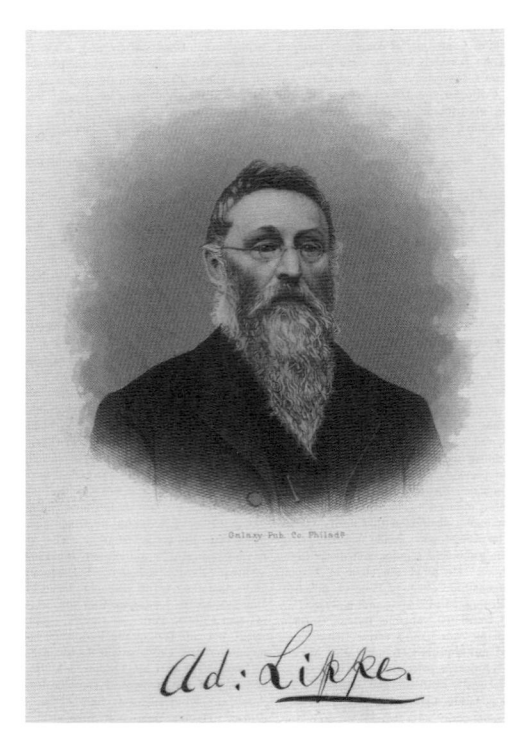

Figure 3.1 Adolphus Lippe (18162-1888)
(From the author's personal collection)

profession of law; finished his academical preparations and was graduated at Berlin. While prosecuting legal studies there, taste and opportunity attracted him to the more congenial pursuits of medicine, and at the close of a year he devoted himself thereto. Emigrating to the United States in 1839, he presented himself to the sole homoeopathic school there sustained, at Allentown, Pa. After a critical examination he was graduated there, and received his diploma from Dr Constantine Hering, the President, on 27th July 1841.

Removing to Pottsville, Dr Lippe practised with success and growing ability until called to a larger field at Carlisle. Here the prevalent epidemics of the Cumberland Valley gave him a new distinction, by means of which he was, six years later, induced to settle in Philadelphia. Here he speedily attained a distinction that needs no publication and cannot be overthrown. Aside from his strictly professional labours, Dr Lippe has been a regular contributor to homoeopathic literature. He filled the chair of Materia Medica in the Homoeopathic College of Pennsylvania from 1863 to 1868 with distinguished success and to an universal acceptance. He also translated valuable Italian, German, and French homoeopathic essays and treatises, that are now standard; and augmented and improved its materia medica, and by his clinical reports has shown how this may be rendered practically available and utilised in the application of homoeopathic knowledge and principles.

Adopting homoeopathy after careful examination, when qualified to institute and conduct it; believing it to be progressive rather than stagnant, and having devoted the best years of a prosperous life to establishing its claims in this country, Dr Lippe has rejected all solicitations that recalled him to Germany. Defending the school in its infancy, and nursing it through a crescent youth, he has had the rare felicity of witnessing the realisation of his best hopes, and enjoying a success to which his labours contributed a full share. Unwilling to abandon results he did so much towards securing; hopeful of further progress and more decisive victory, when all but the last blow seems won, and supported by both pupils and patients, Dr Lippe is continuing his career in the field of its greatest triumphs with undiminished energy and an ability that is increased by every day's labour, study and experience. He is assured of an honourable niche in the American chapter of homoeopathic history, and may eventually challenge a foremost. The peculiar advantages of family and educational discipline in one of the best schools of Germany, that he enjoyed, were thoroughly utilised by original capacity and mental bias. Intellectually rounded and well stored, as well as disciplined, his signal success is a motive as well as a guide to others. He has shed lustre upon German capacity, and identified his native land more closely with the scientific life of his adopted country.

The genius of the homoeopathic healing art[2]
by Samuel Hahnemann

Note by Adolphus Lippe, the translator
This very instructive and logical paper by the founder of our healing art has never been translated before. Why Dr Charles Julius Hempel omitted it we know not. It is, without exception, the most concise and precise rendition of the fundamental principles governing our school of medicine. It requires a study to follow Hahnemann in his logical argument. It has been our aim to give as verbal a translation as possible. Hahnemann's style of writing was quaint, and much of the force of the paper would have been lost by free (much less laborious) translation.

As Hahnemann wrote this paper as early as 1813, we hope that all homoeopathists will accept it, even those who find fault with his later writings, professing to detect in them signs of senility. The liberal-scientific-

peace-offering-reconciliation-and-amalgamation-seeking-men, and such as publicly declare that the laws of our healing art are tolerably good guides, but not applicable in all cases, and that then we are bound to seek other modes of cure, will, by this paper, receive their quietus. Adolphus Lippe.

It is impossible to guess at the internal nature of diseases, and at what is secretly changed by nature in the organism, and it is folly to attempt to base the cure of them on such guess-work and such propositions; it is impossible to divine the healing-power of medicines according to a chemical hypothesis or from their colours, smell, or taste; and it is folly to use these substances (so pernicious when abused) for the cure of diseases based on such hypotheses and such propositions. And had such a course been ever so much in vogue and been generally introduced; had it been for thousands of years *the only, and ever so much admired, course,* it would nevertheless remain an irrational and pernicious method thus to be guided by empty guesswork; to fable about the diseased conditions of the internal organism, and to combat them with fictitious virtues of medicines. In order that we may change disease into health it must be laid open to our senses what is discernibly – clearly discernibly – removable from every disease, and clearly must each medicine express what it can cure with certainty, before it may be applied to the cure of diseases; then the medical art will cease to be a lottery in human life and will then become a certain means of rescuing men from disease.

I will now show what we discern as indubitably curable in diseases; how the curative virtues of medicines can become clearly perceivable, and how then they can be applied for the cure of the sick.

What life is can only be empirically discerned by its manifestations and appearances; but it can never be explained, *à priori,* through metaphysical speculations; what life is, in itself and in its internal essence, can never be comprehended by mortals, and cannot be explained by conjectures.

The life of man, as well as his twofold condition (health and sickness), can never be demonstrated in a manner usual in demonstrating other objects according to definite principles; it cannot be compared with anything else in this world but with itself; it cannot be compared with a wheelwork, with a hydraulic machine, with chemical processes, with decomposition or formation of gases, with a galvanic battery, nor with anything inorganic. Life is in *no respect* controlled by any physical laws, which govern only inorganic substances. The material substances composing the human organism are not governed in their living composition by the same laws to which inorganic substances are subjected, but they follow solely laws peculiar to their vitality; they themselves are animated and vivified, just as the whole organism is animated and vivified. Here reigns a nameless all-powerful fundamental force which suspends all forces of the constituents of the body inclined to follow the laws of pressure, collision, depression, fermentation, and decomposition; and only this force guides and governs by the wonderful laws of life; that is to say, it maintains the necessary conditions for the preservation of the living whole in sensation and action, and that in an almost spiritual dynamic condition.

As the organism in its normal condition depends only on the state of its vitality, it follows that the changed condition which we call sickness must likewise depend not on the operation of physical or chemical principles, but on originally changed vital sensations and actions; that is to say, a dynamically changed state of man – a changed existence – through which eventually the material constituent parts of the body become altered in their character as is rendered necessary in each individual case through the changed conditions of the living organism.

Further, the noxious influences which, as a general rule, create in us from without the various sicknesses, are generally so invisible and immaterial[i] that it is impossible for them to change or disturb the form and components of our body mechanically, nor can they bring into the circulation pernicious or acrid fluids whereby all our blood would be chemically changed or vitiated; an inadmissible crude speculation of material brains which can in no way be proved. The causes producing disease affect, by virtue of their qualifications, the conditions of our life (our state of health) simply in a dynamic (similar to a spiritual) manner; and while at first the higher organs and vital forces become disturbed, there arises through this dynamic alteration of the whole living condition (discomfort, pain) a changed activity (abnormal function) of single or all organs; this necessarily causes secondarily a change of all the fluids in the circulation, and also the secretion of abnormal matter; and this is an inevitable result of that changed condition which is at variance with a state of health.

These abnormal substances appearing in diseases are therefore only products of the disease itself, and as long as the sickness retains its established (present) character, they will necessarily continue to be secreted, and thereby form a part of the signs of the sickness (symptoms); they are only effects, and, therefore, demonstrations of the present internal sickness, and react[ii] on the whole diseased body (while they frequently contain the germs of disease affecting other healthy persons) which produced them, not at all as disease-sustaining or creating matter, not as the material cause of disease. It is just as impossible for a person to infect his body or augment his disease with the poison of his own chancre, or with the

---

i Rare exceptions are some surgical conditions, and complaints arising from indigestible or foreign substances occasionally coming into the alimentary canal.

ii Expulsion and mechanical removal of these abnormal substances, impurities and excrescences, cannot cure the origin of the disease itself, as little as a coryza can be shortened or cured by possibly frequent and perfect blowing of the nose. The coryza does not continue any longer than its stipulated time, if the nose were not cleaned at all by blowing it.

gonorrhœic secretion from his own urethra, as it is for a viper to inflict upon itself with its own poison a dangerous or deadly sting.

Therefore it is obvious that the diseases of mankind caused through the influence of a dynamic (morbid) noxiousness can originally be but dynamic changes (caused almost only in a spiritual manner) of the life-character of our organism.

We perceive easily that these dynamic disorders of the life-character of our organism, which we call disease, inasmuch as they are nothing else but changes in sensations and actions, express themselves only through an aggregate of symptoms, and are recognised only as such by our powers of perception. As the work of healing is such an important one to human life, and as our steps must be guided only by our perception of the condition of the sick body (to be guided by conjectures and improbable hypothesis would be a dangerous folly, yes, even a crime against mankind), it is obvious that diseases, as dynamic disorders of our organism, express themselves only through changes in sensations and actions of the organism, that is, only through an aggregate of perceptible symptoms; therefore they alone must be the object to be healed in every case of illness. If all the symptoms of the disease are removed, nothing but health remains. For the reason that diseases are nothing but dynamic disorders of the condition and character of our organism, they cannot possibly be cured by mankind in any other way than through potencies and forces which are equally able to produce dynamic changes in the condition of man; that is, diseases are cured virtually and dynamically by medicines.[iii]

These efficacious substances and powers (medicines), which are at our command, effect the cure of diseases through the same dynamic changes of the present condition; through the same changes in the character of the organism in the sensation and action as they would in the healthy man; changing him dynamically, and producing in him certain sickness and characteristic symptoms, the knowledge of which, as we shall show, gives us the reliable indication of the diseased condition which can be most surely cured by each particular medicine. Therefore nothing in the world can produce any cure, no substance, no force can effect any such change in the human organism as to make the disease yield; nothing except a power capable of changing dynamically the condition of man, and therefore a power capable also of changing the healthy condition into a sick one.[iv]

---

iii Not by means of ostensibly dissolving or mechanically resolving, evacuating properties of medicinal substances, nor by means of expelling (blood-purifying and secretion-improving) imaginary productions of disease, nor by means of antiseptics (only acting on and useful to purify dead matter), nor through chemical and physical forces of any kind imaginable, in such manner as they affect inorganic material substances; nor in the manner in which the medical schools have always erroneously imagined and dreamt.

iv Therefore none, as, for instance, merely nutritive substance

On the other hand, there is no agent, no power in nature, capable of affecting healthy persons, which does not at the same time possess the capacity of curing certain diseased conditions as well as the power of affecting healthy persons, is found inseparable in all medicines, and as both active powers derive their origin from the same source, that is, from their capacity to change dynamically the condition of man, and as they, therefore, cannot possibly follow different inherent laws of nature in sick persons than in healthy ones, it follows that it must be identically the same power of the medicine which cures the disease in sick persons and possesses sick-making properties in healthy ones.^v

We will, therefore, also find that the healing power of medicines, and what each of them is capable of curing in diseases, can not be expressed in any other possible way, and can never come to our knowledge in greater purity and completeness than through the diseased phenomena and symptoms (a kind of artificial disease) which medicines produce on well persons. If we have before us a record of the characteristic (artificial) symptoms which the various medicines have produced on well persons, it becomes only necessary to let the pure experiment decide what particular symptoms of diseases are invariably quickly and permanently removed by the medicinal symptoms, so that we may know always in advance which of the proved medicines, and which of their known characteristic symptoms, will be the surest curative remedy in each case of disease.^{vi}

---

v The different result in both of these cases depends solely on the difference of the object to be changed.

vi As simple, as true, and as natural as this proposition is – and therefore it would seem as if it should have been made the fundamental means of ascertaining the curative power of medicines – it is evident that, in fact, up to this time this proposition has not been proven even distantly. During these thousands of years, and as far as the history of medicine is known, not one person conceived, *à priori,* the source of ascertaining in so natural a manner the healing properties of medicines before they were applied for the cure of the sick. For hundreds of years, up to the present time, it was surmised that the curative powers of medicines could only be ascertained by the effects they produced on diseases (*ab usu in morbis*). It was attempted to ascertain them in cases in which a certain medicine (and then most frequently a compound of different medicinal substances) has been beneficial in a named given case of disease. It is impossible to learn from the curative effect of a single medicinal substance, even (which not often happened) in an accurately described case of disease, in what case of disease this remedy might again become curative; because (with the exception of diseases caused by fixed miasms, small-pox, measles, lues, the itch, etc., or those consequent on the same disturbing element, as the gout) all other cases of diseases are single cases, that is, they appear under varying and different symptom-combinations, have never appeared in just the same manner; it is on that account that we can not draw the conclusion that the same remedy will also cure another (different) case. The forcible combination of such cases of disease (which nature produces in her wisdom in such an endless variety) under certain named forms, as is done arbitrarily by Pathology, is leading to continuous illusions, and a temptation to a mistaking of various conditions one with another – human guess-work without any reality. Equally seductive and inadmissible, although from times immemorial introduced is the establishment of general (curative) effects, based on occasional results in diseases, which the Materia Medica does when, for instance, in some cases of diseases occasionally during the use of (generally compounded) medicines,

Finally, we appeal to experiment (experience), in order to determine what artificially sick-making powers (observed of medicines) should be applied successfully against certain natural diseases. We ask:-

Whether they be such medicines as are capable of producing on the healthy organism *different* (allopathic) changes from those observed in the disease to be healed.

Or such medicines as are capable of producing on the healthy organism *opposite* (enantiopatic, antipathic) changes to those observed in the disease to be healed.

Or, whether we can expect restoration to health (cure) with the greatest certainty, and in the most permanent manner, by such medicines as are capable of producing on the healthy *similar* (homoeopathic) changes to those observed in the natural disease (there are only these three modes of administering medicines possible); experience most emphatically and indubitably decides for the last.

It is even self-evident that medicines acting heterogeneously and allopathically, capable of producing different symptoms on the healthy organism to those then observed in the disease to be cured, are in the very nature of things incapable of being suitable to the cure, and cannot cure. Their effects consequently must be injurious; otherwise every disease would be cured by means of any imaginable, ever so differently acting, medicine, quickly, safely, and permanently. Whereas each medicine possesses effects differing from all other medicines; and so each disease causes on the human organism, under the eternal laws of nature, different and varying ailments and suffering; this in itself would demonstrate a contradiction *(contradictionem in adjecto)*, and would by itself demonstrate the impossibility of a beneficial result. Furthermore, each demonstrated change can only be produced by a cause especially belonging to it, but not *per quam libet causam*. And experience proves it daily that the common practice of prescribing

---

increased urinary secretions, perspiration, appearance of the menstruation, cessation of convulsions, a kind of sleep, or expectoration appeared; the medicine (which among the rest was honoured with being charged with this effect) was credited with possessing the virtue of being diuretic or soporific, or capable of restoring menstruation, or anti-spasmodic, or soporific, or expectorant, thereby committing a *fallacium causæ* by confounding the terms *with* and *of*. But there was likewise drawn a wrong conclusion, a *particulari ad universale*, in contravention of all the laws of reason, even changing the conditional into the unconditional. Because that which is not capable of causing, in every case of disease, an increase of urinary secretions, or perspiration, or menstruation, or sleep; which can not allay, in all cases, convulsions, or loosen the cough, cannot, without violating common sense, be pronounced unconditionally and absolutely diuretic or sudorific, or emmenagogue, or soporific, or anti-spasmodic, or expectorant.

Furthermore, it is impossible that a medicine in these compound phenomena of our conditions, in such multiplied combinations of a variety of symptoms as are the nameless varieties of the diseases of men, can possibly reveal its original medicinal effects, and that which we expect to know with certainty of its sick-making, sensation changing properties.

for the cure of the sick a compound of medicines, the powers (effects) of each of these unknown, causes a variety of effects, but the least of all – a cure.

The *second method* of curing (treating) diseases with medicines, is the application of means (a medicine acting as a palliative) changing and altering the observed disorder (disease, or the most prominent symptom of it) enantiopathically, antipathically or contrarily. Such an application cannot, as is easily perceived, work a durable cure of the disease, because the disorder is sure to return again, and that in an aggravated form. This is the way it occurs:– It is a marvellous process of nature which orders that organic living bodies are not governed by the same laws by which inorganic substances of (inanimate) physical nature are governed. They do not accept the impressions passively, like the latter; do not follow, like them, external impressions, but they resist and endeavour to oppose these impressions by contraries.[vii]

The living human body can be influenced at first by physical forces; but this impression is not as permanent and lasting as that which is produced on inorganic bodies – (and so it would necessarily be if the medicinal powers, acting by contraries on the disease, could produce a lasting and permanent relief). More than that, the human organism strives to produce the reverse condition through antagonism against the effects of the forces brought to bear upon it from without.[viii] For instance, a hand which has been held long enough in ice-water does not remain cold; nor does the hand only show the warmth of the surrounding

---

vii The green juice of the plant obtained by expressing, no longer an animated organic substance, if spread on linen, soon fades under the rays of the sun, and is destroyed; while the plant bleaching in a cellar for want of daylight soon regains its green colour when exposed to the same rays of the sun. A root which has been dug up, and has been dried, will soon become entirely decomposed and destroyed if laid in warm and moist earth; while a fresh root laid in the same earth will soon bring forth hopeful sprouts. The foaming fresh beer, while in full fermentation, will soon be changed, when bottled, into vinegar, if exposed to a heat of 96 degrees (Fahrenheit). But in the healthy human stomach the same degree of heat will check the fermentation and soon change it into a mild nutriment. Half putrid, already badly-smelling game, and other meats when eaten by healthy persons produce the least smelling evacuations (excrement); while the bark of *Cinchona officinalis*, which possesses the property of checking putrefaction in inanimate animal substances, is affected by the healthy intestines in a contrary manner, so as to cause very offensive flatus. Carbonate of lime destroys all acids in inorganic substances; but when taken into the healthy stomach, is apt to cause sour-smelling perspiration. While the dead animal fibre is preserved from putrefaction with certainty by *Tannin*, healthy ulcers of the living man, if frequently treated with *Tannin*, become impure, green, and putrid. A hand bathed in warm water becomes afterwards colder than the hand which was not bathed; and proportionately colder the warmer the water used for bathing was.

viii This is a law of nature according to which the administration of each medicine causes, at first, certain dynamic changes and abnormal symptoms in the living human body (*primary effects of medicines*), but afterwards, by means of a peculiar antagonism (which in many cases might be termed an effort of self-preservation), it causes a condition entirely the opposite of the first effect (*secondary symptoms*); for instance, narcotic substances produce primarily insensibility, and secondarily painfulness.

atmosphere when taken out of the ice-water, neither does it return to the warmth of the body – by no means – for the colder the water was, and the longer the hand has been kept in it, and thereby affected the healthy skin, the hotter and the more inflamed will it become afterwards.

It cannot be otherwise than thus, that a symptom which yields to a remedy which acts contrarily on the disease does so but for a short time;[ix] and it is bound to yield again, very soon, to the predominating antagonism of the living organism, which causes a contrary; that is, a contrary condition to the one which the palliative has created deceptively for a short time only (a condition corresponding with the original evil) – in fact, a true addition to the returning unextinguished original disease, the original disease in aggravated form. The disorder is always and *surely* aggravated, and as soon as the *palliative* (the contrary and enantiopathic acting remedy) has exhausted its effects.[x]

In chronic diseases, the true test-stone of the genuine healing-art, we perceive the pernicious effects of contrary-acting (palliative) medicines in a high degree; inasmuch as a repetition necessary to cause an illusive effect (a sudden passing appearance of relief), implies a larger and increasingly larger dose, frequently endangering the life of the sick, and not unfrequently causing death.

There remains, therefore, but a third method of administering medicines as a sure mode of relief and cure, and this is the application of a remedy which is capable of causing on the healthy organism an affection (an artificial diseased condition) which is similar, very similar, to the present case of sickness.

It is easy to prove, as has been seen in innumerable cases, and also by those who followed my teachings, by daily experience[xi] as well as by reasoning, that this

---

ix Just as a scalded hand remains cold and painless not much longer than while it is held in cold water; it afterwards burns and pains much more.

x Thus the pain in a scalded hand subsides suddenly, but only for a few minutes, by applying cold water; but afterwards the inflammation and pain become much worse than before (the inflammation, as a secondary effect of the cold water, is an addition to the original inflammation scalding, which the cold water is unable to remove). The painful fullness in the abdomen caused by constipation seems to disappear, as if by magic, after a purgative; but as early as the next day this painful fullness and tension of the abdomen returns worse than it was before. The stupor-like sleep after opium causes a much greater sleeplessness the following night. It becomes evident that this secondary condition constitutes a true aggravation, and is shown by the fact that if the palliative is to be repeated (for instance, opium for habitual sleeplessness or chronic diarrhoea), it must be administered in increased doses, *as against an aggravated disease*, if even then it can be forced to produce, but for a short time, its seeming palliation.

xi We will mention only a few every-day experiences. The burning pain which boiling water causes on the skin is cured by the cook's holding the burned hand near the fire, or by uninterruptedly moistening it with heated alcohol (or turpentine), which causes a still more intense burning sensation. This specific treatment has been followed by varnishers and similar artisans, and has been found reliable. The burning pain caused by these strong and heated spirits remains only for a few minutes, while the organism is homoeopathically relieved of the inflammation caused by the burn. The destruction of the skin is soon repaired by the formation of a thin cuticle, through which

method of administering medicine constitutes the most complete, the best, and only mode of cure.

It will, therefore, not be a difficult task to comprehend by what natural laws the only suitable homoeopathic healing-art is and must be governed.

The first unmistakable natural law is, *that the living organism is comparatively much more easily affected by medicine than by natural diseases.* Many sick-making causes affect us every day, every hour of the day, but they are not able to disturb the equilibrium of our condition, the healthy are not made sick; the activity of our life-preserving principle within us generally resists the most of them, and the individual remains well. If external noxious influences, increased to a high degree, affect us, and if we expose ourselves to them too much, then we sicken, and only to any great degree if our organism, just at that time, shows a weak side (a predisposition), which make us more liable to be affected by the present (simple or complex) cause of the disease. Did the inimical, partly psychical, partly physical forces of nature, called noxious disease influences, have unlimited power to affect and change our condition, then nobody would be well. Inasmuch as they are found everywhere, everybody would be sick, and would not even have a conception of what health is. But, as in general, diseases are only the exception to the condition of men; and as it is necessary that a combination of so many and various circumstances and conditions – partly by the disease-causing forces, partly by the condition of the individual to be made sick – must exist before a disease really follows the effects of the sick-making forces, it becomes evident that man is not easily affected by these noxious influences; that they do not

---

no more alcohol penetrates. In this manner a burn is cured in a few hours by the remedy causing a similar burning pain (by highly heated alcohol or heated oil of turpentine); but if such a burn is treated by cooling palliatives or with ointments, a malignant ulceration follows, which is apt to last many weeks, and even months, causing much suffering. Professional dancers know from long experience that they are momentarily very much refreshed by drinking very cold water, and by taking off their clothing when extremely heated from dancing; but they know also that afterwards they will surely have to suffer from severe, often fatal, diseases. Wisdom has taught such extremely heated persons, without allowing themselves to go into the cool air or remove their clothing, to take a drink which is also heating, either punch or hot tea with arrack or brandy; and under its effects, while slowly walking up and down the room, they are very soon relieved of the hot fever caused by dancing. So even the old and experienced mower never takes any other drink to cool himself from the excessive thirst of labor under a hot sun than a glass of whisky; in an hour's time he is relieved from thirst and heat, and feels well. An experienced person will not expose a frozen limb to the fire, or to a hot stove, or put it in hot water, in order to restore it; covering it with snow, or rubbing it with ice-water, is the well-known homoeopathic remedy for it. The disorders caused by excessive joy (the fantastic mirth, the trembling restlessness, the excessive motion, the palpitation of the heart, the sleeplessness) are soon and permanently removed by coffee, which causes a similar ailment in those not used to take it. There thus exist many daily confirmations of the great truth, that men are relieved from long-lasting sufferings by other short-lasting evils, by a process of nature. Nations, for centuries fallen into apathy and slavishness, elevated their spirits, began to feel the dignity of men, and became again free men, after they had been crushed to the dust by the western tyrants.

necessarily make him sick, and that the organism can only be affected by them under certain predisposing influences.

Quite different are the relations of the artificial dynamic forces, which we call medicines. Every true medicine affects *every* living organic body under *all* circumstances, *at all times*, and causes on it its characteristic symptoms (clearly enough perceivable through the senses, provided the dose is large enough), so that it becomes obvious that *each and every living human organism must become thoroughly affected and seemingly infected by the medicinal disease;* this, as is well known, is not the case with natural diseases.[xii]

All experience proves unmistakably that the human organism is much more predisposed and susceptible to medicinal forces than to diseased noxiousnesses and infectious miasms; or, to express it differently, that the medicinal forces possess an *absolute,* but the diseased affections a merely *limited,* power to change the conditions of the human organism.

This makes it already obvious that a possibility exists of curing disease by medicines (that is to say, that the diseased condition of the sickened organism can be obliterated by means of the most suitable alterations through medicines). But it becomes necessary also to comply with a *second* natural law, if the cure is to be made a reality; that is, *a stronger dynamic affection overcomes the weaker one in the living organism permanently, if the first is similar in kind to the latter;* because the dynamic change of the condition to be expected from the medicine must not, as I believe I have proved, be either differentially deviating from or allopathic to the diseased condition; otherwise a much greater disturbance would follow, as is the case under the common practice; neither must it be *opposite,* so that only a palliative, fallacious improvement, which is invariably followed by an aggravation of the original disease, may be produced. But the medicine must possess the tendency to cause a condition *similar* to the disease (to cause similar symptoms on the healthy person), and observations must have shown this tendency, and then only can it become a permanently curative medicine.

Whereas the dynamic affections of the organism (either by medicines or diseases) can be discerned only by means of expressions of changed sensations and changed functions; and whereas, also, the similarity of their dynamic affections reciprocally can be ascertained only through a similarity of symptoms; and as the organism (much more easily affected by medicines than by diseases) is more submissive to drug-action; that is to say, is more easily affected and changed by it, than from a similar affection of diseases; it follows that, without a possibility of contradiction, the organism must necessarily be relieved from the diseased affections if a medicine is applied which, also entirely different in its nature from

---

xii Even the plague like diseases do not necessarily infect every person; and other diseases leave many more persons unaffected, even if they expose themselves to the changes of the weather, the seasons of the year, and many other pernicious influences.

the disease,[xiii] approaches it as near as possible in its similarity of symptoms, that is, homoeopathic to it; because the organism, as a complete living unit, is not capable of absorbing two similar dynamic affections at the same time without compelling the weaker to succumb to the stronger one; and as the organism is more apt to be affected by the stronger force (medicinal affection), then there will be a necessity created to part with the weaker one (diseased affection), and by that process the organism is healed of it.

It is illusive for any one to think that the living organism under the administration of a dose of homoeopathic medicine, for the cure of its disease, thereby becomes burdened with an addition to its ills; just as if a plate of lead already pressed by an iron weight were the stronger pressed by the adding of a stone to it; or a piece of copper heated by friction, by pouring hot water on it, must become still more heated! Nothing of the kind, not passive, not according to physical laws of inorganic nature is our living organism governed. It reacts with its life-antagonism, so that it, as a unit, as a living whole, submissively permits the diseased condition to be extinguished, if a similarly strong force pervades the organism by means of a homoeopathic remedy.

Our living human organism is spiritually reacting. It excludes by a spontaneous force a less powerful affection, as soon as the stronger force of a homoeopathic remedy produces a different but very similar affection. In other words, on account of the oneness of its life it cannot suffer, at the same time, from two similar general disturbances; but is compelled to part with the previous dynamic affection (disease) as soon as it is acted upon by a second dynamic force (medicine), which is more apt to affect it, provided that medicine possesses the capability of affecting the organism (symptoms) in a very similar manner to the first affection. Something similar occurs in the human mind.[xiv]

---

xiii Without this natural difference between diseased affections and the medicinal affections no cure could be affected. If both were not only similar, but also of the same nature, therefore identical, there would be no effect produced (probably only an aggravation of the evil). In the same manner, it would be vain to expect to cure a chancre by moistening it with the poison of another chancre.

xiv For instance, a grieved girl, lamenting the death of a playmate, becomes solaced through the strong effect of being introduced to a family where she finds half naked children who have just lost their father, their only support. She becomes more reconciled to her comparatively smaller loss; she is cured of her grief for her playmate, because the oneness of the mind can at the same time be affected only by a single similar emotion, and that emotion must be subdued if another similar emotion take possession of her mind which affects her stronger, and in that manner becomes a homoeopathic remedy, extinguishing the former. The girl would not have been relieved of her grief she felt for the loss of her playmate, if, for instance, the mother had scolded her (a heterogene allopathic force). On the contrary, she would have been much sicker in mind by the addition of a different mortification, and again would the grieved girl, had she been seemingly cheered for a few hours palliatively by a jocund festivity (because the emotion in this case was an *opposite*, enantiopathic), have fallen afterwards into deeper sadness when she was left to her solitude, and then would have cried more bitterly than before. What we here see in the psychological condition, we find also

In proportion as the human organism is more easily affected by medicines when in a state of health than by disease, as I have demonstrated above, so is that organism when diseased, without comparison, much more easily affected by homoeopathic medicines than by any other (for instance, allopathic or enantiopathic) – and it is acted upon easily and in a very high degree, as it is already inclined to certain symptoms by the disease, hence it becomes more susceptible to similar symptoms by the homoeopathic medicine – just as our own similar mental suffering causes the mind to become much more sensitive to similar stories of woe. Therefore, it becomes obvious that only the smallest doses become useful and necessary for a cure; that is to say, for the changing of the sickened organism into a similar medicinal disease; and for that reason it is unnecessary to give it in a larger dose, because in this case the object is obtained not through the quantity but through potentiality and quality (dynamic conformity, Homoeopathy). There is no utility in a larger dose, but there is harm done; the larger dose on the one side does not cause the dynamic change of the diseased affection with more certainty than the most suitable smallest does; but it causes and supplants, on the other side, a multiplied medicinal disease, which is always an evil, although it passes by after a certain lapse of time.

The organism becomes strongly affected, and becomes pervaded by the force of a medicinal substance, which is capacitated to obliterate and extinguish the totality of the symptoms of the disease, through its endeavours to create similar symptoms. The organism becomes, as we have said, liberated from the diseased condition at the very time that it is affected by the medicinal power, by which it is decidedly more apt to be impressed.

The medicinal forces, as such, even in larger doses, hold the organism only for a few days under their influence; and, therefore, it becomes apparent that a small dose, and in acute diseases a very small dose, of that medicine (such as it has been proven constitutes the dose for a homoeopathic cure) can effect the organism for a short time only (and in acute diseases the smallest dose is capable of affecting the organism for only a few hours), and that the medicinal affection which now occupies the place of the disease very soon and imperceptibly passes into pure health.

It appears that the nature of the human organism is governed solely by the laws we have here presented, if disease is to be permanently cured by medicines; and really we may say that this action is a mathematical certainty. *There exists no case of a dynamic disease in this world* (with the exception of the death-agony, and, we may so class it here, advanced age and the destruction of indispensable viscera

---

in the organic life. The oneness of our life does not allow itself to be occupied and possessed of two general similar dynamic affections at the same time; because, if the second affection prove itself to be the stronger one, the first will become obliterated, just as soon as the organism becomes affected by the second.

or limbs), which cannot be cured quickly and permanently *by a medicine, which has been found to cause in its positive effects symptoms in great similarity to it.*

The sick person can by no other possible means of cure[xv] be more easily, more quickly, more certainly, in a more reliable and permanent manner, liberated from disease, than through homoeopathic medicines in small doses.

References

1 Cleave, E. *Biographical Cyclopaedia of Homoeopathic Physicians and Surgeons*, Philadelphia, Galaxy Publishing, 1873.
2 Preface to the second volume of Hahnemann's *Materia Medica Pura* 1833. Translated by Adolph Lippe. Published in the journal *Medical Advance* (Chicago), editor HC Allen, and bound into an undated compilation from this journal by a Dr WC Wright probably in 1895.

---

xv Even in the common practice, and in rare cases, the strikingly effective cures are the results of a homoeopathically suitable and homoeopathically acting medicine (accidentally prescribed). It was impossible for the physician to *choose* a homoeopathic remedy for the cure of diseases, as the positive (the positive effects observed on healthy persons) effects of medicines were never thought of, and therefore they remained ignorant of them; and even those medicines, with such as were made known by my writings, were not considered useful for curative purposes. Furthermore, they remained ignorant of the necessary conditions for a permanent cure, and of the effects of medicines on those symptoms of disease which were similar to them (the homoeopathic law of cure).

4

HERING'S PREFACE TO HAHNEMANN'S *CHRONIC DISEASES*

Introduction

Hering was first and foremost Hahnemann's most ardent follower in America. At the same time, being of independent mind, he was also from time to time critical of Hahnemann and so helped Hahnemann develop his theories. This was all done by correspondence, I do not think that they ever met. But so much were they closely aligned that Melanie Hahnemann invited Hering to Paris after Hahnemann's death, to take over his practice, but he declined. His great preface enhances the theoretical introduction to the *Chronic Diseases* of 1828, published in 1845 so soon after Hahnemann's death in 1843 that they must have corresponded about the innovatory rule of the direction of cure.[1]

The following sketch by American physician and historian Dr Thomas Lindsley Bradford (who received his degree from the Homoeopathic Medical College of Pennsylvania (HMCP) in 1869 under the tutelage of Adolphus Lippe) was published in the *Hahnemannian Monthly* shortly after Hering's death.

> **About Dr Constantine Hering (1800–1880)**[2,3]
> Suddenly, at half past ten o'clock, on the evening of July 23rd, Dr Constantine Hering departed this life in the eighty-first year of his age. Thus departed one to whom Homoeopathy in America – yea, in the whole world – will ever remain a debtor. During the past decade the doctor has at times suffered quite severely from asthma, though for several years past the attacks have been less severe, so that he has been enabled to attend almost daily upon a large circle of patients.
>
> East, West, North, and South, Europe and America, have among their busy practitioners many who look toward the home of this truly great man as toward the home of a father. Hundreds have shared with him the entire wondrous store of knowledge which he possessed. Many came; none were

sent empty away. Their capacity to receive, rather than in his willingness to give limited the amount bestowed. Blessings will ever attend name.

Constantine Hering was born at Oschatz, Saxony, on Jan. 1. 1800. From earliest childhood he evinced an extreme desire to investigate all things. Apt as a scholar, he soon mastered the preliminary studies, and was prepared at an early age to enter the Classical School at Zittau. Here he continued his studies from 1811 to 1817. He completed his medical studies, and received the degree of Doctor of Medicine from the University of Wurzburg, March 23, 1826. Soon after his graduation he was appointed by the king of Saxony to accompany the Saxon legation to Dutch Guiana, there to make scientific research and prepare a zoological collection for his government. He continued in this capacity for some years, but his love for the new truth which he had learned impelled him to further study, and finally to the practice of medicine according to Hahnemann's doctrines. Such was his success that he gained great favour with the governor of the province, whose daughter he cured of an affection which the resident physicians had declared incurable.

During his residence at Surinam he was an occasional contributor to the *Homoeopathic Archives*, for which journal he had written as early as 1825, while still a student of medicine. The court physician, learning of this, wrought upon the king sufficiently to cause a notice to be sent Hering, directing him to attend to the duties of his appointment, and let medical matters alone.

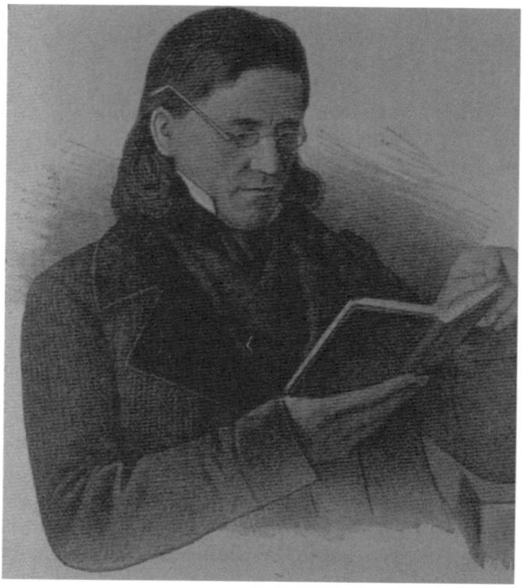

Figure 4.1 Constantine Hering in his early years

Reproduced with permission of National Center for Homeopathy Alexandria VA

His independent nature rebelled at such intolerance, and led him promptly to resign his appointment. Dr George H. Bute, formerly a Moravian missionary at Surinam, and a pupil of Hering, had settled in Philadelphia, and was engaged in the practice of homoeopathy. Learning from Dr Bute that Philadelphia offered a good field; Hering left Surinam and landed at Philadelphia, January 1833. Here he remained for a short season, when he was induced by Dr W. Wesselhoeft to assist in the establishment of a homoeopathic school at Allentown, the North American Academy of the Homoeopathic Healing Art. He laboured in this field until financial embarrassments necessitated the abandonment of the institution.

This led to his return to Philadelphia, where he engaged in practice with Dr Bute, locating on Vine Street, below Fourth. Here he soon acquired a large and lucrative practice.

Though conducting a large practice, he found time to write much, and to superintend the work of many younger and less experienced. His Saturday-night meeting, held for the instruction of students and young practitioners, were prized as a boon. Here he imparted golden truths, reaped from fields of ripe experience such as but few have enjoyed.

Hering's Law of the direction of cure

This law is one of the more mysterious concepts of homeopathy to those who have not studied it, and I have not found any published work that verifies or challenges its existence. Yet to a homeopath it is the benchmark by which to assess the progress of a patient before treatment, and at the second or subsequent follow up consultation. It is mysterious in that most homeopaths learn it from a teacher or a book at two or twenty-two times removed from the original. We are taught that cure comes from the top down, from the inside out, from more to less important organs, and in reverse over time. We are not usually taught that cure is only confirmed when the symptoms are observed to return to the surface with a palpable skin lesion. This is because the essay by Hering had disappeared from the literature. Hering's original explanation appears in this chapter.

We have no evidence that Freud knew of the rule of the direction of cure, but he wrote on the case of Anna, with reference to 'hysteria':

> Thus it was necessary to reproduce the whole chain of pathogenic memories in chronological order, the latest ones first and the earlier ones last; and it was quite impossible to jump over the later traumas in order to get back more quickly to the first, which was often the most potent one.[4]

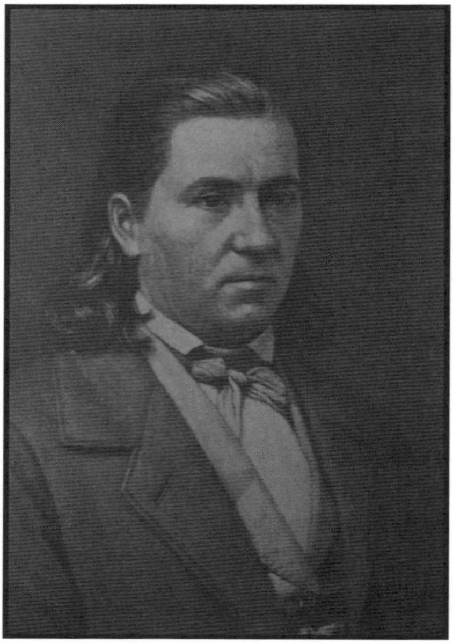

Figure 4.2 Constantine Hering in his later years
Reproduced with permission of National Center for Homeopathy Alexandria VA

Hering presumably wrote his observations at some point between 1828 and 1845, when they were published in a translation of the first edition of Hahnemann's *Chronic Diseases* – 1828 – in English. In 1896 a second edition omitted these observations and the original statement faded from view. As the major scholar and leader of North American homeopathy until his death in 1880, his writings were important and are still used today. He proved the first nosodes, medicines from the products of diseases, of anthrax[5] and of rabies.[6] One can assume that Hahnemann knew of this observation by Hering as they were close correspondents. An account of Hering's life follows,[7] and the story of the direction of cure is here in its original formulation. I should like to see the creation and implementation of a test to verify the truth of this observation, which would also satisfy the supporters of evidence based medicine.

Dr Hering's Preface to *The Chronic Diseases; their specific nature and homoeopathic treatment* by Samuel Hahnemann, 1828[8]

The following article has, been kindly furnished by Dr Constantine Hering of Philadelphia, in German. The Editor (Charles Hempel) is responsible for the translation

Text of preface

Hahnemann's work on chronic diseases may be considered a continuation of his *Organon*; the medicines which will follow the present volume may therefore be considered a continuation of his *Materia Medica Pura*. As the principles and rules of general therapeutics have been developed in the *Organon*, so does Hahnemann develop, in the present treatise, the principles and rules which ought too prevail in the treatment of chronic diseases, whose name is legion. In the *Materia Medica Pura* Hahnemann describes to us the symptoms which the general remedies that he tried upon healthy persons are capable of producing; the present treatise, on the contrary, will be succeeded by an account of those remedies which Hahnemann especially employed in the treatment of chronic diseases, and which he therefore called *antipsorics*. In the *Organon*, Hahnemann tries to establish the fact that the principle "similia similibus curentur" is the supreme rule in every true method of cure, and he shows how this rule is to be followed in the treatment of disease; whereas in his treatise on the chronic diseases, which is based upon the *Organon* and does in the least, modify or alter its teachings, Hahnemann shows that as most chronic disease originate in a common source and are related amongst each other, a special class of remedies designated by Hahnemann as "anti-psoric" should be used in the treatment of those diseases. The common source of most chronic diseases, according to Hahnemann, is *psora*.

The shallow opponents of homoeopathy - and we never had any other - pounced upon the theory of the psoric miasm with a view of attacking it with their hollow and unmeaning sarcasms. Taking *psora* to be identical with itch, they sneeringly pretended that according to Hahnemann's doctrine the itch was the primitive evil, and that this doctrine was akin to the doctrine of the original sin recognised by the Christian faith.*

As it would be absurd for a philosophical Christian to reject the doctrine of original sin, so it is absurd for any one who professes to have a clear perception of homoeopathy to reject the doctrine of hereditary morbific miasm. Both these doctrines must stand and fall together, and, as truth is one and indivisible, they both hold and illustrate each other. If we admit with Rousseau that everything which leaves the hand of God is perfectly holy, then the first created man must have been perfectly pure, and must have appeared in the image and likeness of his maker. It seems to me absurd to suppose that something perfectly pure can, of itself, by its own free and orderly development produce things impure and evil. We do not know how far God permitted an *adaptation to evil* to co-exist in the first man together with an adaptation to goodness. But we certainly know that the evil fruits must be the result of evil forces. In a certain moment man or God through man, permitted the adaptation to evil to prevail in his nature; and instantaneously the forces of evil, be they called serpent, devil, or otherwise, invaded man's nature, engrafted themselves upon it, and have up to this moment perpetuated their existence in it. This is, relatively speaking, a fall, although this fall, having been the first necessary phase of human development, may, in reality, be considered a progress. Man's destiny consists in reuniting himself again with the Divine Life through the universal expansion of all the faculties of his soul, and the realisation of all the celestial harmonies the germs of which God had deposited in his nature and towards the construction of which science and art will furnish him the means. The principle of division, or dissolution, which man had suffered to be introduced into his spiritual nature, must necessarily have embodied itself in a corresponding principle in the material organism. It is this principle which Hahnemann calls *Psora*. In proportion as man's spiritual nature becomes developed and purified, this psoric miasm will be diminished, and will finally be completely removed from the life of humanity. This complete physical regeneration of human nature will necessarily be attended with great changes in all the external relations of man, education, mode of labouring, living. etc. etc.

The principle of division or dissolution existing in the human organism as an established and constituted fact does not preclude the possibility of this organism being invaded by acute miasms. The psoric principle marks the general adaptation to evil, recognised and inherently received by the human organism; acute diseases are violent and sudden invasions of the organism by the forces of evil – which I have named subversive forces in my preface. Those sudden invasions could never have taken place without man having first admitted the psoric principle to be constitutional in his organism.

With the same impudence with which they had, on former occasions, asserted, that Hahnemann rejects all pathology in his *Organon*, they now asserted that he himself advanced a pathological hypothesis, and "that the truth which it contained was not new, nor the new truth."

Equitable judges will not fail to recognise in this treatise on chronic diseases the same carefulness of study and observation which the great author of homoeopathy has shown in all his other writings. Hahnemann had no other object in view except to cure. All the energies of his great soul were directed to this one end. His object was not to overthrow pathology, although the pathology of his time has been set aside as heap of foolish speculations, and has been replaced by other systems that may perhaps suffer the same fate in fifty years; he merely contended against the foolish and. presumptuous applications of pathological hypothesis to the treatment of disease. He rejected and overthrew the foolish belief which had been driven like a rusty nail into the minds of the profession and, by their instrumentality, into the minds of the people, that the remedies should be given against a name, against an imaginary disease, and that the name of this imaginary disease indicated the remedy. Up to this day, physicians have been engaged in accrediting that superstition. Whence should otherwise spring the desire which so many patients manifest, of inquiring into the name of the disease, as if a knowledge of that name were sufficient to discover the true remedy against the disease? Many patients are disconsolate when the doctor cannot tell them what the matter is with them. Do we gain anything by being able to say that the disease is a rheumatism, dyspepsia, liver-complaint? Does it avail the patient any to be able to repeat his doctor's *ipse dixit* "that he is bilious, nervous, etc." Do these words mean anything definite? Are there yet physicians foolish enough to believe that their speculative explanations mean anything? Does not every body acknowledge that they are mere *ignes fatui* flitting to and fro upon the quagmire of the old decayed systems of pathology?

Assuredly, a physician of modern date, who has not remained altogether ignorant, would be ashamed of assuring his patients, with the air of a deep thinker, that one has a disease of spine, another consumption, a third a uterine affection. Every tyro in pathology knows that all this means nothing definite, and that it is only to very ignorant persons that such assertions, can be given as science. Every tyro knows that the question is, to find out what are the symptoms and the nature of that disease of the spine or the uterus. It is moreover known that this more precise knowledge is necessary as respects prognosis, and for the purpose of regulating the mode of life of the patient; but it is also settled that to know merely the variety, to which the disease belongs, is not sufficient to cure it. All the successful and celebrated practitioners of the old school have been such as have constantly modified and individualised the treatment of disease. This is all that Hahnemann has tried to accomplish; with this difference, that he has individualised every case of disease with much more precision than any of the older physicians had done. Hahnemann had courage enough at once to face the contradictions which constantly existed between practice and theory; he declared that the speculative knowledge of physicians was merely learned dust which they were in the habit of throwing into the people's eyes for the purpose of blinding them and inducing them to consider the ignorance of the doctors and the insufficiency of their knowledge as something respectable. Hahnemann dared to lay down this maxim: that, in treating disease, he had nothing to do with its name.

Hahnemann teaches that the remedies should be chosen according to the symptoms of the patient. The physician should be governed by what is certain and safe, not by that which is more or less uncertain and unsafe, and which is changed according to fashion. Both in the *Organon* and in his treatise on the chronic diseases, Hahnemann insists upon the remedies being chosen in accordance with the symptoms.

It is not an easy matter to choose a remedy according to symptoms. This may be inferred from the manner in which tyros in homoeopathy, and physicians in the old school who came over to us, go to work. They constantly rely upon names, giving a certain remedy in scarlet fever, because someone else had found it useful; or a certain remedy in pulmonary inflammation, because it had been successfully exhibited upon a former occasion; whereas Hahnemann teaches that because a remedy has helped before this is no reason why it should help again in a similar disease. The symptoms and not the name are to point out the remedy.

This is also the case in chronic diseases. In the treatment of chronic diseases, Hahnemann has been taught by experience to give preference to anti-psoric remedies. This preference is not theoretical, and is constantly subordinate to the general principle.

Hahnemann has never said that the principal constituents of mountains, which are the most important materials in nature – the metals, for instance – are the most important remedies for the cure of most universal diseases. However, he has pointed out the oxides or salts of *Ammonium, Potassium, Sodium, Calcium, Aluminium, Magnesium* as the most important anti-psoric remedies. Hahnemann has said nowhere that the most important metalloids constitute the most important remedial agents, although he has introduced *Sulphur, Phosphorus, Silicea, Chlorine* and *Iodine*, in one form or another, as antipsoric remedies. In selecting a remedy Hahnemann has never been guided by theories, but always by experience. He chose his remedies agreeably to the symptoms which they had produced upon healthy persons, looking at the same time to their remedial values having been tested by practice. This is the reason why the general views which have been expressed just now did not prevent him from admitting as chief antipsorics, *Borax* and *Ammonium carbonicum, Anacardium* and *Clematis*.

Why, it may be asked, has a great number of homoeopathic physicians, neither recognised Hahnemann's theory of psora, nor the specific character of the antipsoric remedies? Why have some even gone so far as to set the theory sneeringly aside, and to decry the antipsorics as less trustworthy than the other remedies?

For the same reason that the astronomical discoveries of our Herschel are doubted by people who have no faith in the discoverer, and are, not able to verify his discoveries. To do this, knowledge, instruments, talent, care, perseverance, opportunities, and many other things are required. Not one of all these requisites can be found with those who are mere dabblers in practice, scribbling authors opposing their own opinions and imaginations to facts and observation.

Or, for the same reason that Ehrenberg's discoveries cannot be appreciated by those who have either no microscope; or who have one which is not good, or who, have a microscope without understanding the difficult art of using it; or else who know how to use it, but do not use it with same exactness and carefulness as Ehrenberg, who discovered in the chalk dust of visiting cards the shells of new species of animals, by simply making the cards transparent by means of the oil of turpentine.

Or lastly, for the simple reason that physicians find it more easy to write something for print, than to observe nature; that is more easy to impress upon people than to cure the sick, and because the greater number of physicians is affected with the delusion that things which they do not see do not exist.

If such physicians succeed in effecting a cure they are at once ready to boast of their exploits, whereas the cure was due to Hahnemann's doctrine, to the remedies which he has discovered, to the researches of other physicians, to their instructions or example, or to so-called chance. But if they do not succeed they impute their failure to anything but themselves: it is homoeopathy, that is deficient; this or that rule is not correct; the materia medica is at fault; or if something in Hahnemann's system does not suit them, they are prone to say that they have never seen this or that, that they cannot agree with it. And in talking in this way, they really imagine they have said something against the matter itself.

Upon the same ground that Hahnemann carefully distinguished from the disease the symptoms which owed their existence to dietetic transgressions, or to medicinal aggravations; upon the same grounds that he acknowledged as standing and independent diseases the acute miasms, known as purpura, measles, scarlatina, small pox, whooping cough, etc., or that he distinguished the venereal miasm into *syphilis* and *sycosis*, we may afterwards, if experience should demand it, subdivide *psora* into several species and varieties. This is no objection to Hahnemann's theory. Hahnemann has taken the first great step without denying the faculty of progressive development inherent in his system. But let improvements be made in such a way as to become useful, not prejudicial to the patients. We ought to raise our superstructure upon Hahnemann's own ground, in the direction which he has first imparted to his doctrine.

Although it, matters little what opinions the respective disciples of Hahnemann hold relatively to the theory of *psora*. I will nevertheless communicate a short extract from my essay *Guide, to the Progressive Development of Homoeopathy*

As acute diseases terminate in an eruption upon the skin, which divides, dries up, and then passes off, so it is with many chronic diseases. All diseases diminish in intensity, improve, and are cured by the internal organism freeing itself from them little by little; the internal disease approaches more and more to the external tissues, until it finally arrives at the skin.

Every homoeopathic physician must have observed that the improvement in pain takes place from above downward; and in diseases, from within outward. This is the reason why chronic diseases, if they are thoroughly cured, always terminate in some cutaneous eruption. Which differs according to the different constitutions of the patients. This cutaneous eruption may be even perceived when a cure is impossible, and even when the remedies have been improperly chosen. The skin being the outermost surface of the body, it receives upon itself the extreme termination of the disease. This cutaneous eruption is not a mere morbid secretion having been chemically separated from the internal organism in the form of a gas, a liquid, or a solid; it is the whole of the morbid action which is pressed from within outward, and it is characteristic of a thorough and really curative treatment. The morbid action of the internal organism may continue either entirely, or more or less in spite of this cutaneous eruption. Nevertheless, this eruption always is a favourable symptom; it alleviates the sufferings of the patient, and generally prevents a more dangerous affection.

The thorough cure for a widely ramified chronic disease in the organism is indicated by the most important organs being first relieved, the affection passes off in the order in which the organs had been effected, the more important being relieved first, the less important next, and, the, skin last.

Even the superficial observer will not fail in recognising this law of order. An improvement which takes place in a different order can never be relied upon. A fit of hysteria may terminate in a flow of urine; other fits say either terminate in the same way, or in haemorrhage; the next succeeding fit shows how little the affection had been cured. The disease may take a different turn, it may change its form and, in this new form, it say be less troublesome; but the general state of the organism, will suffer in consequence, of this transformation.

Hence it is that Hahnemann inculcates with so such care the important rule to attend to the moral symptoms, and to judge of the degree of homoeopathic adaptation, existing between the remedy and the disease, by the improvement which takes place in the moral condition, and the general well-being of the patient.

The law of order which we have, pointed out above accounts for the numerous cutaneous eruptions consequent upon homoeopathic treatment, even where they never had been before; it accounts for the obstinacy with which many kinds of herpes and ulcers remain upon the skin, whereas others are dissipated like snow. Those which remain do remain because the internal disease is yet existing. This law of order also accounts for the insufficiency of violent sweats, when the internal disease is not yet disposed to leave its hiding place. It lastly accounts for one cutaneous affection being substituted for another.

This transformation of the internal affection of such parts of the organism, as are essential to important functions, to a cutaneous affection a transformation which is entirely, different from the violent change affected by mwans of Authenreith's ointment, ammonium, croton oil, cantharides, mustard, etc. - is chiefly affected by the antipsoric remedies.

Other remedies, may sometimes effect, that transformation, even the use of water, change of climate, of occupation, etc.; but it is more safely more mildly and more thoroughly effected by antipsoric remedies.

This latter is altogether an individual opinion others may have different opinions relative to the same subject; this needs not prevent us from aiming all of us at the same end, side by side, in perfect harmony.

But alas! The rules which the experienced founder of homoeopathy lays down in the subsequent work with so much emphasis are not always practised, and therefore cannot be appreciated. Many oppose them; cures which otherwise might be speedy and certain are delayed; much injury is being done by the wiseacres, who intrude themselves into our literature and mix with it as chaff with the wheat. In all this we may console ourselves with the expectation that also in the history of science there will be those great days of harvest, when the tares shall be gathered in bundles and thrown into the fire.

It is the duty of all of us to go farther in the theory and practice of homoeopathy than Hahnemann has done. We ought to seek the truth which is before us and forsake the errors of the past. But woe unto him who, on that account, should personally attack the author of our doctrine; he will burden himself with infamy. Hahnemann was a great servant, inquirer and discoverer; he was as true a man, without falsity, candid and open as a child, and inspired with pure benevolence and with a holy zeal for science.

When at last the fatal hour had struck for the sublime old man who had preserved his vigour almost to his last moments, then it was that the heart of his consort who had made his last years the brightest of his life was on the point of breaking. Many of us, seeing those who are dearest to us engaged in the death-struggle, would exclaim why should'st thou suffer so much ! So too exclaimed Hahnemann's consort: "Why should'st thou who hast alleviated so much suffering suffer in thy last hour? This is unjust. Providence should have allotted to thee a painless death."

Then he raised his voice as he had often done when he exhorted his disciples to hold fast to the great principles of homoeopathy. "Why should I have been thus extinguished? Each of us should here attend to the duties which God has imposed upon him. Although men may distinguish a more or less, yet no one has any merit. God owes nothing to me, I to him all."

With these words he took leave of the world, of his friends, and his foes. And here we take leave of you, reader, whether our friend or our opponent.

To him who believes that there may yet be truths which he does not know and which he desires to know, will be pointed out such paths as will lead him to the light he needs. If he who has sincere benevolence and wishes to work for the benefit of all be considered by Providence a fit instrument for the accomplishment of the divine will, he will be called upon to fulfil his mission and will be led to truth evermore.

It is the spirit of Truth that tries to unite us all; but the father of Lies keeps us separate and divided.

Constantine Hering, Philadelphia, April 22, 1845

* **Editor's Note:** I beg pardon of my distinguished and learned friend for annexing a few remarks to this passage. In doing so I merely anticipate what I intend to express more fully on this subject some other occasion.

References

1. Raue, CG, Knerr, CB & Mohr, C. *A Memorial of Constantine Hering*, Philadelphia PA, Globe Printing House, 1884.
2. Bradford, TL. *Pioneers of Homoeopathy*, Philadelphia, Boericke & Tafel, 1897.
3. Cleave, E. *Biographical Cyclopædia of Homoeopathic Physicians and Surgeons*, Philadelphia, Galaxy Publishing, 1873
4. Freud, S. in: Strachey, J. ed. *The Standard Edition of the Complete Psychological Works of Sigmund Freud Vol. XI*, Hogarth Press, London, p. 18. (*First Lecture on Psychoanalysis in his Five Lectures.*) 2001. I am indebted to Annette Gamblin RSHom, for drawing my attention to this statement.
5. Allen, HC. *Materia Medica of the Nosodes*, Philadelphia, Boericke & Tafel. 1910, 'The first preparation was made according to Hering's propositions [laid down in Stapf's *Archives*, 1830]'.
6. *Ibid.* 'Introduced and proved by Hering in 1833, fifty years before the crude experiments of Pasteur with the serum.'
7. Knerr, CB. *Life of Hering*, Philadelphia PA, Magee Press 1940; see also: Raue, CG, et. al., 1884.
8. Hahnemann, S. (trans. Hempel, C.) 1828, *The Chronic Diseases, their Specific Nature and Homoeopathic Treatment 1828*, New York, William Radde, 1845. This *Preface* was omitted from the 2nd edition: *Chronic Diseases, Their Peculiar Nature and Their Homoeopathic Cure 1833* (trans. Tafel, LH.), Boericke & Tafel, Philadelphia, 1896.

5

PREFACES TO THE BRITISH AND AMERICAN EDITIONS OF THE *ORGANON*

Introduction

The *Organon* is the first and lasting foundation text of homeopathic medicine, with editions in at least 30 languages: Bengali, Bulgarian, Czech, Danish, Dutch, English, Farsi, Finnish, French, German, Greek, Gujerati, Hebrew, Hindi, Hungarian, Italian, Japanese, Marathi, Norwegian, Oriya, Polish, Portuguese, Romanian, Russian, Spanish, Swedish, Tamil, Telugu, Turkish and Urdu.[1]

Hahnemann set the scene for homeopathy with a principled statement based on a dynamic and vitalist view of health and disease.

> *No disease is caused by any material substance . . . but every one is only and always a peculiar, virtual, dynamic derangement of the health.*[2]

The first translation of the *Organon* into English was of the fourth edition, published in Dublin[3] (see figure 5.1). It was republished in Pennsylvania, with a preface by Hering, where it was titled the British edition, and the reprint as the first American edition.[4] Both prefaces are in this chapter, and together they show a contrast between the more naïve account of a layman - Stratten - explaining his first encounter with the new school, and the already experienced homeopathic physician - Hering - writing en erudite explanation of Hahnemann's ideas in this new edition. Before the famine, Dublin was one of the cultural capitals of Europe, a fitting location for the first exhibition of Hahnemann's work in English.[5]

Pennsylvania became the nineteenth century powerhouse of homeopathy on the Eastern seaboard of America.[6] From this date the epistemology of homeopathy becomes very tangled, as the philosophical underpinnings of the details of homeopathic practice become confused, between different editions and differing translations of the *Organon*.[7,8] The confusion centres round many fundamental aspects, such as the dispensing of medicines as solid or liquid doses, and as a single potency or as ascending potencies; and if so as centesimal potencies, or as succussed daily by the patient using the fifty-millesimal or LM scale. The emergence of the true 6th edition of the *Organon* in 1921, translated in 1922,[9] does not end the controversies, as the new LM scale was not universally adopted[10].

Preface to the Dublin translation of 1833 (known as the 'British Edition')[11]

An accidental interview with a Russian physician, in the year 1828, made me acquainted for the first time with the medical doctrine of homoeopathy; the principle of which is, that certain medicines when administered internally in a healthy state of the system produce certain effects, and that the same medicines are to be used when symptoms similar to those which they give rise to occur in disease. This doctrine, directly opposite to that which hitherto formed the basis of medical practice in these countries, attracted my attention. I immediately procured Hahnemann's *Materia Medica Pura*, in which the doctrine is partially explained, with the view of investigating the system experimentally, and reporting my observations thereon, free from theory, prejudice, or party. The first enquiry was, whether the proposition *similia similibus curentur* was true. This investigation was confined to a single substance at a time. To ascertain the effects of sulphate of quinine, healthy individuals were selected, to whom grain doses of the medicine were administered three times a day. After using it for some days, stomach-sickness, loss of appetite, a sense of cold along the course of the spine, rigour, heat of skin, and general perspiration succeeded. Effects similar to these are often observed when this medicine is injudiciously selected in the treatment of disease. It sometimes happens, that the symptoms of ague are aggravated by the prolonged use of sulphate of quinia, and soon after it is withdrawn the disease gradually subsides. The result of experiments and observations on this remedy elucidate its homeopathic action.

Mercurial preparations, when administered internally, produce symptoms local and constitutional so closely resembling the poison of *lues venerea* that medical practitioners who have spent many years in the investigation of syphilis find it very difficult, nay, in some instances, impossible (guided by the appearances), to distinguish one disease from the other. Of all the medicines used in the treatment of *lues*, mercury is the only one that has stood the test of time and experience. Let us then compare the effects of syphilis, with those of mercury: The venereal poison produces on the skin, pustules, scales, and tubercles. Mercury produces directly the same defoedations of the skin. Syphilis excites inflammation of the periosteum and caries of the bones. Mercury does the same. Inflammation of the iris from lues is an every-day occurrence; the same disease is a very frequent consequence of mercury. Ulceration of the throat is a common symptom in syphilis; the same affection results from mercury. Ulcers on the organs of reproduction are the result of both the poison and the remedy; and furnish another proof of the doctrine *similia similibus*.

Nitric acid is generally recommended in cutaneous diseases; the internal use of this remedy, in a very dilute form, produces scaly eruptions over the surface of

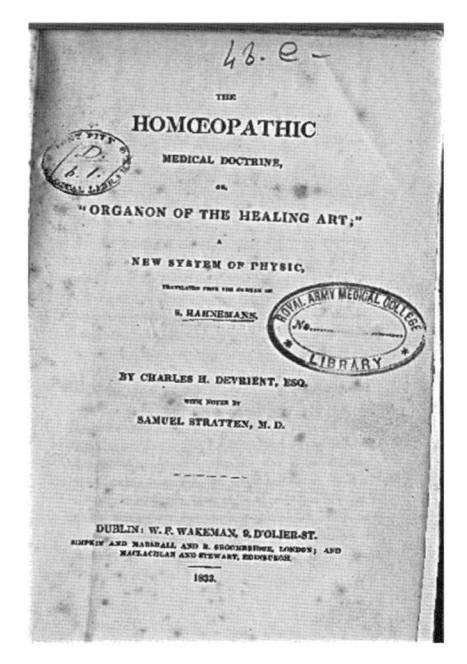

Figure 5.1 Frontispage of the 4th Edition of the *Organon* published in Dublin in 1833 (From the author's personal collection)

the body; and the external application of a solution, in the proportion of one part acid to one hundred and twenty-eight parts of water, will produce inflammation and ulceration of the skin. These observations would lead to the conclusion, that *Nitric acid* cures cutaneous diseases by the faculty it possesses of producing a similar disease of the skin. Nitrate of potash administered internally in small doses, produces a frequent desire to pass water, accompanied with pain and heat. When this state of the urinary system exists as a consequence of disease, or the application of a blister, a very dilute solution of the same remedy has been found beneficial.

The ordinary effects of *Hyoscyamus niger* are vertigo, delirium stupefaction, and somnolency. Where one or other of these diseased states exists, it yields to small doses of the tincture of this plant. The internal use of *Hyoscyamus* is followed by mental aberration, the leading features of which are jealousy, and irascibility. When these hallucinations exist, this remedy is indicated.

Opium in general causes drowsiness, torpor, and deep sleep, and yet this remedy in small doses removes these symptoms when they occur in disease.

Sulphur is a specific against itch; notwithstanding which, when it is administered to healthy individuals it frequently excites a pustular eruption resembling itch in every particular.

These observations corroborate the statements of our author as to the value and importance of homoeopathy, and were not the limits of a preface too confined

I could bring forward the actual experiments from which these deductions have been drawn.

On the subject of small doses of medicines a few observations will suffice.

A mixture composed of one drop of hydrocyanic acid and eight ounces of water, administered in a drachm dose, has produced vertigo and anxious breathing. Vomiting has followed the use of the sixteenth of a grain of emetic tartar; narcotism, the twentieth of a grain of muriate of morphia; and spirit of ammonia, in doses of one drop, acts on the system as a stimulant.

On the homoeopathic attenuation of medicines, many are sceptical, and presume that the quantity of the article extant in the dose cannot produce a medicinal effect. I refer to the pages of the *Organon* for an elucidation of this proposition, and will relate an experiment, which may serve to explain the degree of dilution substances are capable of. One grain of nitrate of silver dissolved in 1560 grains of distilled water, to which were added two grains of muriatic acid, a gray precipitate of chloride of silver was evident in every part of the liquor. One grain of iodine dissolved in a drachm of alcohol and mixed with the same quantity of water as in the preceding experiment, to which were added two grains of starch dissolved in an ounce of water, caused an evident blue tint in the solution. In these experiments the grain of the nitrate of silver and iodine must have been divided into 1/5360 of a grain.

A few particulars connected with the discoverer and founder of the homoeopathic system of medicine, cannot but prove interesting to the readers of this volume. Samuel Hahnemann was born in 1755, at Meissen, in Upper Saxony. He exhibited at "an early age traits of a superior genius; his school education being completed, he applied himself to the study of natural philosophy and natural history, and afterwards prosecuted the study of medicine at Leipzig and other universities. A most accurate observer, a skilful experimenter, and an indefatigable searcher after truth, he appeared formed by nature for the investigation and improvement of medical science. On commencing the study of medicine he soon became disgusted with the mass of contradictory assertions and theories which then existed. He found every thing in this department obscure, hypothetical and vague, and resolved to abandon the medical profession. Having been previously engaged in the study of chemistry, he determined on translating into his native language the best English and French works on the subject. Whilst engaged in translating the *Materia Medica* of the illustrious Cullen, in 1790, in which the febrifuge virtues of cinchona bark are described, he became fired with the desire of ascertaining its mode of action. Whilst in the enjoyment of the most robust health, he commenced the use of this substance, and in a short time was attacked with all the symptoms of intermittent fever, similar in every respect to those which that medicine is known to cure, being struck with the identity of the two diseases he immediately divined the great truth which has become the foundation of the new medical doctrine of homoeopathy.

Not contented with one experiment he tried the virtues of medicines on his own person, and on that of others. In his investigations he arrived at this conclusion: that the substance employed possessed an inherent power of exciting in healthy subjects the same symptoms which it is said to cure in the sick. He compared the assertions of ancient and modern physicians upon the properties of poisonous substances with the result of his own experiments, and found them to coincide in every respect; and upon these deductions he brought forth his doctrine of homoeopathy. Taking this law for a guide, he recommenced the practice of medicine, with every prospect of his labours being ultimately crowned with success.

In 1796 he published his first dissertation on homoeopathy in Hufeland's *Journal*. A treatise on the virtues of medicine appeared in 1805, and the *Organon* in 1810. Hahnemann commenced as a public medical teacher in Leipsic, in 1811, where, with his pupils, he zealously investigated the effects of medicines on the living body, which formed the basis of the Materia Medica Pura, which appeared during the same year.

Like many other discoverers in medicine, the author of the *Organon* has been persecuted with the utmost rigour; and in 1820 he quitted his native country in disgust. In retirement he was joined by several of his pupils, who formed themselves into a society for the purpose of prosecuting the homoeopathic system of physic, and reporting their observations thereon. Several fasciculi detailing their labours have been since published.

In 1824 the homoeopathic doctrine was embraced by Rau, physician to the Duke of Hesse Darmstadt; by Bigelius, physician to the Emperor of Russia; by Stegemann, and many other names celebrated in medicine.

We find, from a published letter of Dr Peschier of Geneva, that Hahnemann resides at Köthen (capital of Anhalt-Köthen), in the enjoyment of perfect health and spirits. He is consulted by patients from almost every nation, who have been attracted by his fame as a physician.

Of the doctrine of homoeopathy generally, I have little more to add in this place; time will develop the truth or fallacy of the principle on which it is founded; but in the mean time let us not lose sight of the fact, that this new system of physic is spreading throughout the continent of Europe with the rapidity of lightning. Germany, Austria, Russia, and Poland, have already done homage to the doctrine, and physicians have been appointed to make a specific trial of its effects, the results of which are unequivocally acknowledged to be of a favourable nature. The writings of the illustrious Hahnemann have appeared in five different languages, independent of the present version of his *Organon*, and in France alone, a translation of this work, from the pen of AJL Jourdan, member of the Academie Royale de Médécine, has reached a fourth edition.

Convinced, from reflection and observation, of the value of homoeopathy, the first step in the propagation and dissemination of this doctrine, in Britain, was to obtain an English version of the *Organon*.

Samuel Stratten Dublin 14th June 1833

Preface to the first American edition of 1836[12]

First impressions commonly determine our judgment of books as well as men. If, on a first interview, a person be repulsive to us, and those who for years have had familiar intercourse with him, admit that we are excusable for first impressions, but nevertheless assure us that he is possessed of very valuable qualities, and that a nearer acquaintance with him may be useful to us, when, in addition, our informants give us a key to a more correct judgment, we are no longer justifiable in maintaining our original impressions. Still more would our opinions be influenced, if, before seeing the person, we were furnished in advance with a short and impartial representation of his character by one who knew him intimately. If this rule of judgment be applicable to persons, wherefore should it not apply to books?

The *Organon* contains much that is peculiar and different from the views hitherto entertained by the prevailing school of medicine. Most readers of the

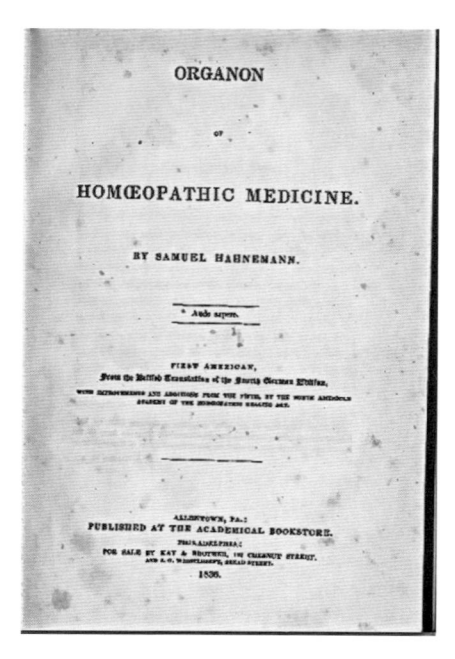

Figure 5.2 Frontispage of the 4th Edition of the *Organon* published in Philadelphia in 1836 (From the author's personal collection)

medical profession, therefore, conceive prejudices against it, and fall into the vulgar error of rejecting the whole, merely because they do not justly regard it as a whole, they reject the main propositions, because they are offended at the subordinate.

The reader needs no elaborate introduction to the following work, and it is requisite, perhaps, only to apprise him of the different classes into which its several paragraphs may be divided; and this being done, we shall submit each separate class to his own judgment.

The entire contents of the *Organon* may be easily arranged under the four following divisions, which, indeed, do not occur in the order in which they are here given, but they might easily have been designated in accordance to it, by causing them to be severally printed in a different type. They consist, 1, of discoveries – experimental propositions, or the results of actual experiment; 2, of directions or instructions; 3, of theoretical and philosophical illustration; 4 of defences and accusations.

Of discoveries

Among men of deliberate and acute reflection, no difference of opinion can exist relative to the truth of a discovery, which rests upon the basis of actual experiment. When the author appeals to such experiments, they must be led to a repetition of them, and not oppose their own opinions to the dictates of experience; in fine, they have no other way in forming a judgment, than that of accurate and careful experiment.

It may be said that every charlatan in extolling his nostrums in like manner appeals to experience, and no one is required for that reason to investigate the merits of his compounds; but it will not be denied that, although the person of the quack may deserve little forbearance, yet the remedy with which he dupes the public, may in some cases prove beneficial. The old school has received many remedies, mercury among others, from the hands of the quack.

But, in the *Organon*, experience is not referred to for the purpose of lauding any individual remedy; far more, it has relation to an entire method of cure. None but a vulgar dealer in calumny of the grosser sort, would attempt to degrade Hahnemann to a level with the charlatan; because he promulgates his views and the peculiarities of his method, as a learned physician, and in a manner that is sanctioned by custom, and fully recognised in the history of medicine.

But his method, as we have already intimated, appeals to experience. Not to mention the example of Brown, we need only refer to that of Broussais, and the reports received strikingly in favour of his doctrines, or even to the contra-stimulus of the Italians, which incessantly appeals to the same experience as the test of its value.

It is, indeed, desirable that every learned physician – professors, hospital physicians, and others in prominent stations should carefully study, and so far as the experiments are innocuous, prove his new method; nay, Hahnemann and his adherents often and ardently desire that every physician would learn, investigate, and prove homoeopathy for himself.

But homoeopathy is not only a new method, but much more.

This method does not rest upon new views, like every other hitherto promulgated, but upon new discoveries, which appertain to the departments of natural philosophy, the natural sciences, physiology and biology.

The doctrine that every peculiar substance – every mineral, plant, animal, in fact every part of them, or every preparation derived from a preceding one, produces a series of peculiar effects upon the human organism, manifestly belongs to the natural sciences, and only so far to the *materia medica* as the latter calls these properties into requisition. But it is a science in itself, a science which treats of the effect of a diversity of substances upon the human frame. Whether such a science, in point of fact, be capable of formation, and whether it have any value, can be determined only by experiment. It were equally foolish to deny this without trial, as it was formerly to deny, without exploring, the way which Columbus opened to the west. It would be inexcusable in the present condition of the *materia medica,* confessedly imperfect, and deficient in all the attributes of a science, to despise this new way of Hahnemann, before knowing, by careful experiment, that it conducts to nothing better.

The doctrine of the preparation of the remedies into the so-called dilutions belongs to natural philosophy, in common with the doctrines of magnetism, electricity, and galvanism. Nor is it more a subject of wonder than the latter, except that these sooner came under investigation by the natural philosopher. The repetition of the new electro-magnetic experiments requires great accuracy; those concerning the operation of minute doses require just as much, nay even more. To deny the results of the electro-magnetic experiments, previous to repeating them, were ridiculous, and it is equally so to deny the results of these. But no hasty, superficial, partial, or wholly perverted experiments must be instituted.

The doctrine that such dilutions or potencies are capable of curing diseases according to the law 'similia similibus,' is a proposition, which belongs to biology, and there finds its confirmation; it likewise can only be investigated by experiment, and cannot be estimated without it.

The cautious investigator will not pass judgment upon all these discoveries, until he shall have performed a series of rigorous experiments. Then only will he be prepared either to reject or accept the method founded thereon, or, at least, learn the useful part of it.

Directions
These appertain to the method of cure, are derived from the long continued application of the law previously referred to, and acquire their principal value from its

truth. No one can judge of them but he who has tested the truth of the experimental propositions, and in doing so, adhered to these directions. By this means only can he become convinced of their great value, which is entirely lost on those who deny the discoveries.

We enumerate under this head, directions for the examination of the sick, for the preparation of the medicines, for trying them on the healthy subject, for the selection of the remedies, dietetics, and directions for the psychical treatment.

Illustrations
Hahnemann has appended certain theories to the laws of nature discovered by him, by which these laws are illustrated and brought into unison with other laws already acknowledged, or with other theories received as true. This has never been reckoned a subject of reproach to any discoverer. Man will and must seek to illustrate the phenomena which he observes, and bring individual parts into co-aptation – the new into harmony with that previously known. In this endeavour, not only is he liable to err, but actually does err in the great majority of cases; accordingly, few hypotheses and attempts at explanation have endured long, and it is a fact of daily acknowledgment, that one hypothesis gives place to another in all sciences. Columbus himself entertained numerous conjectures which time has verified or overthrown. Whether the theories of Hahnemann are destined to endure a longer or a shorter space, whether they be the best or not, time only can determine; be it as it may, however, it is a mailer of minor importance. For myself, I am generally considered as a disciple and adherent of Hahnemann, and I do indeed declare that I am one among the most enthusiastic in doing homage to his greatness; but nevertheless I declare also, that since my first acquaintance with homoeopathy, (in the year 1821), down to the present day, I have never yet accepted a single theory in the *Organon* as it is there promulgated. I feel no aversion to acknowledge this even to the venerable sage himself. It is the genuine Hahnemannean spirit totally to disregard all theories, even those of one's own fabrication, when they are in opposition to the results of pure experience. All theories and hypotheses have no positive weight whatever, only so far as they lead to new experiments, and afford a better survey of the results of those already made. Whoever, therefore, will assail the theories of Hahnemann, or even altogether reject them, is at perfect liberty to do so; but let him not imagine that he has thereby accomplished a memorable achievement. In every respect it is an affair of little importance.

Defences
Opinions upon this head are also things of secondary consideration, inasmuch as the entire polemical matter is of subordinate estimation in forming a judgment concerning new discoveries. Had Hahnemann the right to defend himself as he

has done, and thereby promote the progress of his doctrine, or had he not? We cannot judge concerning it, but justly commit the decision of the question to future history. The entire polemical part may be stricken out, without in the slightest degree changing the principal matters, or without having any influence either to ratify or invalidate the doctrine itself.

Is there a physician who feels that individual expressions will apply to him, let him take heed to the truth; but if they do not reach him, then is he unaffected by them. He who is offended at the polemical part, let him reflect that it is the first step towards an unjust estimate of the rest.

A just judgment is all that we wish from every reader of the *Organon*, and to contribute something to this end was the design of these preliminary remarks.

Constantine Hering, Academy at Allentown, Penn.,
10th August 1836.

References

1. Treuherz, F, *Library Catalogue*, unpublished.
2. Hahnemann, S. Boericke, W. trans. *The Organon of Medicine 6th edition*, Philadelphia, Boericke & Tafel, 1922. Introduction, p. 22.
3. Hahnemann, S. *The Homoeopathic Medical Doctrine, or Organon of the Healing Art. A New System of Physic translated from the German of S. Hahnemann by Charles H. Devrient, esq., with notes by Samuel Stratten, MD*, Wakeman, Dublin, 1833.
4. Hahnemann, S. *Organon of Homoeopathic Medicine. 1st American from the British translation of the Fourth German Edition with Improvements and Additions from the Fifth by the North American Academy of the Homoeopathic Healing Art*, Allentown, PA, Academical Bookstore, 1836.
5. Treuherz, F. *Homoeopathy in the Irish Potato Famine*, London, Samuel Press, 1995.
6. Treuherz, F. The origins of Kent's homeopathy, *Journal of The American Institute of Homeopathy*, 1984 77:4.
7. Hahnemann S. Dudgeon, RE. trans. *The Organon of Medicine, 5th edition*, London, W. Headland & New York, Radde, 1849.
8. Hahnemann, S. Wesselhoeft, C. trans. *The Organon of the Art of Healing 5th edition*. 5th American Edition, Philadephia, Boericke & Tafel, 1876.
9. Hahnemann, S. Boericke, W. trans. *The Organon of Medicine 6th edition*, Philadelphia, Boericke & Tafel, 1922.
10. Schmidt, P. Hahnemann's *Organon* and its Hidden Treasures, *Homoeopathic Recorder*, 1955 & 1956, 70 & 71.
11. Hahnemann, S. *The Homoeopathic Medical Doctrine, or Organon of the Healing Art. A New System of Physic translated from the German of S. Hahnemann by Charles H. Devrient, esq., with notes by Samuel Stratten, MD*, Wakeman, Dublin, 1833.

12 Hahnemann, S. *Organon of Homoeopathic Medicine. 1st American from the British translation of the Fourth German Edition with Improvements and Additions from the Fifth by the North American Academy of the Homoeopathic Healing Art*, Allentown, PA, Academical Bookstore, 1836.

6

HOMEOPATHIC REMINISCENCES

Introduction

The essay in this chapter forms part of the writings of Hahnemann that, together with a quantity of furniture, were ceded to Mr Peter Stuart in 1878 by Madame von Boenninghausen (the adopted daughter of Melanie Hahnemann and married to Dr Carl von Boenninghausen). The translation from German was made by a Herr Kroeber.[1] The documents remained with the Stuart family until they were donated to the UK Faculty of Homeopathy early in the 20th century.

Here Hahnemann states what may be his real reasons for moving to Paris. In homeopathic circles, a version probably going back to Haehl, suggests Melanie married Samuel for selfish ends, abducted him to Paris and then persuaded him to practice there.[2] A more humane and modern version of events is that of Rima Handley.[3] Would it be impossible to consider that Hahnemann wrote with conviction in the first three paragraphs of this manuscript?[1]

Also notable is Hahnemann's statement that those whose cases have been spoilt by the predominant medicine of the day, have little chance of homeopathic cure. We should always remind ourselves of this fact and not put homeopathy itself in doubt, when patients who have been under the influence of strong-acting medicines for years do not recover speedily or perhaps not at all. He also emphasises the need for daily study of materia medica to memorise the characteristic symptoms. He considers repertories as subordinate in this context. How should we consider the situation today, where the repertories have such a dominant role? Are these lines still relevant?

The final few paragraphs are startling in the light of modern ethics and practice. It is the practice of members of the Society of Homeopaths to inform their patients of the name of the remedy. Homeopathic practitioners and patients do not view homeopathy as a cult, which is a common view of the enemies of homeopathy. I suggest that in the last paragraph Hahnemann is writing with humility about a physician as a priest and healer, with a sacred vocation to help the sick humanity.

JH Clarke (see Chapter 12) commented as editor of *Homoeopathic World* in which journal the piece was published in 1908 :

this article will be read with pleasure for the valuable practical points it contains. I have taken the liberty to add cross-headings; and I have left out some critical passages referring to the practice in vogue at the time.[4]

Dedicated to the day of the Union between the two Homoeopathic Societies, the Gallic[5] *with the Parisian.*[6]

Homoeopathic reminiscences[7]
By Samuel Hahnemann

When I fancied that I should quietly pass the evening of my strenuous and laborious life in pacific retirement in the small town of Köthen, I was again launched into activity by the news that in beautiful France – that country which in recognition of humanity and the rights of mankind seems destined to be a light to be copied by the rest of the world – the only true new healing science, called homoeopathy, was beginning to be eagerly adopted and practised by the more erudite doctors, more energetically almost than in any other land.

The less prejudiced mode of thinking of the Frenchmen, and their talent more easily to assimilate new truths, and allow them to develop in their Country, made it appear to me extremely probable that this healing art would develop far more rapidly in France than anywhere else, and that only a guiding hand was wanting in order to give France the complete superiority over all other lands, also in the practice of the medical science.

This consideration made me decide to go to Paris.

As always during my long life, as also now, almost visibly led by the kindly providence of the Supreme Being, I arrived some time ago in France, and certainly saw that a large number of doctors in Paris practised homoeopathy, even diligently, but also that very few of them had penetrated deeply enough into the true healing spirit of this new real healing art to enable them to exercise the same with good results, and allow me to acknowledge them as my genuine successors. From the majority of the others, on the other hand, I saw that they had not given much deep study to this so difficult as well as beneficent art, and tried to make their practice of it far too easy, only treating their patients in a superficial manner, and therefore perfectly curing but a small number of them, which, of course, would diminish the confidence of the public in this sole helpful healing art, and, as a matter of fact, has weakened it.

I should be glad if they would pay due attention to my exhortations, and conscientiously follow the example of the best real disciples, as well as mine, and so show to the world that France, and especially Paris, is ahead of all other lands in the deep study of homoeopathy and in the practice of the only real and right, helpful, and indispensable true method of saving and healing our sick fellow-creatures.

I call this new and sole true healing art indispensable, because it was high time that the same should be made known, as the elder medicinal art, which so far has imposed itself on the world for more than two thousand years as a help in sickness, simply raged like a destroyer amongst the peoples, always under some new disguise of systems which contradicted each other, and of which not one could produce a principle based on nature and experience, and so simply went on their old destructive way in their torturing of humanity under delusions and illusive representations.

In opposition to this methodical barbaric extermination of the pitiable invalids, the great creator and preserver of mankind allowed a mild true healing art to be found, not built up on sophistical mistaken school doctrines of ancient academies and faculties, but on clear and simple observation of nature, and of what is established by her inexorable laws for the welfare of sick humanity.

Homoeopathy appeared and maintained its place with its true practitioners for more than thirty years' experience in nearly all parts of the world, as a saviour of sick humanity.

The peoples themselves were and remained so far in striking danger of being at least decimated, if not altogether exterminated, through the so-called art of the then obtaining school of medicine.

That, however, this heavenly mild help, called homoeopathy, when properly learned and conscientiously carried out, has almost miraculously, quickly, mildly, and permanently cured sicknesses – i.e., not of those already ruined by the hitherto obtaining school of medicine – has brought upon itself the bitterest most implacable hate and unceasing persecution from the obtaining school of medicine, which must first die off before homoeopathy can spread its blessings over sick humanity.

That homoeopathy can save and restore to good health those predestined to a certain death by the misuse of *Mercury* in all shapes and forms, *Lapis infernalis* (*Caustic*), *Iodine, Prussic acid, Quinine, Digitalis,* &c., or restore those who, through innumerable cuppings, have lost blood – that sap absolutely necessary to life, consequently to those sick people who are radically ruined, can save and reconstitute – no sensible person would ascribe this power to homoeopathy. It is not permitted to any mortal to do the impossible.

But even the most difficult cases, excepting those already hopelessly spoilt by wrong treatment, are cured by homoeopathy without any difficulty and with apparently the most insignificant remedies, which, however, have been discovered to be the most efficacious for the illness, i.e., through specific homoeopathic medicine, administered in the minutest doses, and the restoration to sound health follows quickly and imperceptibly, often incredibly quickly and unperceived.

Homoeopathy not an easy art
I consider it my duty, however, to draw the attention of my disciples in all earnestness to the labour and difficulty connected with the proper execution of the homoeopathic curing art, with a view of frightening off all such doctors from the exercise of it, who think it to be a superficial matter, with which one can make healing very easy, as the doctors of the old school have done, up to now, as well as those now obtaining, who can only find 'Irritation' and 'Irritation' everywhere, and consequently do not know what to prescribe other than diet, starvation, calf's-foot jelly, bleeding, re-bleeding with applications of leeches, until the last breath of life has evaporated.

That is certainly an easy, although a destructive method, because it requires no trouble or thought, but only a pitiless audacity, combined with a lack of conscience, exactly the reverse of what is necessary to the successful practice of the only true healing art, homoeopathy.

Individualisation
No one can be looked upon as a real and true homoeopathic doctor who does not give the most exhaustive attention to each individual case of illness, combined with a knowledge of healthy mankind, and of those extraneous things which affect people, but principally endowed with a good sound understanding, which rejects all and every prejudice, and a philanthropical heart completely dedicated to the welfare of his suffering fellow creatures. He must, alike with rich or poor, find out what the cause or the promotion of his present sickness is, also with chronic sicknesses note their changes, and find out the nature of the previous illnesses, take into consideration, and put in writing, the age of the patient, his visible bodily state, the condition of the sexual functions, as well as that of the intellect and temper, and lastly, carefully weigh the possible influence exercised on him by his home and business associations and by the people who surround him, in his attack of illness, so as to possibly eliminate any cause for protraction of the sickness. He must obtain a full and explicit account of all the present ailments from the patient himself for choice, complete the rest by questions, and carefully write down all that he knows of him, has heard of him, and himself observed, so as to be able to regulate him accordingly during the future treatment.

Note-taking essential, as well as memorising
As it is impossible for a doctor to remember all these details regarding his sundry patients, one who does not write down this necessary examinations of his patient must be accounted a thoughtless man, and cannot be regarded as a true and conscientious homoeopathic doctor, and therefore nowise deserves the confidence of the Public.

When the true homoeopathic doctor is fully cognisant of the efficacy of all the medical mediums employed, which may rightly be expected and demanded from him; when he has fully learnt and impressed upon his memory, through daily studying and learning of all given in the best and true publications connected with the true mediums of medicine, the characteristic and special signs of each most thoroughly approved of medicines (an indispensable study which repays itself enormously), then he can always, and almost without any augmentary help from the well-known Repertories, hit upon and apply the homoeopathic (specially helpful) curing means for the then existing state of sickness, in the necessary small doses.

After subsequent research he will, no less than before, put down in writing the result of the working of the medicine taken on the state of the patient, and comparing this state with the previously annotated condition, be able to determine whether the medicine given has still any necessity for working on the organism, or whether a fresh dose has to be ordered, either of the same medicine in a different grade of potency, or of a different and now more suitable medicine, and all this the true homoeopathic doctor will carry out in cold blood and after ripe consideration – without any haste, and then he will reap the sweet recompense – the curing of his patient. In this solely helpful treatment of a patient by homoeopathy, in order to attain a thorough cure, the frequently appearing local maladies are generally never treated externally by homoeopathic doctors with medicinal applications (as the doctors of the old school do, just as if the illness were only located in that particular spot), because through such local applications they are often only driven from that spot to invariably reappear in a worse form in another more important and vital part, to the greater detriment of the patient. On the contrary, the homoeopath, in order to attain a radical cure, will only work through inwardly taken medicine on the incapacitated vitality, that is to say, on the whole organism at once, because this with every one, even with an only locally appearing disease, is still generally seized and afflicted – this general sickness consequently only showing itself in that particular spot, usually the weakest.

Since our organism combines in the sound as well as in the sick state an inseparable whole, composed of material parts which are dependent for their feeling and action solely on that animating unceasingly active force – which in itself is inscrutable – called vital power, therefore, upon this immaterial human vital power (because the material body is only the vehicle of vitality) an impression can only be made by extraneous matters in nature, and also by medicines only in their immaterial force, i.e. only in potency, and in this way bring about changes in the condition of the man, and only thus can he be healed.

Proved remedies only, and one at a time

The homoeopathic doctor gives no other medicine to his patients than such as have already been adequately proved in their working, by application in healthy people, so that he knows beforehand what changes they can make in the human state, and consequently could cure homoeopathically. He makes no blind trials with strong unknown substances in all sorts of illnesses, as the doctors of the old school do, through which, with Iodine, Prussic Acid, Creosote, &c., they have uselessly, and as if it were fun, killed off numbers of innocent patients in hospitals! And still kill them. The true homoeopathic doctor, in order to ascertain what he is doing, and what he has to expect, never gives his patients more than one single medicinal substance at a time, never two or more medicines mixed together, or with each other, or one remedy internally, and a different one externally. He leaves it to the doctors of the existing school to issue prescriptions of various things put together – which goes against sound common sense – the separate effects of, which on the condition of the patient they did not even know, and nevertheless allow their patients to absorb such mixtures indiscriminately, blindly, in frequent strong doses – to their ruin.

The true homoeopathic doctor gives with his own hand his simple medicines, which for security he has prepared himself or obtained from a trustworthy preparer of homoeopathic medicines, in order to be certain that his patient has got the right medicine, and this matter he relegates to nobody else; otherwise he must every time with his own eyes see that the assistant has certainly found the right medicine and really administered it. Whoever leaves this business to the apothecary is no true, conscientious homoeopath, and can never be certain of the consequences.

Homoeopathic dietary and regimen

The homoeopath orders diet and living regimen according to the nature of the illnesses, but does not try to make himself important by forbidding a large quantity of immaterial things, and so make the patient nervous. He therefore prescribes only such things as we really know act medicinally, or could otherwise retard the cure. But he may forbid, and rightly so, the simultaneous employment of household remedies, such as cosmetics, tooth-powders and washes, clysters, warm baths, &c.; he may alter deleterious covering, clothing and dwelling, and forbid the reading of harmful periodicals to the mentally disordered and diseased, and obtain for them practical conversation with rational people. He enjoins his chronic patients to enjoy the fresh air, combined with as much exercise as possible on foot without tiring themselves, also to washing in cold water or to short plunges. He strives to cheer their spirits and to remove their grief.

No boasting but keep the name of your remedy to yourself

The true homoeopath never boasts about his cures, does not promise his patient a quick cure, but knows how to obtain and hold their respect and obedience by kind, dignified, and straightforward dealing. To endeavour to win over the patients by telling them the name of the medicine they are to take, is a degrading conduct on the part of the doctor. No one proclaims himself a homoeopathic doctor who robs his patient of a single drop of blood (be it through blood-letting, cupping-glass, or leeches), who gives them aperients, or applies to the skin painful drawing-out remedies, puts on blisters or mustard poultices, opens Fontanels or keeps them down. His excuse for this - that he has not yet got so far in the new and difficult art of homoeopathy - is by no means an excuse for such a betrayal of the same. He should rather in such cases where he does not know how to help himself homoeopathically, call in another homoeopath who has progressed further than himself in the acquisition of this helpful art, for help and advice, until he himself, through zealous application, has equally progressed therein and possibly even further than his present adviser.

He who has once, by his own grand experiences, arrived at the conviction that homoeopathy is the only true way to heal human ills, must - if he has still a sensitive conscience - where his homoeopathic knowledge does not suffice for curing, rather strike out in a better way, than infamously bed pernicious alms with the old medical bungling work which is rightly called allopathy. When he who has morally gone astray has once become converted to virtue and uprightness, then he should rather give up his life than take refuge again in scoundrelism, even in his greatest need.

Real homoeopathic curing is a cult, a holy action in which the good homoeopathist takes the place of the creating Godhead to reform the human creature spoilt by sickness, and he restores to him, through the true healing art, his health, that inestimable gift at last bestowed by the All-bountiful to Mankind, which was vainly yearned for during all the past centuries.

References and notes

1 Hahnemann, S. Gypser, K-H. ed. Ein Manuskript Hahnemanns aus seiner Pariser Zeit, Homöopathische Erinnerungen von Samuel Hahnemann, in *Zeitschrift für klassische Homöopathie*, Heidelberg: Karl F. Haug, [1836], 1987:2, 65-73
2 Haehl, R. Grundy M. & Wheeler, C. trans. *Samuel Hahnemann, His Life and Work*, 2 vols., London, Homoeopathic Publishing Company, 1922.
3 Handley, R. *A Homeopathic Love Story: the Story of Samuel and Melanie Hahnemann*, North Atlantic Books, Berkeley, CA, 1990.
4 What has been omitted are mainly descriptions and assertive condemnations of the common allopathic practices of the times. There is also an exhortation that the homeopath should permit 'a moderate satisfaction of the sexual urge within marriage, and the reduction of unmarried celibacy'. I am indebted to Suse Moebius RSHom for assistance with reviewing the German.
5 The journal has 'Gaelic' but I am convinced that *Gallic* was the intended meaning, from *Société Gallicane*.

6 This 'day of the Union' never happened; the manuscript was prepared by Hahnemann, but he never read it in public. Denis Fournier cites 1835 as the probable date that it was written; Dr K-H Gypser suggests 1836–1837, and Dr Olivier Rabanes suggests 1836 for what he names as the 'non-fusion' (personal communications).
7 Hahnemann, S. Clarke, JH. Ed. Homoeopathic Reminiscences, *Homoeopathic World*, 1905; 40:4; 1st April, published to mark the 150th anniversary of the birth of Hahnemann on 10th April 1855.

7

MEMORIAL

Introduction

The title of this essay written by the American homeopath Carroll Dunham is Memorial, but it could well have been intended to mean what we now call a 'Memorandum'. It concerns the controversy engendered by the publication of a spurious or forged *Organon* edition in 1865 by a Dr Lutze in Germany, containing the heretical idea of the simultaneous prescription of more than one medicine.

> **About Carroll Dunham**[1]
> Dunham was born in the New York City, the son of a prosperous merchant. His mother died during the 1834 cholera epidemic, shortly after the family moved to Brooklyn.
> As a schoolboy he was reported to have a quiet, studious disposition, more given to reading than play, especially of the rough and noisy sort. At 15 he matriculated at Columbia College, graduating with honours in 1847.
> After leaving college, he studied medicine, placing himself under Dr Whittaker, an old school physician. Having been helped through an illness by homeopathic treatment, he investigated its claims and became a firm believer in its principles and practice. Nevertheless, he attended the course of instruction at the New York College of Physicians and Surgeons and at the various clinics to which he had access. Dunham received his medical degree in 1850, and left for Europe to continue his studies.
> He visited Dublin, where he served a term in the lying-in hospital, as well as Paris, Vienna and other centres of medical science. At Munster, he became a pupil of von Boenninghausen, daily attending at his office and making careful and elaborate notes of the cases he saw, their treatment, and the results.
> Dunham returned to the United States a year later and commenced practising in Brooklyn, New York. In 1845, he married Harriet Kellog. After

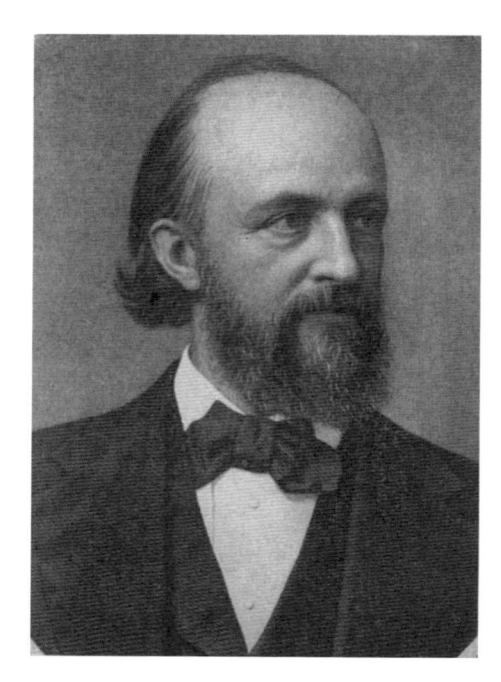

Figure 7.1 Carroll Dunham (1828-1877)
Reproduced with permission from The Institute for the History of Medicine of the Robert Bosch Foundation.

practising four or five years in Brooklyn with good success, not withstanding some interruptions from sickness (one instance lasting several months) it was deemed necessary for health reasons to take a vacation. He returned to Europe, and again spent several weeks renewing his studies with Boenninghausen, passing the greater part of every day with him.

On returning to the United States he moved to Newburgh, New York and practised for six years before his poor health forced him to retire again. He visited the West Indies and other foreign parts searching for health or relief. Finally he settled in Irvington-on-the-Hudson, where he lived until his death.

In 1865 Dunham accepted the professorship of materia medica in the New York Homoeopathic Medical College. He also served as the college's dean. In 1874, in such poor health, he resigned all positions and went to Europe. Upon returning a year later, his health had substantially improved.

The 1876 AIH meeting in Philadelphia was a turning point for homeopathy in the United States. On one side were the stalwart homeopaths like Hering, Lippe, Wells, Wessellhoeft. On the other were the 'mixers', those already teaching allopathic therapeutics and 'this for that' prescribing. Dunham's efforts to combine the factions was a severe strain on his health.

> Always of a weak constitution, he died shortly after the 1876 Congress and was buried in Greenwood Cemetery in Brooklyn. His wife died about a year later.

Memorial

by Carroll Dunham MD[2]

To the American Institute of Homoeopathy, the National Representative Organisation of the Homoeopathic physicians of the United States, this memorial respectfully showeth:

- That there has recently been issued in Germany, from the private press of Mr Arthur Lutze, and under his editorship, what purports to be a sixth edition of Hahnemann's *Organon*, with alleged additions from the pen of Hahnemann, and with annotations by the editor, Mr Lutze.
- That his alleged sixth edition of the *Organon*, thus edited and printed by Mr Arthur Lutze, appears to contain unwarranted alterations from the original text, as Hahnemann left it, together with suppressions of important parts of the text. And these changes are of so important a character that the editors of all the homoeopathic periodicals of Germany, differing widely as they do, on many points of doctrine and practice, have united in a solemn and earnest *protest* against the reception of this edition of the *Organon* as authentic.
- In this *protest* they earnestly beseech all homoeopathic physicians throughout the world, and especially all societies, institutes, and organised bodies of homoeopathic physicians, after due investigation of the subject, to unite with them.
- And that the object of this memorial is to lay before the American Institute of Homoeopathy this unanimous *protest* of the German homoeopathic press, and likewise to present such additional history and testimony bearing on the subject, as may be necessary to a full comprehension of it.

The protest of the German Homoeopathic Press is in the following words:[3]

Protest

In view of the fact that A. Lutze, of Köthen, has undertaken to publish a sixth edition of Hahnemann's *Organon of the Healing Art*, the *undersigned*, in the interests of their science, and as the present representatives of the German homoeopathic press, feel it their duty to make the following explanations.

Homoeopathy has always excited the interest of the laity in a far greater degree than any other system of medicine, and to this very interest it is largely indebted for its expansion and recognition. Even now, many places, in which the number of its representatives is far from corresponding to the needs of the public who confide in it, are dependent upon practitioners who are not regularly educated physicians (not doctors) and whose true devotion to homoeopathy must, in part, compensate for their lack of a scientific study of it. It would be ungrateful to wish to conceal this fact, and not to lay aside all spirit of caste, and recompenses with the most public recognition the services of very many of these persons in the matter of the propagation of homoeopathy.

But it is no less true, that there are *limits* within which an *active* and *independent participation* by *laymen* and *dilettante* becomes an *impossibility*, unless one would reduce the science to a piece of mechanism, and make the healing art a handicraft. It is the duty of every honourable representative of homoeopathy to keep a zealous watch, to the end that no unqualified hand grasp and jostle its inner sanctuary, whether it be the hand of an opponent or of an adherent.

The *Organon*, that work of Hahnemann's, which comprises the collected principles of homoeopathy and establishes them on a scientific basis, has already, with great propriety, been called the *Bible of Homoeopathy*. A new edition of this work, which, it is well known, has long been out of the book trade, must be a welcome circumstance to every homoeopathician.

But, assuredly, every one will feel constrained to ask, how comes Mr Lutze to undertake this honourable duty? And, still more, how comes Mr Lutze to introduce this new edition of Hahnemann's work, with *his own name* upon the title page; since, assuredly, he can have exercised no function but simply and purely that of a publisher and bookseller.

But this reasonable question is completely silenced in the face of an incomparably more important and weighty fact, which nothing short of a complete misapprehension of his own position, and the greatest self-conceit on the part of Mr Lutze, could have rendered possible.

Lutze has permitted himself, not only to add to Hahnemann's work a new and emphatic dedication and several annotations and an appendix, but he has even removed several paragraphs of Hahnemann's work (sections 272–274 of 5th edition), and has substituted for them a new paragraph, which expresses directly the opposite of what was heretofore said therein; and he has, by so doing, deliberately and without any right, annihilated one of the three cardinal principles of homoeopathy.

The annulled paragraphs contain the precept that, in homoeopathic practice, *only one single, simple remedy should be given at one time* to the patient; they contain the reason for this precept, and, moreover, an impressive warning against the dangers of ever combining remedies. Instead of all this, the paragraph which has been smuggled in, sanctions the administration of the so-called double and triple remedies for certain alleged cases.

Everyone who is only tolerably familiar with homoeopathy must know that the exclusive administration of simple and un-combined remedies, is one of the principal pillars on which the entire edifice of homoeopathy rests. To take this away, means nothing less than to entirely overturn homoeopathy itself.

And how does Mr Lutze justify this outrage, or, at least, cloak it with the semblances of a title? In this way: He perpetrates a falsification of history, and he confounds with one another events that occurred in former years, in that he appeals to a letter written by Hahnemann in 1832, and from which it appears that Hahnemann, at the instance of Dr Ægidi, had, at one time, been ready to introduce into the 5th edition of the *Organon*, a paragraph in favour of 'double remedies.' But, to a right understanding of this circumstance, and in justice to the history of homoeopathy and to the name of Hahnemann, it should not be concealed, that, upon the unanimous representation of his followers, Hahnemann immediately reconsidered this momentary weakness towards a dear friend (Ægidi), and that he *not only did not* introduce the unwholesome paragraph into the said 5th edition, but even thought it his duty to repeat more impressively than ever, the before mentioned warning against combining remedies.

And in this conviction he remained true and firm; for, up to the day of his death, ten full years, he did and published nothing which could be alleged as contradicting this statement.

But can any one who has any knowledge whatever of Hahnemann's character, suppose, for an instant, that he could be turned back by any except the *most conclusive* reasons, or that, for the space of ten years, he could have failed, through hesitancy or indecision, to recall this 5th edition, if he had been really convinced of the correctness of other views than those therein stated?

No! Hahnemann, that iron-headed, was not the man of cowardly compliance or passive sufferance, who would have let that which he did not deem to be *the right* befall in regard to his own homoeopathy! And now, twenty-two years after his death, there comes an officious, meddling fellow, who would make us believe – as though he had only soft-heads and neophytes to deal with – that Hahnemann had, "like Saturn, devoured his own children!"

Have we then said too much, when we speak of falsification of history and of a perversion of the facts? Truly, even were Lutze quite another than, in fact, he is, we should be compelled to fling in his face the charge of the boldest assumption, the most unheard-of self-exaltation, and of falsification, and we should, without mercy, tear him down from the dictatorial chair which he has usurped. He, least of all, is the man who should offer to do such things. Out of such timber (as he is) may indeed be hewn *lubbers for the masses*, who are incapable of reflecting and of calling to account, but *never* the *reformers of medicine*.

In view of these facts, we, the representatives of the scientific homoeopathic press of Germany, hereby *solemnly protest* against this alleged 6th edition of Hahnemann's *Organon,* and we declare the same to be spurious and apocryphal; and, at the same time, we repudiate all fellowship with such conduct and with its perpetrators, and we denounce it and them. Confident of the entire support of all true representatives of homoeopathy, we anticipate, first of all, from all parts of Germany and from foreign lands, from individuals and from societies, a *formal concurrence* in this *protest;* and we look forward with special confidence to the next meeting of the Central Union of German Homoeopathic Physicians, expecting that this body will then adopt more positive regulations against such compromisings of homoeopathy, and will go to work energetically against all spoilers of our science.

Signed
Dr Bolle, *Ed. Pop. Hom. Zeitung.*
Dr Hirschel, *Ed. Zeitschrift fra Hom. Klinik.*
Dr Meyer, *Ed. Allg. Hom. Zeitung.*
Dr Cl. Muller, *Ed. Hom. Veirteljahrschrift.*

In order that the allusion in the above *protest* to Hahnemann's 'dear friend,' Dr Ægidi, as well as the documents which are to follow in this memorial, may be more clearly understood, a few words of a historical nature may here be introduced.

Mr Lutze published, in 1860, a popular *Manual of Homoeopathic Theory and Practice;* a translation of which into English, by Dr Hempel, was published in New York in 1863. In this Manual Mr Lutze authorises the use of two or even three different *drugs in combination in one and the same dose.* He claims to have for this practice the sanction and encouragement of Hahnemann, Ægidi and Boenninghausen.

He says:

> This important discovery of the combination of drugs was first announced, twenty-four years ago, by Dr Julius Ægidi. This discovery was communicated to Hahnemann in 1833, corroborated by two hundred and thirty-three cures with combined remedies, and was joyfully received by Hahnemann, but kept secret from the public by the imbecility of the foes of truth, whereas the worthy discoverer was insulted and derided by those who were unworthy of unloosing his shoe-strings.

Mr Lutze then gives a letter from Hahnemann to Dr Ægidi, dated May 15, 1833:

> Dear friend and colleague – do not suppose that I reject anything good from mere prejudice, or because it might lead to modification in my doctrine. I am rejoiced that you should have such a happy though, at the same time confining its execution to proper limits. Two remedies should only be given in combination in a highly potentised form, provided each is, in its own way, Homoeopathic to the case. In such a case, this

proceeding is an advantage to our art, which should not be repudiated. *I shall take the first opportunity of making a trial, and I doubt not it will be successful.* I am likewise glad to hear that Boenninghausen approves of the plan.

Lutze further says:

In another letter to Dr Ægidi, Hahnemann writes, date, June 19, 1833: 'I have devoted a special paragraph to your discovery of a combination of drugs, in the 5th edition of my *Organon*, &c.'

What, says Lutze, what has become of this paragraph?

We search the *Organon* from beginning to end without finding it. Here is the explanation. Hahnemann laid the new discovery, which he had kept heretofore secret, before the meeting of the homoeopathic physicians of the 10th of August, 1833. Their number was as yet small, but, instead of meeting with open hearts, he found stubborn minds," &c., &c., "who, instead of accepting the blissful truth, assailed it with all sorts of persecutions, comparing it to the mixtures of allopathic practitioners, and persuading Hahnemann to abandon the publication of the discovery, and to allow one of his friends to suppress the paragraph, which had been already printed.

Lutze goes on to say

Ægidi was shamefully abused, and that he preferred to remain silent rather than expose himself to abuse and insults." He adds, "The time for requital has come; the hitherto suppressed discovery rises like a phoenix from its ashes, and the name of its author, Dr Julius Ægidi, shall be snatched from oblivion.

Three or four years ago, the discoverer first acquainted me with the combination of remedies." [Therefore about 1856–57.] "Our excellent Boenninghausen has informed me, orally, that he has obtained equally fortunate results.

It will be seen that Mr Lutze defends his use of combined drugs by the testimony of Drs. Ægidi and Von Boenninghausen.

But it happens that Dr Ægidi, who is still living, has placed himself on record in terms which directly contradict the above statement of Mr Lutze, while a letter quoted below, from Dr Von Boenninghausen to your memorialist, is equally conclusive touching the decided *disapproval* with which the practice of combining drugs was regarded by Dr Von Boenninghausen, who, moreover, far from having been likely to "communicate" anything "orally" to Mr Lutze, clearly intimates that he does not know, and has never met, Mr Arthur Lutze.

May 12, 1857, Dr Ægidi published, in the *Allgemeine H. Zeitung*, an explanatory note, disavowing and disapproving the practice of combining drugs. Yet, in 1860, with this note of Ægidi's published and before him, Lutze hails Ægidi as the discoverer of a "blissful truth," and claims thereby to "snatch his name from oblivion!"

Now, again, April 12, 1865, on seeing the *protest* of the German Homoeopathic Press against Lutze's edition of the Organon, Dr Ægidi publishes a second card (*Allg. H. Zeitung*, 70, 17), in the following words:

> The *protest* of the honoured representatives of the homoeopathic press of Germany, against the alleged 6th edition of the *Organon of the Healing Art*, published in the *Allg. Hom. Zeitung* of April 10, (Hahnemann's birthday,) having embraced the mention of my name, yet having omitted to mention – that I also participate in the conviction which it is the purpose of the writers of the *protest* to express – that, years ago, I, loudly and publicly, made known my disapproval of the administration of so-called *double remedies*, as an abuse and a mischievous proceeding.
>
> I find myself compelled to republish my explanation (which seems to have been forgotten,) as it originally appeared in the *Allgemeine Homoeopathische Zeitung* 54, 12, May 18, 1857, and thence was copied into the *Neue Zeitschrift fur Homoeopathische Klinik*, II. 12, June 15, 1857. It was in the following words:
>
> 'The undersigned finds himself compelled to join his voice to the reproaches that have been made, particularly of late, against the administration of the so-called *double remedies*; the more inasmuch as it is he who is charged with having taken the initiative in this mode of prescribing, which is the subject of reprobation.
>
> 'Entirely agreeing with all the arguments adduced against it by competent persons, and the refutation of which must be impossible, the undersigned desires to make known, publicly and emphatically, his decided disapproval of such an abuse of our most excellent and serviceable art, as has lately been recommended in an apparently systematic manner, and as a rule, to the end that person may forbear to take his supposed authority, as a *sanction* of a mode of treatment which, even as *he* (Stapf's *Archiv.*, 1834, 14,) thought he might recommend a modification of it for very rare and exceptional cases, is very far from being the abuse and mischief which it is now made and is being made.'
>
> I add to this, that I thoroughly agree with the contents of the above mentioned *protest*, and that, in my opinion, the practice therein rebuked is not dealt with even as severely as, in the interests of the science, it should have been.
>
> *Signed*
> Ægidi."
> *Freienwald, April 12, 1865.*

Thus it is clear, that at the time when Lutze's *Manual* appeared (1860), advocating double or combined remedies, naming Ægidi as the author and champion of the practice, and kindly promising to snatch Ægidi's name from oblivion, Ægidi's disavowal and rebuke of the practice had already been published (1857). It is a matter of surprise (!) that no notice was taken of these facts in the *American* translation!

When the American translation of Lutze's *Manual* appeared (1863), your memorialist wrote, under date March 2, 1863, to Dr von Boenninghausen, quoting to him the passages which refer to him, and asking for information. The following reply was promptly received:

Munster, March 25, 1863.

My very dear friend and colleague – I have received your letter of 2nd instant. The passage which you quote concerning the 'combined doses containing two different remedies,' imposes on me the duty of replying without a moment's delay.

It is true that, during the years 1832 and 1833, at the instance of Dr Ægidi, I made some experiments with combined doses; that the results were sometimes surprising, and that I spoke of the circumstances to Hahnemann, who, after some investigations made by himself, had entertained, for a while, the idea of alluding to the matter in the 5th edition of the *Organon*, which he was preparing in 1833. But this novelty appeared too dangerous for the new method of cure, and it was I who induced Hahnemann to express his disapproval of it in the 5th edition of the *Organon* (1833), in the note to section 272. After this period, neither Hahnemann nor myself made any use of these combined doses. And Dr Ægidi was not long in abandoning this method, which resembles too closely the procedures of allopathy, opening the way to a relapse from the precious law of simplicity – a method, too, which is becoming every day more entirely superfluous from the augmentation of our *Materia Medica*.

If, consequently, at the present day, a homoeopathist takes it into his head to act according to *experiments* made thirty years ago, in the infancy of our science, and subsequently rebuked by unanimous vote, he clearly *walks backwards*, like a crab, and shows that he has not kept up with nor followed the progress of science.

Supposing that it may interest you to know the origin of the above named method, I add a few words. There was, about this time (1831–1832), at Cologne, an old physician named Dr Stoll, himself a constant invalid and hypochondriac, who, distrusting the old medical doctrines, but having only a superficial smattering of homoeopathy, had conceived the idea of dividing the remedies into two classes, *the one of which should act upon the body* and the *other* upon the *soul.* He thought that these two kinds of medicines should be *combined* in a prescription, in order to supplement each other.

His method making some noise in Cologne, and Dr Ægidi, who then lived at Düsseldorf, having in vain endeavored to discover the essential secret of its novelty, the latter induced me to try to find it out. I succeeded in doing so. Although the idea of Dr Stoll was utterly devoid of foundation, it nevertheless induced us to make experiments in another way, namely, the before mentioned, but which, as I said before, was utterly rejected long, long ago.

Yours very sincerely,
Signed
C. von Boenninghausen.

It thus appears, even from Hahnemann's own letter to Ægidi, which is the only authority Lutze had, in 1860 for claiming Hahnemann's approval of this practice, that Hahnemann only *promised* to *"take the first opportunity of making a trial."* And although he subsequently speaks of a purpose to allude to the subject in the *Organon*, he nowhere states that he *did* make *successful* "trials." But he *does* say, in that same letter that, "he would not reject *anything good* from *mere prejudice."* From the fact, then, that he *did* reject this method, and that he concluded not even to allude to it in the *Organon*, we are forced to the conviction that he did not regard it as *"anything good!"*

Moreover, Ægidi, its reputed author, and von Boenninghausen, who is alleged to have favoured it, are most emphatic in its reprobation.

The Homoeopathic Medical College of Pennsylvania, having carefully considered this subject, have issued the following:

A protest
At a meeting of the Faculty of the Homoeopathic Medical College of Pennsylvania, the following Preamble and Resolutions were unanimously adopted:

Whereas, A book, purporting to be the 6th edition of Hahnemann's *Organon*, has been published at Köthen, Germany; and

Whereas, The representatives of homoeopathic journalism in Germany have issued their earnest protest against this unwarranted 6th edition of said work, and have *pronounced and declared it to be mutilated and perverted*, in that the paragraphs numbered 272-274, in the 5th edition of the said work, treating on the simplicity of the remedy to be administered, have been omitted, and spurious and false ones have been inserted in their place, recommending double and triple mixtures.

Resolved, That we fully endorse the '*protest*' published in Vol. 70, No.15 of the '*Allgemeine Homoeopathische Zeitung.*'

Resolved, that we protest against the introduction of any translation into English of said spurious and false edition, as a standard work of homoeopathics.

Resolved, That we call the attention of the 'American Institute of Homoeopathy,' at its next meeting in Cincinnati, on the 6th proximo, and of all other State and County Homoeopathic societies, to the above protest; and that we solicit their co-operation in endeavouring to protect our science from perversion by false and spurious interpolations into its standard literature.

Resolved, That we request this, our protest against said book, to be published in all the American, British, and German, and other homoeopathic journals, and a copy thereof to be transmitted to each of the state and county homoeopathic societies in the United States.

In testimony whereof, we have hereunto affixed our signatures, this twentieth day of May, AD 1865.

Signed
Constantine Hering MD, *Prof. Inst. and Prac.*
Adolphus Lippe, MD, *Prof. Materia Medica.*
HN Guernsey, MD, *Prof. Obstetrics.*
Charles G Raue, MD, *Prof. Pathology.*
George R. Starkey, MD, *Prof. Surgery.*
Pusey Wilson, MD, *Prof. Anatomy.*
JHP Frost, MD, *Prof. Physiology.*

With these citations and statements, the subject is respectfully submitted to the American Institute of Homoeopathy, and their considerate action upon it is earnestly invited.

Carroll Dunham, MD, New York, June 3, 1865.

References

1 Winston, J. *The Faces of Homeopathy*, Tawa, Wellington. Great Auk Publishing 1999, p 75.
2 Dunham, C. Memorial, *Proceedings of the Eighteenth Annual Meeting of the American Institute of Homoeopathy: Held in Cincinnati June 7, 1865*, 77–86. Chicago, American Institute of Homoeopathy, 1865.
3 *Allgemeine Hom. Zeitung.*, 70, 15, April 10, 1865.

8

ECCE MEDICUS

Introduction

Ecce Medicus was the title of the first of many annual lectures about Hahnemann, given by James Compton Burnett in his unique style with verve, and with scholarship.

Then as now, homeopathy and Hahnemann were ridiculed. Burnett mentioned the enemies of homeopathy and recommended countering them with a robust defence or even attack, with the truth about Hahnemann and his life. Burnett can tell us more than many of his contemporaries, as he learned German and studied in Vienna, and so was able not only to pepper his writings with German quotations, but also to read original sources. Burnett was a prize-winning anatomist. He was able to bring into Anglophone homeopathy the work of Rademacher and so indirectly of Paracelsus, especially the knowledge of the affinity of certain medicines with different human organs.

While Burnett does not always give detailed information about his medicines in his own work, they have been well documented by JH Clarke in his *Dictionary* where they are referenced with a (B).[1] In this combination of skill and knowledge Burnett must have been unique in his time. His lecture focuses on the details of Hahnemann's life before he went to Paris and is reproduced together with lengthy footnotes.

To assist in understanding Burnett, part of an obituary published in *The Homoeopathic World* follows.[2] For more about Burnett readers are referred to biographical essays by Clarke.[3] and Spurling.[4]

About James Compton Burnett

James Compton Burnett belonged to an old Scots family, the younger branch of which came south, notably Gilbert Burnett, afterwards created Bishop of Salisbury, from whom James Compton is directly descended. The name Compton was taken about the year 1770, on the marriage of his grandfather with a Miss Compton of Hampshire, a lady of large fortune, at whose desire the addition was made. There were several sons of this marriage, one of whom, Charles by name, married a Miss Sarah Wilson, and James Compton Burnett was their son. He was born at Redlinch, in Wiltshire, July 21, 1840, his father being a considerable landowner in that neighbourhood.

He had an ordinary English education until he reached the age of sixteen, when he went to school in France for a term of about three years. After this he travelled for several years, principally on the Continent, studying philology, the love of which in him amounted almost to a passion, and he had serious thoughts of devoting his life to that object.

Deciding later on to study medicine, he became a student of Vienna, and was so absorbed in the study of anatomy, that he devoted two years more of his time than the ordinary curriculum demanded to that branch of science. He prepared many valuable specimens for his professors during that term, most of which are now preserved in the Pathological Museum of Vienna. It was doubtless this long course of study, with his own great gift of perception, which enabled him in after life to diagnose complicated disease with almost absolute certainty. Having taken the Vienna M.B. in 1869, he entered Glasgow University and studied there until in 1872 he took the M.B. of that University, taking the M.D. in 1876. Passing through a brilliant examination in anatomy, lasting one hour and a half, the professor shook hands with him, saying that he had never examined a student with so brilliant and thorough a knowledge of anatomy. The same professor, on hearing later that he had decided to become a homoeopath, entreated him to alter his mind, saying he was convinced that he would reap all honours in the medical world, and that he was throwing his life away. His reply was, "that he could not buy worldly honours at the cost of his conscience," and he continued to fight the good fight of homoeopathy to the last day of his life. The reason graduating M.B. was that he wrote his first thesis on "Specific Therapeutics," and the homoeopathic flavour was too strong for the examiners, who rejected in spite of its merits. His next essay evaded such dangerous ground and was duly accepted.

He began practice in Chester, and afterwards practised for a short time in Birkenhead, from whence he came in 1877 to London, where he has carried on a large consulting practice for twenty-three years.

Beloved by all his friends, in his home he was idolised. The helpful sympathy and kindly interest always shown to his patients makes realistic in a high degree how vast would be the love and tenderness lavished on those who were dearest to him; the loss to all who were brought in contact

> with him is truly great, to them irreparable. He leaves a widow and family, for whom the deepest sympathy must be felt.

Ecce Medicus, or Hahnemann as a man and as a physician and the lessons of his life[5]
Being the first Hahnemannian Lecture, 1880.

By James Compton Burnett 1840–1901

> *Es liebt die Welt, das Strahlende zu schwaerzen.*
> Schiller

This first Hahnemann lecture is dedicated to William Bayes Esq. MD in admiration of his public spirit and far-seeing wisdom, as shown in the establishment and maintenance of the London School of Homoeopathy.

Preface

On sending this *Hahnemannian Lecture* to press, it is right to remark that, in deference to the expressed wish of valued friends, certain expressions that were made use of in delivering it have been omitted. The substance, however, remains the same. To say a thing in simple homely Saxon is often apt to shock; such is better told with the tamed tongue of a Talleyrand, and with . . . *surtout point de zèle*.

It has not been deemed wise to extend the subject by following up Hahnemann's history at Köthen and Paris: that would have involved a consideration of his tripartite pathology; and the Parisian episode has but little scientific interest so long as his latest writings are beyond our reach.

The following pages, therefore, contain the first *Hahnemannian Lecture* essentially as it was delivered at the London Homoeopathic Hospital in Great Ormond Street last October.

JC Burnett
Gentlemen,

At a meeting of the authorities of the London School of Homoeopathy, held in this building on July 12th, 1880, it was proposed by Major Vaughan Morgan, and seconded by the Earl of Denbigh, "That it is desirable that a Lecture be delivered explanatory of the *History of Hahnemann's Discovery of Homoeopathy*, illustrating its Principles and the *Life and Works of its Founder*, that such Lecture shall be delivered annually, in place of the Introductory School Lecture, by a lecturer to be appointed each year by the Committee of the School in accordance with Rule V."

This was passed unanimously, and the speaker was asked to deliver the first lecture under arrangements to be made by the sub-committee consisting of Drs. Bayes, Hughes, and Yeldham.

This, Gentlemen, I stand before you today to carry out the intention of the London School of Homoeopathy in this regard.

May this first Hahnemannian Lecture be the starting-point of a genuine, free, and manly appreciation of him whom the Earl Cairns, not long since, very justly designated the greatest benefactor of his age.

We, whose duty it is to hand on a *true* history of Samuel Hahnemann to our children and to posterity, could not well adopt a better plan than that of a yearly Lecture on the subject of his Life and Labours; and it is with the desire of bearing my share of this sacred duty that I beg leave now to address you.

Some account it a shameful thing to be a believer in homoeopathy or in its founder, because, forsooth, the powers that be have decreed the former a delusion and the latter an unworthy outcast from the fold of the *Ecclesia medica catholica*. As for me, I count it the proudest day of my life to be permitted to stand here and endeavour to vindicate the honour of the master, than whom a kinder or purer man, a greater *savant*, a profounder thinker, or a truer physician the world has but very seldom seen.

It is not unknown to you that the very vilest slanders have been hurled against him; the highways and by-ways of all the languages of Europe - nay, of the world - are literally strewn with these slanders, in order thereby to damn the man and make his name a by-word in the mouths of the people.

Medicine mongers and leeches, worshipful companies of apothecaries, colleges of physicians and surgeons - royal and imperial - have all united to do him to death; the serial journals of the world, medical and surgical, have with on accord combined to bespatter his name with dirt, or they have entered into a conspiracy of silence to mum him and his homoeopathy to death.

For eighty-one years Hahnemann has been thus treated, and yet there are some six or seven thousands of physicians and surgeons in the world who swear by him as by a holy prophet, and millions of the human race have cause to daily bless his memory; and I venture to predict that in the ripeness of time the peoples of the world will unite to give him a high place, not merely in the *Panthéon* at Paris, or in our own Westminster Abbey, but in the great Valhalla of mankind.

But that time is not yet; and no one here, not even the youngest, is likely to live to see it. Ours is the seed time; let us see to it that we sow the sound seed of truth, and tend it carefully, and root up the weeds of hatred, ignorance, slander, and prejudice, in the sure and certain hope that such time will come although we may not be there to witness it.

To this end it is of vast importance, alike in the interest of medical science and of our common humanity, that the *real* Hahnemann and the labour of his life should be held up in the clearest possible light.

It is also needful that the labour of his life should be frequently examined afresh for the benefit of successive rising generations, who do not always know much of what was done even a few decades ago, and that we may have a standard whereby to measure the fashionable foibles of the hour.

For there is fashion in physic, and the pigmies of the day are very apt to appear might giants, unless the deeds of the great dead be present with us. Hence, I take it, the far-seeing wisdom of a yearly Hahnemannian Lecture, so that we may learn and re-learn the lessons of his life.

Much misconception of Hahnemann's labours and teachings exists even amongst some of his disciples, and it will be the privilege of the Hahnemannian lecturers, from time to time, to throw as much light as they can thereon; and may we all catch the true spirit of the mighty man and fervid physician, that it may not be said of our lesson-learning what the *Jaeger* said of the *Wachtmeister* in Schiller's *Wallensteins Lager*:

> "Sie bekam euch übel, die Lektion. Wie er räuspert und wie er spuckt, Das habt ihr ihm glücklich abgeguckt; Aber sein Schenie, ich meine, sein Geist Sich nicht auf der Wachparade weist."

No, Gentlemen, the genius of the great general does not show itself on parade, when playing at soldiers is going on, but in battle. So the genius of Hahnemann's teachings cannot be found by the dandy doctor *á la mode*, or by the mere scientist or book-worm or dead-house pathologist, but rather in reading the book of nature with a humble, receptive mind, and with the aid of Hahnemann's biopathology; and in treading the living sick according to his law. Did I say *his* law? I mean Nature's law, which he first saw in a clear light, and which he practically elaborated for us, thereby firmly fixing the treatment of the sick upon a scientific groundwork.

The boy Hahnemann

Will you come with me now and let us scrutinise the boy Samuel Hahnemann?[i,6] But, before doing so, just go over in your minds the early preparatory history of any of the heroes of our race, and you will most invariably find that *before* the real life-work began there had been a trialful preparation, then a *Sturm und Drang-Periode*, and then comes the working out of the individual redemption.

Hahnemann was destined to meet with enormous difficulties, to encounter unheard-of opposition, and then to come out victor over all. So he was not born

---

i Born 10 April 1755.

of rich parents or nursed in the lap of luxury. He was not "swaddled, rocked and dandled"[ii] into his life's work. Great reformers do not come that way. Scions of noble houses are often great leaders of men, but not because they are scions of noble houses, but because they still retain the pith and marrow of the original founders of their families.

Hahnemann was, however, not the offspring of vulgar or illiterate parents; his parents were indeed poor, but they were, nevertheless, people of taste and refinement, notably his father, who was a painter on porcelain in Saxony; for poverty, happily, neither excludes genius nor culture.

We should expect the son of an artist to become a man of refinement and taste: such was Hahnemann. He was of small stature and of a delicate constitution; not a man of muscle, but of iron will and indomitable perseverance. Yet he must have been well knit, for he lasted nearly ninety years.

You know the old saw – *She who rocks the cradle, rules the world* – and hence I wish I could draw you a word-picture of Hahnemann's mother, for mothers make our men; but the material necessary for such a delineation was not at my disposal: yet, perhaps, it matters little, as the real history of a mother is written by the lives of her children.

Of Hahnemann's father we know sufficient to be sure that he was no ordinary man, inasmuch as he taught the young Samuel *to think* for himself, for which purpose he is said to have shut him up alone, and *given him a theme to think out.* How many fathers show such a knowledge of what true education means in its etymological sense, viz., a leading or *drawing-out?* Without these lessons in thinking the young Hahnemann would never have studied medicine, for he did so in the teeth of parental opposition, and without them he would never have discovered scientific homoeopathy.

The great anatomist Hyrtl was wont to relate how as a little boy he used to study the anatomy of his throat with the aid of a hand-glass; and he was fond of exclaiming at the close of the story – *Was Essig warden soll, muss fruh sauer werden!*[iii]

So with Hahnemann: as a lad he wrote an essay on the human hand. He had an excellent education, first at the communal school till he was twelve years of age, and then at the Grammar School of his native place,[iv] and was moreover the pet pupil of his master (the Rector) from whom he received friendly instruction in his free time; and so well did he profit by this large-hearted instruction, that he was an accomplished linguist at the age of twenty, when he left Meissen for Leipzig, to study medicine.

---

ii "I was not swaddled, rocked, and dandled into a legislator." – Burke.

iii "What is to be vinegar, must soon get sour!"

iv Meissen also has the honour of being the birthplace of the two brothers Schlegel. The little town is in the kingdom of Saxony, at the confluence of the Elbe and the Meisse.

Hahnemann began already at the grammar school to be a teacher of his fellows; and already at the age of thirteen he was so far advanced in his knowledge of Hebrew as to be able to give lessons in that tongue[v,vi,vii]

He was not permitted to go away to the universities to study medicine without having first been subjected to parental opposition, for we are told that his father compelled him to take a situation in some business; or, rather, his father's poverty made it an apparent necessity. But trade was so distasteful to the ambitious and gifted boy Hahnemann that he fell ill in consequence, and then he was permitted to follow the bent of his noble mind. We have here the key to his subsequent successes; for what greater opposition can there be offered to the onward career of any man that that of his own parents and poverty combined? When a lad has the stuff in him to conquer father and mother and poverty combined, what possible concatenation of adverse circumstances in after life is likely to thwart him? And so we find him, then, at twenty *en route* for Leipzig University, and already at that age thoroughly acquainted with German, Arabic, Hebrew, Greek, Latin, French, Italian, and English. To know eight languages already at the age of twenty is, you will admit, not a bad preliminary education.

The Student Hahnemann

It was his extensive knowledge of languages that enabled him to gain a livelihood while studying medicine and after taking his degree. It was this same linguistic knowledge that subsequently was the means of his great discovery, as we shall presently see.

History tells us that Hahnemann had not the means to pay for his classes at the University of Leipzig, and that he enjoyed the privilege of free instruction. It is right to explain that this has been a common thing in German universities from time immemorial, and it is not there thought by any means an undignified thing to receive gratuitous instruction, as it is the right of poor students, especially such as matriculate with honours, as Hahnemann evidently did. Many of the most renowned professors in Germany were thus educated; for instance, Skoda, Oppolzer, and Hyrtl. Such students are not regarded as receivers of alms, but as being educated by the State, which pays and pensions its professors to educate its promising young citizens. Such men, also, most frequently fill the professorial chairs in after years. To this is largely due the astounding erudition of the German

---

  v *Biographie universelle ancieanne et moderne*, par M. Michaud. Paris. Art. S. Hahnemann.
  vi *Treue Bilder aus dem Leben der verewigten Frau Hofrath Johanne Henriette Leopoldine Hahnemann, geb. Küchler.*" Berlin, 1865.
  vii Hahnemann's grandson, Dr Süss Hahnemann, of London, informs me that this statement is strictly correct.

professorate that is justly a source of pride for the German fatherland and the admiration of the world of science and letters.[viii]

Thus Hahnemann was already, as a student, a man of great acquirements. Not the least of his acquirements was that of the autodidact in its grandest sense. Who in this world ever rose to eminence in learning other than autodidactically?

No doubt it is immensely important to receive sound instruction at school and university, but those who mount the ladder of life begin to learn where teachers cease to instruct: so did Hahnemann. In Leipzig he earned his living by translating scientific works from the English and French, for which he was paid by the publishers.

It might, not unnaturally, be asked how it was possible for the young Hahnemann to study medicine and gain his daily bread at the same time. He managed it in this wise: he sat up all night at this translation work every third night, and this became such a habit that he continued to do so for more than forty years. This also explains how he found time for his enormous literary labours in after years.

And, oddly enough, he not only managed to live during the two years he heard lectures at the Leipzig university, but he also contrived to save a little money, and thus became enabled to extend his field of observation; so we find him at the end of this period passing from the University of Leipzig to that of Vienna, one of the most renowned schools of medicine of the world, where he enjoyed the friendship of Professor von Quarin, by whom he was treated as a son, and who took great pains to teach him the practice of medicine. What was there, then, in this poor young Saxon that endeared him thus to his teachers? Clearly he was an extraordinary youth.

After a stay of an *annus medicus*, he accepted the post of librarian and family physician to the Governor of Transylvania, at Hermannstadt, the new home of his Saxon fellow-countrymen.

The learned Dr Dudgeon, in his biography of Hahnemann,[7] tells us that Hahnemann resided two years at Hermannstadt; but this can hardly be, for, as Dr Dudgeon himself states, Hahnemann removed to graduate in Erlangen in 1779, and this was in August.

It is to be remembered that Hahnemann practised in various parts of Lower Hungary during this period. He was either not altogether, or else not all the time attached to the Governor's service, or the Governor must have resided in various places. This is clear from Hahnemann's remark on page 114 of the second volume of his translation of Cullen's *Materia Medica*, where he says, in regard to Cullen's

---

viii Some ten or a dozen years ago Professor Billroth, of Vienna, proposed to arrange the medical curriculum, in Austria, with the avowed object that only students of some means could possibly enter the profession. In the heated controversy that ensued it transpired that nearly all the noted, then teaching, pro-professors of the Vienna School (Rokitansky, Hyrtl, Skoda and Oppolzer) had been poor students!

opinion that engorgements of internal organs do not constitute a contra-indication for the bark in ague – "The author (Cullen) is wrong; he would appear to have been unacquainted with the stubborn intermittents of hot fenny countries. I (Hahnemann) observed such in Lower Hungary, more particularly in the fortified places of that country, which owe their impregnability to the extensive marshes around them. I saw such in Carlstadt, Raab, Comorn, Temesvar, and Hermannstadt," &c., &c. And from the subsequent detailed remarks it is clear that he must have had practical experience in these places of sufficient extent to observe the courses of the various kinds of ague of the very worst types, and also their concomitants and sequels. Those of us who have seen the human wrecks that even at this day come in large numbers from the low-lying marshy plains of Hungary to the *Allgemeines Krankenhaus* in Vienna, will have a very concrete conception of the enormous practical advantages which Hahnemann enjoyed in observing the worst forms of disease that can ever fall to the lot of any physician; for in malarial districts such as those in which Hahnemann spent these two years in active practice, and of which he thus gives an account, we have in the wake of their pernicious intermittents the most severe forms of heart, lung, liver, spleen, kidney, and abdominal affections, with all varieties of dropsy, and to have gone to school in such a place means, at the very least, much practical experience.

Be it noted that this was all before he graduated as doctor of medicine at the ripe age of twenty-four years and not quite four months.

Thus we have seen our youthful Hahnemann at the communal and grammar schools of his native place, Meissen, until he was twenty years of age, and then we find him studying medicine, first in Leipzig and then in Vienna – my own dear old *alma mater* – and then in practice in a district full of disease, and finally graduating at the age of twenty-four. And, be it remembered, earning his living and paying his way during the whole of his medical curriculum.

I dwell somewhat on the practical professional education of Hahnemann because some of his detractors try to persuade us and themselves that he was not a physician at all, but some else – a librarian, a teacher, a translator, a book-worm, a chemist, anything, but not a physician. You have seen that his farewell grammar school thesis was *On the Human Hand*, and if you only read the footnotes to his very earliest translations, you will agree with me that he was already at twenty-five a notable physician. Notable, I say, for some men see more in a year than others in a lifetime. Many a man has grown gray in the wards of hospitals, and yet has never seen anything.

We have made the acquaintance of the schoolboy Hahnemann, and of the student Hahnemann. Gentlemen, I beg you will now come with me and take a look at: the Doctor Hahnemann.

The Doctor Hahnemann

I have seen a painting of the young doctor Hahnemann painted by his father on a fan representing the young Æsculapius giving physic to his first patient, a shoemaker. Little did his good father then dream what a son he had begotten; let us study him a little closely. He is one of the *chefs d'œuvre* of the Creator.

By the way, why did Hahnemann go to Erlangen for his doctor's hat rather than to Leipzig? Because the graduation fees at Erlangen were much less there than at Leipzig. This information I have from his grandson, Dr Süss Hahnemann, who resides in our midst. The subject of Hahnemann's inaugural thesis was "*Conspectus affectuum spasmodicorum œtiologicus et therapeuticus.*"

We come at once to his wanderings, and to the *Sturm und Drang* period of his life.

First he goes to a little place called Hettstädt, and then to the small capital of Dessau, where he devoted himself particularly to the study of chemistry and mineralogy, and also as it would seem to the no less agreeable occupation of courting the fair German maiden, Miss Henrietta Küchler, the daughter of an apothecary at Dessau. He afterwards became medical officer of health at Gommern near Magdeburg, and there in 1782 he led the young lady to the altar.

We owe much to this noble woman, who was a beautiful character, and stood by him as a true companion and a faithful loving wife in the many terrible trials that were in store for him; but for her love and encouragement he would often have found the burden of his life an unbearable one. In after years he would often take her endearingly by the hand and exclaim, "Darling, but for thy loving support I could not bear it."

Mankind thus owes much to this noble Deutsche Frau, and in connection with our great medical reform she deserves our grateful remembrance.

Learned colleagues, do not think that in this hall the mention of a woman is out of place, for the influence of Hahnemann's wife has been a blessed one in the life of her illustrious husband, and has thus helped to bring health and happiness into many hearts and homes all the world over. Honour then to her who loved and helped him when well nigh all were against him.

But Gommern soon became unbearable for Hahnemann, and he left it after a two years' stay, and betook himself to polite and polished Dresden, the home of learning and culture. Here Hahnemann soon became a favourite with the leading men, and particularly with the eminent chief surgeon of the hospital, Dr Wagner, who formed such a high opinion of his abilities that he chose him to take his place – the highest medical post in the country – during a long illness.

Remember, gentlemen, this was the pre-homoeopathic Hahnemann who was thus chosen to temporarily fill the place of the highest medical functionary of his country. He was no longer the poor struggling student or the obscure parish doctor, but his professional position was one of which any physician at any period of life would be proud. I do not mean merely because he was thus, for a time, as a very young man called to such a responsible position, but he had also by this time made a name for himself in the world of medicine and of science, and his literary labours had carried his fame far beyond the confines of this own immediate country.

In 1786 he published his work *On Arsenical Poisoning* that is even now authoritative.

If you want to know Hahnemann's frame of mind at this period, you will find it in the introduction to this book *On Arsenical Poisoning*, which is dedicated *"To the Majesty of the Good Kaizer Joseph,"* and called by the author his firstling. You will see it is full of the bitterness of despair at the miserable condition in which he found practical medicine, and in it he appears to us as an expert medical jurist and practical toxicologist. He evidently had his back to practical medicine at this period (1786), for he says: "A number of causes, I care not to count them up, have for centuries been dragging down the dignity of that divine science of practical medicine, and have converted it into a miserable grabbing after bread (Brodklauberei), a mere cloaking of symptoms, a degrading prescription trade, a very God-forgotten handiwork, so that the real physicians are very hopelessly jumbled together with a heap of befrilled medicine-mongers. How seldom is it possible for a straight-forward man by means of his great knowledge of the sciences and by his talents to raise himself above the crowd of medicasters, and to throw such a pure bright sheen upon the Healing Art at whose altar he ministers that it becomes impossible even for the common herd to mistake a glorious benign evening star for mere vapoury skyfall! (Sternschnupfen). How seldom is such a phenomenon seen, and hence how difficult it is to obtain for a purified science of medicine a renewal of her musty letters of nobility."

In 1787 he wrote a treatise on the advantages of using coal as a means of warming, there being at that time much prejudice against its use.

1789 he wrote a work entitled *Instruction for Surgeons in the Treatment of the Venereal Disease*, and at this same period he wrote many important articles in Crell's *Chemical Annals* on chemical subjects, and amongst these: *Chemical Investigations on the Nature of Gall and Gallstones*, and another *On Antiseptics*. And he also published about this time in Baldinger's *Magazin* the mode of making the preparation of quicksilver that to this day is known in Germany as the *Mercurius solubilis Hahnemanni*.

Then he occupied himself with the question of the *Insolubility of Certain Metals*.

Hereupon he wrote in Blumenbach's *Bibliothek On the Means of Avoiding Salivation and other Ill Effects of Mercury*, and in Crell's *Annals: On the Preparation of Glauber's Salt*.

His enormous literary activity, coupled with his practical work in the chemical laboratory and his extraordinary knowledge, both in medicine and chemistry, began at this time to fix the attention of men of science and practice upon him, and he was accordingly elected a Member of the *Oekonomische Gesellschaft* in Leipzig, and a Fellow of the Academy of Sciences of Mayence.

Hahnemann in the Slough of Despond

Gentlemen, we are still in the presence of the pre-homoeopathic Hahnemann; he is thirty-five years of age, and thus barely in the prime of his years and mental development; he has already practised a dozen years as a physician, and it is fifteen years since he left his father's roof to go to study at Leipzig; he is happily married, the head of a large family, and enjoys a considerable reputation as a physician and as a man of science and letters. He returns to that Leipzig which had been the seat of the early student life and labour.

And what next? He suddenly gives up the practice of physic in disgust. He has lost all faith in physic, and believes ordinary medicine worse than nothing; not only no good, but a positively hurtful art.

From the frame of mind in which he wrote the introduction to his book *On Arsenical Poisoning* (in which he had already his back to the practice) to a total giving-up of such practice is a very great distance *for a poor man* with nothing else to fall back upon.

And then he had practised medicine with more than ordinary success. His detractors ask us to believe that he had no patients, and that it was practical medicine which gave him up, and not he it. But this is merely a falsehood; he absolutely refused to continue to treat those who had long been his patients, declining to live by practicing a system of medicine that experience at the bedside had taught him was far worse than useless.

At this period of the world's history a revolutionary spirit was in men's minds, and a medical revolution was brewing in Samuel Hahnemann's brain. Was he conscious of it? I think not. Was God's hand leading him in this mighty matter? So it seems to me.

You will agree with me that a violent storm of doubt and fear was raging in this man's mind; it raged to some effect, for it swept everything before it except his uprightness, his honesty of purpose, and his mighty manhood.

We shall have a concrete conception of the terrific nature of this psychic whirlwind when we bear in mind that he had no fortune beyond his practice, for his literary labours at this period were purely scientific, and mostly un-remunerative; he had comparative monetary ease in his practice, could give an elegant home to his loved ones and an adequate education to his children, who, with his exemplary wife, were the sweetness of his life, but nothing could withstand the force of this whirlwind, and he abandoned his practice entirely, and once more, but this time voluntarily, became a bookseller's hack, a translation-slave!

To get a living as a translator was hard enough for a young student with only himself to care for, but to keep a wife and a large family all accustomed to plenty and comfort was quite another matter. At one stroke he reduced himself and his wife and children to penury and want, and this for conscience' sake! And yet he knew but too well the pinch of poverty and the weirdness of want.

What a contrast this with some of the young men of our own day, whose doctrine is expediency and fashion, and who deem the chance of a hospital appointment or a professorship a fair exchange for their modicum of conscience, and who coolly say, "Homoeopathy is true, of course, I know that well enough, but *if I say so*, what chance have I of becoming surgeon to the infirmary, or lecturer at the medical school?"

Well, we must remember that there is the wrong, and the nemesis of wrong, too. These men (save the mark! I mean these social eunuchs) who thus deny or ignore the truth for mere expediency and supposed social advantages will, nevertheless, attain to nothing. Why? Because I find it written in the Big Book that "whatsoever a man soweth that shall he also reap."

But to return. Hahnemann removed, we saw, to his old Leipzig that was not specially propitious to him at any time, and again took up his old book-making drudgery; read his foot-notes to his translations from this period, and behold the bitterness in his soul.

When some of *us* feel bitter and downcast at being debarred from some coveted social or professional preferment for conscience' sake, let us just look at this period of our master's life, and we shall feel that ours are as the piping times of peace to the horrors of war.

Are you weary of the story of these dismal days of doubt and despond? Bear with me yet a little, and let us see how he bore his burden.

After a certain time he found that he no longer earned sufficient to pay the expenses of town life in Leipzig, and so we find him removing to a village outside of the town, in the hope that his literary earnings might suffice to keep the wolf from the door. He there clad himself in the garb of the very poor, wore clogs of wood, and helped his wife in the heavy work of the house, and kneaded his bread with his own hands! And the blatant ignoramuses who forge medical history, and who rule the rostrum in medical societies, ask the world to believe that Samuel Hahnemann was a lover of lucre, and a man given to gain! But poor Hahnemann had not yet drunk the dregs of his misery; as things got worse and worse, and his daughters and wife began to reproach him for sacrificing the amenities and comforts of life for seemingly chimeral dreams, his cup was full. Yet his firmness of character and his rooted steadfastness in his consciousness of right kept him up, and he worked on, perhaps with a faint inkling of a great something to come. But his cup of misery, though full, had not yet run over, but even this was to be. *Several of his children fell ill.* Now he was in the slough of despond indeed. He, the accomplished physician has given up physic as worthless and see his own children fall ill! In despair he cast about for the right remedies and found them not; yet he seemed certain they must exist. Writing to Hufeland, he exclaimed, "Oh! I cannot believe that the almighty and fatherly good of Him whom we cannot even call by a name worthy of Himself, Who so freely cares even for the tiniest of His animate beings that are invisible to our eyes, Who freely lavishes life and plenty throughout His whole creation, I *cannot* believe that He should inevitably deliver over His dearest and highest creatures to the pangs of disease." We thus see that he did not despair of a Healing Art; but, on the contrary, was firmly convinced that nature was replete with elements and forces for such an art, and that they were present in plenty all around. He also did not deny the possibility of a science of medicine, but the then existing methods and systems were demonstrably and in his own experience false; on the contrary, he evidently did believe in a science of medicine that was yet to be found, but how to find it he did not see.

This brings us to the threshold of the discovery of homoeopathy. Here we have the soil tilled ready for the seed; an invisible power sowed the seed, and the harvest is sure. We are about to part with the pre-homoeopathic Hahnemann, but before we do so let us just run back over the ground we have traversed; let us picture to ourselves the boy studying in his father's house by the light of a little lamp made of clay with his own hands; let us follow him from the national school up to the grammar school; let us realise him at the age of thirteen giving lessons in the mystic language of the Hebrews, and let us go with him, the accomplished youth, to Leipzig, silent in eight tongues, and watch how he toiled for bread, and studied amid such difficulties a system of medicine that he was destined in the full ripeness of manhood to cast away as worthless.

But enough; time presses, so we must hurry on to that point in his history whence arose a thought that grew so mightily that it has revolutionised medical society; and cast down the old idols from the high places to make room for a truer Æsculapian cultus.

A French biographer tells us that chance led Hahnemann to the discovery of homoeopathy. Nay, I cannot believe it; chance never did such a mighty thing. Chance may roll up a bit of clay, or perpetrate a daub, but chance does not mould such an exquisite model or paint such a perfect picture. I see the hand of providence in this thing; if chance did it, I, individually, have lived in vain.

Dawn of Homoeopathy

The renowned Scotch professor Cullen once wrote a remarkable work on *Materia Medica* that has gained much in reputation by having been rendered into German by Hahnemann. Perhaps the world does not owe much to South America, but it owes *Cinchona* to it, and we are not usually specially grateful for the benefactions of the Jesuits, but for once we may think kindly of them for bringing us over *the bark which has immortalised them in every marsh of the world.*

Cinchona[ix] has probably saved more lives than any other remedy in the pharmacopœia, and to it we owe the discovery of homoeopathy. Hahnemann went to Transylvania, as you know, and studied ague in the Danubian marshes; he not only studied it in others, but he had it himself. When Hahnemann was living in the country near Leipzig, clad in homespun and clogs, he got an order from a publisher to translate this *Materia Medica*[x] of Cullen so our own tongue had a share in the great discovery, and I think Cullen had more to do with paving the way for it than is generally thought. In all his translations Hahnemann had the habit of writing footnotes, often sitting heavily on his author's shortcomings; and it is in one of these footnotes to his translation of Cullen's *Materia Medica* that homoeopathy dawns upon us. Not the homoeopathy of Hippocrates, nor the homoeopathy of the writers of the 16th and 17th centuries, but the scientific homoeopathy that is based upon the proving of drugs on the healthy as shadowed forth by the genial Stoerck, and incidentally taught by the immortal Haller.

I believe it has been asserted that the Irish Physician, Crumpe, was before Hahnemann in trying drugs on the healthy. This statement is not correct. I beg leave to show you Crumpe's most interesting and scientific *Inquiry into the Nature and Properties of Opium*, which you will see was published in this city in 1793. (Antonius Stoerck was, however, before Hahnemann, in this respect.)

Hahnemann's Translation of Cullen's *Materia Medica* bears on its title-page the date 1790, that is ninety years ago (and three years before Crumpe's work). It was published in two volumes, and these two ragged old books I take the liberty of showing you also, both on account of their great historic interest as the birthplace of homoeopathy, and because of their being decidedly rare books. Here arose a therapeutic thought that has not so much *reformed* the practice of medicine as *revolutionised* it.

There is a slight indication of a crude kind of homoeopathy in this Translation anterior to the *Cinchona* episode. If you look at p. 17 of Vol. ii. You will find this foot-note in regard to the use and utility of astringents:- "*Acids* have likewise the power of bettering a weak stomach that has a tendency to produce a morbid acidity, as, for instance, *Sulphuric acid*." The influence of the great Cullen upon the ripe mind of the discoverer of scientific homoeopathy has not been, I think, sufficiently dwelt upon.

---

ix Proud science owes its knowledge of *Cinchona* really to the Indians, and these first ascertained its antiperiodic property by drinking the water of the swampy pools in which the Cinchona trees stood; so they really got a natural cold infusion.

x William Cullen's *Abhandlung über die Materia Medica nach der Nunmehr von dem Verfasser selbst ausgearbeiteten Originalausgabe Übersezt und mit Anmerkungen von Samuel Hahnemann, der Arzneikunde Doktor*. In 2 vols. Leipzig, 1790.

Cullen, at the beginning of his work, gives us an exhaustive history of *Materia Medica* as found in pharmacological works, and comes to the conclusion that the writings on this subject are in great part "a collection of errors and falsehoods." We can readily imagine how consonant this was with the feelings of the translator at that period.

At the end of his *History of the Materia Medica,* Cullen faintly apologises for his almost wholesale condemnation of the writers on that subject, and says that a number of the public may be dissatisfied with his judgment thereon. To this Hahnemann remarks:-

> "The translator does not belong to this number. For having himself read, compared and thought over most of the older writers and many of the new ones quoted by Cullen, so that the *non habet osorem nisi* might not be applied to him, he is constrained in a general way to subscribe to Cullen's opinion *with all his heart*. Dioscorides and Schröder, with all their shallowness, indefiniteness, old women's stories, and untruths, have all along been slavishly worshipped (with but few exceptions); and neither the old fathers themselves nor their weak disciples deserve to be spared." "We must," continues Hahnemann, "tear ourselves by very force away from these worshipped authorities if we in this important part of practical medicine are ever to be able to cast off the yoke of ignorance and superstition. It is indeed high time that we did!"

So you see the sceptic Cullen had found a congenial translator in our Hahnemann, and we can fancy with what eagerness the latter went on from the iconoclastic to the re-constructive Cullen. Hahnemann was looking with keen pleasure on the idols that Cullen had cast down and smashed. Now said he to his hero Cullen, give us something better; let us have a really scientific *Materia Medica.*

Hahnemann was already hungering and thirsting after a scientific therapeutics, and translating Cullen rendered him starving and famished: Hahnemann was longing for the bread of science; Cullen gave him the stone of hypothesis!

Thus he still craved for something better. For it must not be lost sight of that Hahnemann *had never for a moment lost faith in the efficacy of given drugs,* but he yearned for a fixed unalterable law according to which drugs in general might be used. He was sure it existed somewhere close by, but where? How was it to be found?

Yet Cullen came very near the proving of drugs on the healthy; he discussed all possible ways of finding out the remedial properties of drugs, and cast them all away one after another just as Hahnemann does six years later in his *Essay on a New Principle.* He enters into the question of the trial of drugs on animals, and rightly remarks that this mode can have but a very limited application; our allopathic friends still cling to this method, which their own Cullen for the most part condemned ninety years ago.

Cullen even went so far as to mention the trial of drugs on the human body, but he merely mentions it in passing, and he seemingly meant the ordinary way of trying them on the *sick*. After he had upset every thing he simply put up a counterpart of the old idol he had himself but just demolished. Yet I think Cullen's *tabula rasa* greatly helped Hahnemann in his discovery of scientific homoeopathy, inasmuch as it cleared the ground for the homoeopathic edifice. Hahnemann himself would most probably not be conscious of this; great minds read books and nature, and often build up new structures with very old material. Then it is the trite old story of Columbus and his egg.

Homoeopathy looming through the ages

Gentlemen, will you allow me here to interpose a somewhat long parenthesis by way of setting forth some forecastings of homoeopathy. I fear I shall have to trouble you with a few rather dry quotations, but the line of thought which I am following necessitates it.

It is often said that homoeopathy existed before Hahnemann. So it did, just as gravitation existed before Newton. Even a little more than this, for the formula *similia similibus curantur* may be found in authors, from Hippocrates onwards, from some of whom Hahnemann himself quotes (*Organon*). Nay more, I have myself works from the 16th and 17th centuries in which the question is clearly argued, viz., whether are diseases best cured by similars or by contraries? There is a whole literature on the subject principally in the 16th and 17th centuries. I have read quite a number of these works with avidity, and have been more than once on the point of declaring that this was the pit whence Hahnemann dug his homoeopathy. How true it is: Die Welt liebt, das *Strahlende zu schwärzen!* More than once I have gravely doubted Hahnemann's honesty in this particular, but wrongly, as I now know. The subject is too vast to be largely entered upon here,[xi] but I will give you the conclusion to which I have come. The homoeopathy of Hahnemann has nothing whatever to do with the homoeopathies of the Paracelcists, hermeticists and iatrochemists, *i.e.*, nothing whatever beyond the *mere notion* of healing by similars; yet I shall submit that the suggestive value of these other homoeopathies was great to him in thinking out his own scientific system. You will therefore see that those who quote triumphantly from these various authors to show that our homoeopathy was an old affair, and needed no Hahnemann to discover it, have merely skimmed the surface, and run away with an entirely false impression. Honesty compels me to confess that I was myself, for a time, in doubt. Let me ask, if it was already there, why did not somebody use it and *teach* it? Scientific homoeopathy was not there, but only its foreshadowings.

---

xi For a masterly contribution to this subject see *Lectures on the Theory and Practice of Homoeopathy*, by RE Dudgeon, M.D. London, 1854. This incomparable savant here traces the homoeopathic idea all through medical literature beginning with Hippocrates. I cannot, however, subscribe to several of his conclusions. By the way, nothing gives one such an exalted conception of literary labour as trying to do it one's self! And still better than Dudgeon's is de Gohren's.

Just to give those younger colleagues, who may not be familiar with the details of this part of our subject, an idea of what the homoeopathies of these other consisted in, it will suffice to state that their homoeopathies were of various kinds, and principally of these four –

Firstly. The doctrine of signatures,[xii] for instance the juice of the *Chelidonium majus* is yellow; the bile is yellow; like cures like, *ergo*, *Chelidonium majus* is a remedy for bad bile; a *remedium ictericum*. If you take a walnut and remove the hard shell carefully, and take a thoughtful look at the surface of the kernel, and note its *sulci* and *tyri* and hemispheres, you will get a simile of the brain surface. Therefore walnuts are good for the brain and reliable *remedium encephalicum*; and so on.

Secondly. Parts of the macrocosm (the world) as compared to supposedly similar parts of the microcosm (man's body). For instance, the sun in their pharmacology was the metal gold, which was therefore called *sol*.

In the microcosm, or man's body, the heart is the sun, or *sol microcosmi*. Like cures like; therefore gold is a good cardiac. Silver is the moon – *luna*,[xiii] the *luna microcosmi* is the brain; therefore, silver is a brain medicine. And so forth.

Thirdly. Animal parts to cure similar human parts: for instance, a fox's lung, in pulmonary affections. This is the crude prototype of Schüssler's clever notion with his tissue remedies, and the lamented Grauvogl a few years since recommended the *Pulmo vulpis* for asthma. This idea is as old as the hills.

Fourthly. Certain types of disease prevail in certain regions of the earth; in these same or similar regions their remedies are to be found ... *ubi malam, ibi remedium*. Thus in cold, damp places we find the *Solanum dulcamara*, therefore *Dulcamara* is remedial for the diseases of such places. *Cinchona* has a malarial habitat: it cures malarial diseases.[xiv] A modern example of this might be found in the undoubtedly anti-rheumatic virtues of the willow,[xv] which grows in wet places where rheumatism abounds, as some of us know but too well.

---

xii A modern supporter of the practical value of the Doctrine of Signatures is M. Chassiel: *Des Rapports de l' Homoeopathie avec la Doctrine des Signatures, Lettre à M. le Dr F. Fredault*. Paris, 1866. This is an honest work, seemingly aimed at M. Teste, who had entrevu the principle of ubi malum ibi remedium, without referring to Porta or Crollius. Chassiel starts a fifth notion of healing by similitudes, viz. (p. 48), diœcious plants cure contagious diseases: "La similitude avec le mode de propagation." But this is not all homoeopathy. The best historical essay on the subject with which I am acquainted is:- *Medicorum Priscorum de Signatura imprimis plantarum doctrina*, author F. L. A. H. de Gohren. Jena, 1840. This is an inaugural thesis, giving a faithful account of it, and, of course, ridiculing it.

xiii The curious in etymologies will note that this old designation of silver (luna) survives to this day in our lunar caustic – the nitrate of silver.

xiv We may laugh at this anthropoteleological contemplation of natural things; but suppose we had the ordaining of nature, where would we have put the *Cinchona* tree?

xv The willow (*Salix* whence our *Salicin*) was of old in good repute as a febrifuge.

Now Hahnemann had *evidently* read these sixteenth century homoeopathies, no other hypothesis is conceivable in one of his extensive reading, and they enlightened him no doubt very considerably by setting him thinking about a law of healing, and as to whether diseases are best cured by likes or by contraries, but they could not have taught him more, they could not have given him *his* homoeopathy for the best of all reasons, viz., that the scientific homoeopathy of Hahnemann has nothing to do with either the doctrine of signatures, the relationships of the macrocosm to the microcosm, the cure of human organs by giving the corresponding organs of animals as remedies, or with the apparent fact expressed by the words: *ubi malum, ibi remedium.*

Thus we see that Hahnemann's homoeopathy (our scientific homoeopathy) has really nothing in common with those which flourished in the sixteenth century and thereafter (as well as before) but the formula *similia similibus curantur.*

To *prove* this to you *in extenso* would carry us too far away from our present purpose.

But a consideration of this subject is, I submit, here not out of place, as it helps to shed light upon the dawn and rise of our own Hahnemannian homoeopathy, the more so as I am not aware that *this view* of the subject has ever been propounded; these various homoeopathies having been usually confounded, and regarded as identical with Hahnemann's.

That certain of these authors come *very near* to it, I freely admit; and it will be right, even at the risk of wearying you, to show how near they came. Therefore I beg to bring to your notice one or two of the works bearing on *these* more or less *crude prototypes* of homoeopathy that have led many sound scholars away with the idea that *our* homoeopathy existed before Hahnemann.

For instance Fernelius argues *against* the principle of healing by similars (Joannis Fernelii Ambiani, *Therapeutices Universalis*, 1574. p. 6, c. ii. *De Remedii Inventione*). He says in effect that every disease is driven out by its contrary, but that many evert this great law, and affirm that diseases are cured by their similars. He then discussed the mode of action, of exercise in fatigue, of the vomiting which cures vomiting, and of the purgation which cures dysentery, and maintains that they are in truth examples of healing by contraries. Here Fernelius comes very near indeed to true homoeopathy, yet only in arguing against it, and without comprehending its real essence.

We may affirm that, with his crude conception of disease and of remedies, homoeopathy would indeed be an impossibility.[xvi]

---

xvi Morbus omnis contrariis profligandus: contraria erim sunt morborum remedia. Remedium est quod morbum depellit: quicquid autem morbum depellit, id illi vim infert: quod vim infert, contrarium est: omni ratione igitur rememdium morbo contrarium esse necesse est, omnemque morbi depulsionem atque curationem contrariis perfici . . . Rata igitur constansque manet curandi lex per contraria. ARBITRANTUR PLERIQUE, MEDENDI SUMMAM LEGEM EVERTI, DUM

I will not, however, stop to argue the points which he raises, as I merely wish to show that the *idea* was prevalent, and I quote from Fernelius as an out-and-out opponent of it.

That he was a staunch adherent of the principle *contraria contrariis curantur* may be seen from his introduction to the fourth book, p. 136: "Nullus igitur affectus subsistere potest in nobis, cui non partier contrarium quiddam tanquam remedium illa protulerit."

He nevertheless discusses the use of *Pulmones vulpecularum* in asthma, and explains their action on the ground of *similitude* and *affinity for the offended parts;* and Dr Sharp, FRS, will be interested to learn that Fernelius terms their *mode* of action *antipathia*.

Dr Dudgeon quotes Rivière on the side of the law of similars, but Rivière argues hotly *against* it. Dr Dudgeon also credits Paracelsus with being in possession of enough knowledge of drug pathogenetics to lead us to suppose that he (Paracelsus) had conceived and taught our Hahnemann homoeopathy; this is decidedly erroneous. It is quite true that Paracelsus was a very close observer, and an original and deep thinker, but he nowhere teaches that his notion of similars was based on knowledge of the pathogenetic effects of drugs. And not only so, but he clearly inculcates the doctrine of signatures and similitudes of the macrocosm with the microcosm. No doubt he understood and taught organopathy, *i.e.*, local drug-affinity, though, of course, somewhat crudely.

Riolanus was also an opponent of the idea of healing by similars; the gist of what he says in his *Ars Bene Medendi*, Parisiis, 1601 (*De Remedio*, s. iv. c. l, p. 12), amounts practically to this, that all diseases are necessarily cured by contraries, and then he indulges in a little innocent fun at the expense, as he supposes, of Paracelsus, and of the Paracelsic signatural homoeopathy.[xvii]

Having given one or two opponents of the principle of *similia*, I will ask you to listen to me while I adduce a couple of advocates of it.

MORBOS QUOSDAM AUDIUNT REMEDIIS DEPELLI SIMILIBUS. At ejusmodi omnia morbolicet similia sint, ejus tamen causae primum ac per se adversantur, morbo autem ex accidenti: huncque tollunt non per se, sed sublata ejus causa. Sic ehrumbarbarum quamvis calidum febrem solvit, dum ipsius materiam expurgat. Et lassitudinem exercitatio lenit, quod humorem per musculos effusum discutiat. Et vomitionem sedat vomitio, quae proritantem umorem excutiat. Et dysenteram purgatio levat, noxia materia ejus efficiente causa detracta. Ad eundem prope modum frigidae larga perfusio convulsionem (ut est apud Hippocratem) (Aph. 25, lib. v.) solvere putatur . . . Sunt autem ejusmodi omnia curando affectui vere contraria, etc.

xvii Ergo morbid omnes contrario curantur. Sit hoc primum inveniendi remedii principium, quod in genere breviter declaratum sequentibus libris singulorum morborum et remediorum comparatione fiet notius. Velim interea lectorem observare quam sapienter Paracelsus suae medicinae contrarium jecerit fundamentum, Morbos omnes sanari similibus. Quod si contrariorum contraria sint consequential, sanitas autem servetur similibus, quis non videt morbos abigendos esse contraries? Nonne morbus cum sit hostis naturae se depellendum indicat! at simile non agit in simile, contrario igitur profligandus.

The following article was copied verbatim by Mr. WH Heard, of St Petersburg, as it appeared in the *Daheim*, No. 16, of 17th January, 1880, under the heading, *Zur Geschichte der Homoeopathie*:

"So far back as the seventeenth century Homoeopathy was understood and preferred to Allopathy by Paul Fleming, a celebrated poet, who was at the same time a physician."

In his poem to his friend Dr Hartmann the following passage occurs:

"'A clever physician takes his remedies from substances which cause the harm: removes a craving for salt with salt, puts out fire with flames, a thing not understood by many. You contract the art by doing so little with much; you ought to make much out of little. A grain should be more efficacious than a long draught capable of doing harm to a butcher. We have got rid of the old fancy. Who is there now who will commend the doctor simply for his deserving the thanks of the chemist who prefers the latter mode to the former and must then the poor patients weakness be redoubled by a heavy potion?' etc."[xviii]

And Mr. Heard in a letter to me observes:

"This remarkable extract deserves a place by the side of an equally interesting acknowledgement made about the same time by Johan Faramund Rumel, physician to the Duke of Anhalt, and evidently a disciple of Paracelsus, in his work entitled, 'Medicina Spagirica.' The passage is brought forward in the Populäre Homoeopathische Zeitung, 1871, No. 10."

So you perceive, gentlemen, that every one locks upon all these various notions of healing by similars as identical with the scientific inductive homoeopathy bequeathed to us by Hahnemann.

Now let us glance at the author thus introduced by Mr. Heard; he says:

"For every spirit must be modified by that which is the most intimately related to its own nature (*simile a simili curare*), and herein we see the difference between the Hermetists and the Galenists." Then:

---

xviii Schon im XVII. Jahrhundert kannte Dr Paul Fleming, der berühmte Dichter, der zugleich auch Arzt war, die Homoeopathie und gab ihr vor der Allopathie den Vorzug. In seinem Gedichte an Dr Hartmann, seinen Freund, findet sich folgende Stelle:-

'Ein kluger Arzt der nimmt, Da seine Hilfe her, von was der Schade kömmt
Lös't Salzsucht auf durch Salz; löscht Geuer aus mit Flammen.
Was mancher nicht begreift. Ihr zieht die Kunst zusammen,
Macht wenig aus so viel. Ihr wirket viel durch wenig
Von Euch thut ein Gran mehr, als jener langer Trank,
An dem ein Fleischer wol sich möchte heben krank
Wir sind nun überhoben
Der alten Fantasey. Wer will den Arzt noch loben
Um dass er nur verdient des Apotheker's Dank
Der doch dies setzt vor das. Soll man die armen Schwachen
Durch einen schweren Trunk noch doppelt schwächer machen?' etc."

> "And this it is with the diseases in the elemental fire, air, and water, and in like manner must these same be helped and *ever must like help its like*.[xix]

We have already seen that Rhumel was a Paracelsist, and we note that he puts the date of Hermes in the time of Moses, when the law of similars was (he says) first committed to writing.

Rhumel's homoeopathy (like that of his master Paracelsus) consists in the doctrine of signatures, and generally in the similarity (and equality) of the *major mundus* to the *minor mundus*. This he makes perfectly clear; indeed of all the Paracelsists, he is, perhaps, the least mystic, and his writings constitute a good introduction to those of Paracelsus himself. Thus he says (c. vi., De Curatione Morborum, pp. 82-83):

> "With regard to the cure it is either general or special, and takes place either in the common, or the Galenic way, or else after the manner of the new Hermetic or Paracelsic medicine, in which we must include natural *Magia*. As for the ordinary Galenic mode of treatment, I will pass it by in silence rather that make much ado about it, so that I may not open the would aftresh. This consists in stubbornly maintaining: *contraria contrariis curare debeant*.

But on the other hand the old Hermetic method of treatment is far preferable, as daily experience teaches us, for by it the human body may often be cured (with the help of God) even of diseases commonly considered incurable, as we can sufficiently testify from our own humble experience.[xx] This consists in the formula *similia similibus curentur*. He then goes on to enlarge upon the *sympathia*, and *antipathia*, and the concordance of the macrocosm with the microcosm.

There are a number of other authors, some of whom are quoted by Dudgeon, who write in the same strain, but these examples suffice for our present purpose. Rhumel's remark about not being willing to "open the wound afresh," shows that

---

xix *Medicina Spagijrica Tripartita*, oder *Spagijrische Artzneij Kunst in dreij theil getheilet*. Authore, Joanne Pharamundo Rhumelio. Franckfurt, 1662. Editio Secunda (date of first, 1630).

In the *Compendium Hermeticum*, c. ii. p. 3, we read: Dieweilen ein jeder Spiritus allein begehrt von demjenigen mutirt zu werden das seiner Naturam hefftigsten verwandt ist (Simile a simili curari) dardurch der Hermetisten Galenisten Uneterschied kund und offenbar. Then (c. iv., p. 11) . . . Also auch wird eine Krankheit im elemento ignis, aëris, vel aquae microcosmi, so müssen ihr dieselbig auch zu hülff kommen, und ALLEZEIT MUSS GLEICHES SEIN GLEICHES HELFFEN.

xx Die curation belangend, ist dieselbe generalis oder specialis, und geschieht entweder auff die gemeine oder Galenische Weise, oder aber nach Art der newen Hermetischen und Paracelsischen Medicin, neben welchen auch die naturliche Magia, was bisshero durch die gemeine Galenische Art zu curiren verrichtet, will ich lieber stillschweigend vorbeij behen, als davon viel Klagens machen, DAMIT ICH DIE WUNDE NICHT ERFRISCHE. Welche darinn beharrlich besteht: contraria contraries curare debeant.

Was im Gegentheil die alte Hermetische art zu curiren praestiret, lehret die tagliche Erfahrung, und wird der Menschliche Leib so dadurch vielmals glücklich von auch unheilbar gehaltenen Kranckheiten (mit Göttlicher Hulffe liberiret), wie auch unsere weiwol geringe experientz genugsam bezeugen. Diese beruhet in dem: quod similia similibus curentur.

a bitter controversy had been carried on between the Galenists and Hermetists about the principles of similars and contraries.

Dudgeon (op. j. cit.) shows that even popular preachers referred to the controversy in their sermons.

Gentlemen, I much fear you are finding these arid quotations a little tedious, but I want to prove not only that these old authors had crude inklings of a law of cure by similars, but that the coming event did cast a shadow before it, and that this shadow led Hahnemann to the substance.

It is very important to dwell a little on this foreshadowing, because it has been urged by no less a man than Sir Robert Chistison as an argument against our scientific homoeopathy, that no such shadow had been cast before the coming event; so Sir Robert's objection falls to the ground. You know this had already been amply proved by Hahnemann, and since by Dudgeon.

You will, perhaps, ask the very pertinent question: Did Hahnemann himself claim to have originated the *notion* of healing by similars? No, he did not. He rightly claimed to have seen the substance of the various fitful and flickering foreshadowings, and to have transformed a semi-superstition inkling into an inductive science. Let us see what he says on the subject in his *Organon*.

The copy which I have at hand is the fourth Leipzig Edition (1829), and from this I quote. On page 51 he gives examples of involuntary homoeopathic cures wrought by the physicians of the old school. He mentions the palliative mode of treatment according to the law *contraria contrariis*, and then remarks:

> "By observation, reflection, and experience, I found that, on the contrary, the true, right, and best way of healing is to be found in the formula: *similia similibus curentur*. In order to cure gently, quickly, certainly, and enduringly, you must in every case of disease choose a remedy that is itself capable of producing a complaint like the one it is to cure (ὅμοιον πάθος).

> "This homoeopathic way of healing has thus far been taught by no one, nobody has carried it out [in practice]. [The italics are Hahnemann's own.] But if the truth lie solely in this proceeding, as you will see with me, then it may be expected that, admitting that it had not been acknowledged for thousands of years, nevertheless traces of it may be found in all ages. And thus it is."

He then goes on to argue that all real cures by remedies in every age have been according to the law of similars, although the physicians who prescribed the remedies were not aware of the fact.

And in a footnote he says: "For truth is co-eternal with the all-wise beneficent Godhead. Man may long leave it unnoticed until the time comes when, according to the decree of Providence, its bright sheen shall irresistibly penetrate the fog, and appear as the aurora of the morn and the dawn of day to shine brightly, for the weal of mankind for evermore."

Further on (p. 102) he quotes real *inklings* of scientific homoeopathy; but they were mere inklings, and remained such and no one *taught them* or *put them into practice*. Hahnemann remarks in the foot-note (p. 102) that he gives these examples of inklings of homoeopathy not as proofs of a really founded homoeopathy; but *so that he may not be reproached with having purposely ignored them in order to secure for himself the priority of the idea*. Thus you clearly perceive that he does not lay any claim to having *originated the idea of healing by similars*.

To my mind all these historic inklings very much enhance Hahnemann's great merit as an original thinker, and as the founder of scientific homoeopathy. I do not, however, think that Hahnemann was himself acquainted with *all* these inklings at the time of his great discovery, most probably he hunted many of them up afterwards. I also question very much whether he had himself a clear conception of *how* the idea *first* came to him. He must have gradually *thought it out*, and applied the result of his experiment with *Cinchona* to the *idea*, or conversely.

Hahnemann's position with regard to the *notion* of healing by similars is also very prettily and clearly indicated *by himself* in his historical communication to Guiznot. Writing to this great man in 1835, on the question of homoeopathy, Hahnemann quotes the following lines from Béranger:

> Combien de temps une pensée, Vierge obscure, attend son époux!
> Les sots la traitent d'insensée; Le sage lui dit: cachez-vous.
> Mais le rencontrant loin du monde, Un fou qui croit au lendemain,
> L'épouse; elle devient féconde, Pour le bonheur du genre humain.

Till Hahnemann, homoeopathy was an obscure, wandering and despised maiden thought, awaiting marriage with a male mind; this thought became united with Hahnemann's mind, and fecundity followed for the weal of mankind.

You will readily admit that familiarity with these sixteenth century writers in their homoeopathies, and on the question of whether diseases are best cured by contraries or similars would prepare Hahnemann's mind for his own scientific induction. Nay, perhaps you will even admit, with me, that had he been unacquainted herewith, his historic proving of *Cinchona* might not have eventuated as it did in the establishment of scientific homoeopathy.

For we admit that Hahnemann did not *originate* the *conception* of *a* law of cure by contraries or by similars; neither did he *originate* the *idea* of the trail of drugs on the healthy human organism.

Baron von Stoerck tried medicines on himself; Haller, and possibly others also. Crumpe's[xxi] trial of opium on himself and others, in health, is, as you have seen, subsequent to Hahnemann's.

---

xxi Before venturing to publish his work on *Opium*, Crumpe submitted the MS. to Dr Gregory of Edinburgh. Dr Gregory "read it with attention," and considered that "as a book of medical science it possessed considerable merit." But Gregory was led to no law by it more than Crumpe himself.

Haller's position may be seen in the Preface to his *Pharmacopoeia*, where he clearly enunciates the principle of trying drugs on the healthy in these words...

"Primùm in corpore sano medel tentanda est, sine peregrina ulla miscela, exigua illius dosis ingerenda et ad omnes, quæ inde contiguas affections, qui pulsus, qui calor, quae respiratio, quaenam excretions attendum. Indè adductum phaenomenorum in sano obviorum transeas ad experimenta in corpore aegroto".[xxii]

Let us just now glance at a veritable forerunner of Hahnemann: I mean the Danish regimental surgeon Stahl, whom Hahnemann refers to in his *Organon* (p. 104).

The passage runs thus: "The rule that is generally accepted in the medical art, to cure by means of oppositely-acting remedies (*contraria contrariis*) is quite false, and the very reverse of the truth; on the contrary, he (Stahl) is convinced that diseases yield to and are cured by a remedy that can produce a like affection (*similia similibus*) – burns, by being brought near a fire, frost-bitten limbs by the application of snow and very cold water, inflammation and bruises by distilled spirits; and thus he was in the habit of treating a tendency to acidity of the stomach by a very small does of sulphuric acid with the most happy results, in case in which a number of absorbent powders had been used in vain."

But Stoerck also seems to have come very near to it.

Anton Stoerck (Libellus quo demonstratur: *Stramonium, Hyosciamum, Aconitum* non solum tuto posse exhiberi usu interno hominibus, verum et ea esse remedia in multis morbis maxime salutifera. Vindobonae, MDCCLXIJ.) tried drugs on himself on June 23, 1760[xxiii] by rubbing some fresh stramony on his

---

So we see that the mere fact of carefully conducted experiments with drugs on the healthy did not of itself lead to the discovery of homoeopathy, any more tan did the various inklings of real homoeopathy, or the various notions of healing by similitudes already alluded to.

xxii This is the birth place of the modern physiological phase of allopathy, to which the rank of a science cannot be denied, i.e., the science of palliative medicine; homoeopathy being the science of curative medicine.

xxiii But Stoerck had already previously tried remedies on the healthy. See his *Libellus de Cicuta*, Vindobonae, 1760 (c. i. p. 8). He first gave cicuta to a dog, and:–

"His audacior redditus, in me ipso experimentum feci. Mane ac vesperi sumsi granum unum hujus extracti, et vasculum unum infusi theae hausi desuper. Diateam tunc Paulo strictiorem observavi, ut ilico (sic) adverterem, si quid insoliti in meo corpore fieret." It did him no harm. Then he increased the dose, but still obtained only a negative result. What was his conclusion? "Jam ergo optimo jure et salva conscientia hoc in aliis mihi licuit tentare."

That was the extract. "Quae autem radici cicutae vis inesset? quoque scire volui."

The significance of this question is seen in Stoerck's answer to it. He says: "Radix recens dum in taleolas discinditur, fundit lac, quod gustu amarum et acre est. hujus lactis unam alteramve guttulam linguae apice delibavi. Mox lingua facta est rigida, intumuit, valde doluit, et ego nec verbum loqui poteram. Sinistro hoc eventu terrefacturs multum timui."

This was much relieved by lemon juice, so that th epain and tension were so far better that he could just lisp a few words (balbutire). In two hours, he was all right.

hands to see whether the dictum of the botanists – *Si tantum olfeceris stramonium, ebrietatum facit* – was correct, but no ebriety followed. This emboldened him. Then he and his famulus cut up a quantity and rubbed it up in a mortar, and expressed a *succus*. Then he slept in the same room with it and got a dull headache. Then he made an extract and put a grain and a half on his tongue, and pressed it against the palate, and so on.

But his object was *not to discover* an explanation of its *modus in morbis operandi*, but to find out whether such a poison could be safely exhibited as a remedy. That is a very different thing to Hahnemann's first trial with cinchona thirty years later.

Stoerck's next step after determining that the extract of *Stramony* might by safely exhibited to human beings (I beg to show you the work, you will find this narrated on pp. 7, 8, and 9) – his next step was this:

> "Agebatur" (says he) "tunc de morbo, in quo conveniret, et de aegris, quibus prodesset." To this end he consulted both the older and more recent writers,[xxiv] but found nothing favour its use as a remedy.

He exclaims:

> 'Etenim omnes scribebant:
> "*Stramonium* turbare mentem, adferre insaniam, delere ideas et memoriam, producere convulsiones."

All this, says he, is bad, and forbids the internal use of stramony. Here comes a memorable sentence – memorable, that is from our present scientific standpoint:

> "Interim tamen ex his formavi sequentem quaestionem:
> "Si *Stramonium* turbando mentem insaniam sanis, an non licet experiri: num insanientibus et mente captis turbando, mutandoque ideas, et sensorium commune adferret mentem sanam, et convulses tolleret contrario motu convulsiones?"

These are the nearest approaches to our scientific homoeopathy with which I am acquainted, and *how* near too! Yet they resulted in nothing beyond enunciating *the* ODD *notion*[xxv] of healing by similars, and establishing the fact that moderate doses of stramony may be safely given in disease, and that it cases and cures insanity and convulsions.

Then he took the dried root, reduced it to powder, and found it "minus nociva." He therefore prepared a dry extract... "tunc fit extractum minus efficax, attamen utile."

Did this lead to Stoerck to use cicuta (*Conium maculatum*) for a painful tumid tongue with loss of speech? By no means, but for indurated glands!

xxiv Thus you see he made no attempt at induction.
xxv Not a law.

Stoerck[xxvi] here came so near to discovering scientific homoeopathy, that, with our present light, we may marvel that he did not do so.

Is submit that these near approaches of Stoerck and many others to the discovery of our great law, with the trial of drugs on the healthy, and the very question formulated by Stoerck himself in such clear language, prove how much was necessary for its discovery. Stoerck (and most of the others) wanted three things:

1. The true spirit of philosophy.
2. The requisite leisure and the habit of *thinking deeply*
3. A knowledge of the history of theories of drug action

Stoerck came to the very verge of the discovery of scientific homoeopathy, and nevertheless did not see it; this is *proved* by reference to his later works. Thus if you refer to his "Libellus, quo demonstratur: Herbam, veteribus dictam Flammulam Jovis," etc., Vienna, 1769, you will find that he had rather retrograded, as he there only tried it very superficially on lower animals, and not on man at all, by way of proving it.

These facts give us, better than anything I know, an adequate conception of Hahnemann's true greatness. Had Hahnemann stumbled against homoeopathy, as so many did, or formulated Stoerck's question in 1790, he would have infallibly discovered scientific homoeopathy. Had Stoerck been a better read man, with a little more of the spirit of philosophy, and been also an impecunious physician who had given up practice for conscience' sake, he, too, must infallibly have discovered *the* therapeutic law that leads us, and we should have to-day met at an Stoerckian Address. But Stoerck was a baron of the empire, and court physician, and too much success does not conduce to mental progress and development.

It is fortunate for mankind that Hahnemann's noble conscientiousness had reduced him to beggary. Had he too been a baron of the Holy Roman Empire, and court physician, we should not have been here to-day, for the doctrine of healing by similars had been freely discussed for centuries, and yet homoeopathy was there only as a portentous shadow.

Progress in science is not made by big bounds with great gaps between, but rather bit by bit, one succeeding another unconnectedly, and then comes a third connecting the two. So was it, I submit, with the scientific homoeopathy of Hahnemann. Drug physiology had just dawned, and may be said to have existed as an odd notion. The question of *a* law of similars was there looming through the ages, and awaited, in the language of Béranger, as an obscure maiden thought for a husband; this she found in the male mind of Hahnemann.

---

xxvi Oddly enough, Stoerck's bitter foe, de Haen (*Ratio medendi*, Tom. iv. p. 228), almost stumbled against our scientific homoeopathy, for he says: "Dulco-amarae stipites majori dosi convulsiones et deliria excitant, moderata vero spasmos, convulsionesque solvunt." Well may Hahnemann remark, "How near de Haen was to recognising nature's law of healing!" (*Organon.*) Yet he did not. The mighty genius of a Hahnemann is not often found in nature's children.

For what was the use of these two without the connecting link? None, and the absolute proof of this lies in the fact that although they were there, still there was no scientific homoeopathy.

This ends my long parenthetic chapter; let us now return to Cullen.

Homoeopathy as a scientific induction

We can readily imagine how Hahnemann would receive any new hypothesis anent the *modus operandi* of *Cinchona*. He knew well enough that this remedy *did* cure certain forms of ague, just as he knew that arsenic would cure other forms of the same disease, *but according to what law, how?*

Cullen said the bark cured ague because it was a bitter and an astringent combined, and at the same time somewhat aromatic, a tonic and roborant. It strengthens the stomach and thus cures ague as a roborant stomachic. Thus, for Cullen, *Cinchona* is a bitter, astringent, aromatic, roborant, stomachic tonic!

Surely it was not needful to clear away all his predecessors from the pharmacological field in order to set up such a worthless hypothesis; no wonder Hahnemann in his turn dealt with Cullen as Cullen had dealt with his predecessors. Here is Hahnemann's historical footnote: "By uniting the strongest bitters with the strongest astringents, you may get a compound that in a small dose shall possess much more of both qualities than the bark, and yet you will in all eternity never obtain a fever specific from such a compound. Our author should have settled this point. It will not be such an easy matter to discover the still lacking principle according to which its action may be explained. Nevertheless, let us reflect on the following: Substances such as very strong coffee, pepper, *Arnica, Ignatia*, and *Arsenic, that are capable of exciting a kind of fever*,[xxvii] will extinguish the types of ague. For the sake of experiment I took for several days four *quentchen* of good cinchona twice a day; my feet, the tips of my fingers, etc., first became cold, and I felt tired and sleepy, then my heart began to beat, my pulse became hard and quick; I got an insufferable feeling of uneasiness, a trembling (but without chill), a weariness sin all my limbs; then a beating in my head, redness of the cheeks, thirst, in short, all the old symptoms with which I was familiar in ague appeared one after another, yet without any actual chill or rigor. In brief, also those particularly characteristic symptoms such as I was wont to observe in agues, obtuseness of the senses, the kind of stiffness in all the limbs, but especially that dull disagreeable feeling which seems to have its seat in the periosteum of all the bones of the body – they all put in an appearance. This paroxysm lasted each time two or three hours, and came again afresh whenever I repeated the dose, but not otherwise. I left off, and became well." (pp. 108, 9, Vol. II.)

---

xxvii   You observe Hahnemann already knew something of the pathogenic effects of drugs.

On the next page, Cullen seeks to defend his hypothesis against all comers, and hereto Hahnemann adds this remarkable footnote. By the way, Hahnemann's footnotes are very like the traditional postscripts to ladies' letters – they are the most important parts of the whole. Well, the note is this:– "We readily see how sorry our author is, not to be able to fell his opponents to the ground with all their objections to his mode of explanation. His zeal seems particularly directed against those who always have the vague word *specific*[xxviii] in their mouths when they discourse of the Bark; without knowing what they really mean by it. But had he for a moment reflected that one can prepare from an extract of quassia and oak apples a far more powerful astringent bitter than cinchona is, but which nevertheless cannot cure a quartan fever that is half a year old; had he scented in the Bark *a power of exciting an artificial antagonistic fever* (&c.), most certainly he would not have zealously stuck to his own hypothesis."

You will note, gentlemen, that here, at the birth of scientific Homoeopathy, ninety years ago, Hahnemann's conception of homoeopathic drug action in disease is that of *antagonism* to it; he speaks of the cinchonic fever as artificial and *antagonistic, i.e.,* antagonistic to the ague which it cures by reason of its similarity. This has been lately presented to us as something new, with vain verbosity; but the babe is no more, having succumbed to antipathy. The fact is, the number of men who persist in burning farthing rush-lights of their own, is verily not small. Another reason this for an *annual* Hahnemann Lecture, so that the old lamp may not be allowed to choke up with the soot of neglect. For we cannot afford to give up the grand electric light of homoeopathy for the faint flickering of these tiny tapers.

Two or three pages further on we already find Hahnemann individualizing, for he speaks of the cinchonic fever as of a particular find (*von besondrer Art*, p. 177).

We now proceed to take leave of the pre-homoeopathic Hahnemann, to learn how he thought out his Homoeopathy from this cinchonic artificial fever which he had produced in himself.

Before doing so, let me express a hope that no one here is yawningly saying to himself:–

"Hier auf diesen Bänken Vergehen mir Hören, Sehen, und Denken."

In 1795 the renowned Hufeland began his "*Journal der practischen Arzneikunde und Wundarzneikunst,*" in Jena. Hahnemann and Hufeland were of the leading

---

xxviii There is too great a tendency amongst us now to degenerate into mere homoeopathic Specifiker; witness Dr Yeldham's Presidential Address at the Leeds Congress, 1880. No doubt it is good, nay very good to be a homoeopathic Specifiker, but it is better, very much better, to be an individualising homoeopath. I do not claim to be any better than my neighbours: almost daily I find myself slipping back into the royal road of treating the disease in lieu of the patient. Individualising is so laborious, and still too far in advance of the hodiernal medical mind.

medical men of the day, and personal friends; the latter was then professor of physic in Jena. In the first volume (1795) Hahnemann is quoted on the treatment of an important affection. In the second volume (1796) the historic cure of Klockenbring is mentioned.

In this same volume we find Hahnemann's celebrated *"Versuch über ein neues Prinzip zur Auffindung der Heilkräfte der Arzneisubstansen, nebst einigen Blicken auf die bisherigen,"* which must be regarded as the starting point of the greatest revolution in medicine that the world has ever witnessed. In this masterly Essay he undermined the whole then existing fabric of practical medicine, and laid the corner stone of scientific therapeutics, by enunciating the law of healing by similars, based on the effects of drugs on the healthy human body. I feel it is utterly impossible for me to do justice to this wonderful Essay, or to the majestic modesty of its style. You all know it well; and, although it was published eighty-four years ago, our very presence here to-day is its echo.

Hahnemann the homoeopath

We have at last come into the presence of Hahnemann the homoeopath. Of course a little country village like Stötteritz was not the place in which the founder of a new system of practical medicine was likely to be content to remain. Not because a physician's skill should be measured by the number of inhabitants of the place he lives in, but because a village does not offer the requisite material for testing a new doctrine of practical physic.

The iconoclastic Hahnemann goes *pari passu* with his upbuilding of a new teaching, and herein lies his vast superiority over all other medical reformers. He does not merely knock everything down, and then leave everybody staring hopelessly about in anarchic chaos as did Cullen, but he skilfully uses the *débris* of the demolished edifices for the erection of his own. Having been set thinking by his trial of cinchona that grew out of his translating Cullen's *Materia Medica*, he returned to his old love, the practice of medicine. Very fortunately he obtained a post as medical superintendent of an asylum for the insane at Georgenthal in the Thuringian forest, which was offered him by the Duke regnant of Saxe-Gotha. Here he wrought the cure of the wonderfully gifted Hanoverian Minister Klockenbring, who had been driven mad by a withering satire of Kotzebue; an account of the case was published (you will find it in the *Lesser Writings*), and it very naturally created a considerable stir in Germany, where Klockenbring was at the time a kind of Lord Beaconsfield. Perhaps the most remarkable part of this case lies in the fact that Hahnemann gave bodily freedom to his maniacs, and in general treated them with kindly benevolent mildness.

Thus we see that Hahnemann must be regarded as the pioneer of a rational treatment of the mentally afflicted. He has left on record that he never allowed any insane person to be punished by blows or any other pain-giving bodily inflictions, inasmuch as there cannot possibly be any punishment, properly so-called, where there is no real responsibility. For when the law shuts up an individual in an asylum, such person thereby receives the stamp of irresponsibility.

Hereupon we find Hahnemann again on the wander again after a stay of only a few months at the asylum; he is first at Walschleben, then at Pyrmont, then at Brunswick, then at Wolfenbüttel and finally at Königslutter where he remained till 1799.

You remember that his famous experiment with cinchona was in 1790; and during the nine years that elapsed between this and his being driven out from Königslutter he had tried his new notion, and found it the basis of a scientific therapeutics. It is no wonder that Hahnemann was restless, and given to roaming during these nine years, for he must then have begun to realise the immense range of his new idea, he must have foreseen that it would bring about a total *bouleversement* of time-honored physic.

At Königslutter he gradually ripened into a scientific practitioner, for he gave one medicine at a time, and that according to the law of similars. And he, moreover, made use of only comparatively small doses; of course, these were material and appreciable; but, remember, this was eighty odd years ago, when physician who dared to give one medicine at a time was looked at askance both by his colleagues and by the apothecaries – especially by the apothecaries. It is still a very suspicious thing to give but one medicine at a time. At that period an orthodox prescription was half a foot long, and contained a score of invaluable ingredients, and a mysteriously occult art lay supposedly in the mode of combining them in such proportions and degrees that they should be at any rate a mighty mystery to the less canny colleagues. We are told that in these latter days *nous avons changé tout cela*, and that the allopaths and homoeopaths are now all alike in their mode of practice.

Well let us compare the prescriptions of our most eminent allopathic practitioners; we have them daily in our hands, and we see them in our literature; judging from these I must affirm that the general run of allopathic practice of to-day is, taken for all in all, no better than it was a century ago, and that because their principle is wrong. I have taken the trouble to compare the papers on practical medicine that appear now-a-days in the *Lancet* with those that appeared eighty years ago in Hufeland's *Journal*, and with the single exception of bleeding I prefer those cases in Hufeland's Journal as less hurtful and less complicated, and some of them as at least empirically commendable.

But I am wandering away from my text; yet having wandered so far, permit me to say before returning to it that when I speak of the "general run of allopathic practice," I mean allopathically, and not homoeopathy on the sly, or crypto-homoeopathy that some of the writers in the "Practitioner" impose upon the credulity of their ignorant readers as discoveries of their own. For along the corridor of time I hear the voice of the sage of Köthen echoing the words, "*Hos ego versiculos feci: tulit alter honores.*"

Homoeopathy is homoeopathy, whether openly and honestly taught within these walls or elsewhere, or slily smuggled into the student's skulls at certain colleges and schools. Professor Bathyllus[xxix] has carried on this smuggling business for a good many years, and his pupils are beginning to fill the other chairs of medicine throughout the country; but I have yet to learn that plagiarism is so far condoned as to be converted into honesty by social success.

Gentlemen, do not misunderstand me; I am *not* pleading for privileged schism and narrow sectarianism, as do the allopaths by crying themselves out from the very rooftops as the Levites of the Ark of the Medical Covenant. No; I am merely maintaining that homoeopathy is the mental property of Samuel Hahnemann, and of such of his disciples as have contributed to its development and propagation, and honestly give honour to whom honour is due. Science is the common property of mankind; the *honour of her discoveries* is private property.

The mean-souled Bathylluses of our medical colleges may impose upon beardless boys raw from the schools, but they cannot, in the very nature of things, own what belongs to another man, although that other man be dead. Hahnemann *is* dead, it is true, and cannot appear in the flesh to claim his own; but he has followers still, who dare stand up and maintain that with all respect for professional unity, with all regard for professional brotherhood, there cannot be any real unity in the professional so long as common honesty is banished from its portals, and the premium of professional rewards is put upon plagiarism. In my opinion the man who knowingly appropriates another man's discoveries, and debits them as his own, is to all intents and purposes dishonest; and *the more so* as he is beyond the reach of ordinary laws.

Gentlemen, you are perhaps shocked at my making use of such a strong expression. Be shocked rather at the thing not at the word. I would I could call it by some other name that, being more euphemistic to your ears, were still as true to fact; but I cannot. Throughout the profession – may God forgive them – the great name of Hahnemann is shamelessly maligned, while at the same time his life's labour is being appropriated by the pilfering professors of our schools. And the worst thing about it is that the present generation of students are thus deliberately demoralised by being taught to sacrifice moral principle for mere expedience; taught at the very threshold of life to gain a cheap pseudo-success, to crown themselves with tawdry tinsel in lieu of earning a really golden crown that comes only to honest truthful labour.

Tell me, you with hoary heads, and you who have only the silvery streaks of time to mark the years which have gone, what has helped *you* most in the march of life

---

xxix Quamobrem donatus honoratúsque á Cæsare fuit.

thus far? Was it public applause, or the still small voice within that kept you up in the most trying hours of your life's battle? Have you unexpectedly triumphed over disease and death at your isolated posts with the aid of the doctrine of expedience? I trow not.

Alas! that the brightness of the honour of our students should be tarnished by the example and precepts of their own teachers before the trials and temptations of real life begin. *C'est le premier pas qui coûte*, and hence the future of such is not bright. Of the original Bathyllus we read that after awhile . . . *Romae fibula fuit, Maro verò exaltatior*. So it will be in this matter; if not, it will be the fault of our future Hahnemannian lecturers.

Militant Homeopathy

I come back now and ask you to fix your attention for a moment on the beginning of *militant* homoeopathy, and the hatred that is as alive to-day as it was eighty-one years ago, when bigoted ignorance and a degrading trades-unionism drove the enlightened and learned Hahnemann out of Königslutter. You know certain wiseacres say that the founder of homoeopathy had himself to blame for this hatred by violently attacking his medical peers. Gentlemen, this is not correct. Permit me to point out that Hahnemann's violent language is found at a later date than 1799. Just turn to his *Essay on a New Principle*, and point out one single unbecoming word, or one flash of passion: it is modest and dignified, and respectful to his fellows. I find nothing anterior to his departure from Königslutter that betokens even the slightest anger or hatred of a blamable nature against his fellow practitioners. I maintain that up to the departure from Königslutter Hahnemann was filled with love and respect for this worthy fellow-physicians.

We are also told it was *the small dose notion* that set the medical world against him. This is impossible, for the best of all reasons, viz., that when the opposition to him began, Hahnemann had not yet enunciated his doctrine of drug dynamisation, and he himself was still using certainly small, but nevertheless moderate, material doses.

Then we are told that it was his notions about pathology, his doctrine of psora more particularly.

But, gentlemen, Hahnemann was driven out of Königslutter twenty-eight years *before* he called Stapf and Gross to Köthen to announce to them his theory of chronic diseases. We, therefore, come to the inevitable conclusion that it was neither his vituperative language, nor his doctrine of drug dynamisation, nor his psora doctrine, *because* none of these existed when the bitter persecution set in.

You probably remember the sweet little story of the lamb and of another quadruped that, I believe, was not a lamb; in that celebrated tale the water flowed up-stream.

So it must be with *militant* homoeopathy in Hahnemann's person: for his personal persecution began in 1798, and in a most violent manner. If therefore his violent language, or his small doses, or his psora doctrine set the medical world against him, they must have done so by anticipation, and the effect preceded its causes by a good many years.

Then it has been flaunted in his face that he went to the lay public with his discovery, and thus set the profession against him. This is equally untrue: Hahnemann published his *Essay on a New Principle* in the leading *medical* journal – I hold it in my hand. There it is. (Hufeland's.) Moreover he kept within the most strict code of medical ethics.

Thus we see that the separation of Hahnemann from the profession did not come from him but from his beloved professional brethren, who thrust him out, as they thrust you out, by forbidding freedom to openly and honestly practise according to the law of similars.

The vulnerable point with Hahnemann was this: at Königslutter he gave his own medicines to his patients, though gratuitously.

The physicians at Königslutter became jealous of his rising fame, and they incited the apothecaries against him, and these latter brought an action at law against Hahnemann for dispensing his own medicines, and thus encroaching on their rights. It was decided against him: he was forbidden to give his own medicines, and this of course rendered his further stay impossible.

That was what these unprofessional brethren wanted. The letter of the law was no doubt against Hahnemann, but the spirit of the law was in his favour, as were also justice and common sense. The injustice of the decree against him was all the more glaring because he was a recognised authority on the apothecary's art, and had thoroughly qualified himself as an overseer of chemists, and had actually been in such a position before. Then already, in 1787, Hahnemann had published a kind of adaptation of a pharmacological work from the French of Van den Sande (Brussels, 1784), entitled *La falsification des medicamens dévoillée.*

But this work is completely put into the shade by his "learned and laborious *Pharmaceutical Lexicon.*"

It is important to know that in Germany the pharmaceutical chemists are under the control and supervision of the medical officers of health, the *Stadtphysici*, who are necessarily medical men. The *Stadtphysikus* of a given district, must visit the chemists' shops of his neighbourhood at stated intervals to see that the proper drugs are in stock and good. Now Hahnemann had years before held such a post, and his books were actually the authorities for the chemists and their respective overseers. I dwell on this because it explains to us how flagrant the injustice done to him was: he the great authority in pharmaceutical chemistry was prohibited form even giving away his medicines for nothing! Nay more, he was *such* an authority on all matters pertaining to the apothecaries' art that some of his detractors on that very account maintained, and maintain it still, for I have heard it with my own ears, that he was not a physician at all in reality, but an apothecary!! The fact is, Hahnemann was a master in *materia medica*, whether such medical material be on the chemists' shelves, in their original habitats, in the laboratory, in the healthy human body, or in the sick.

Driven out of Königslutter in 1799 by the persecution of the profession, he wended his way to Hamburg. Of course in those days there were no railways or any of the furniture-removing vans that render *our* flittings comparatively small affairs. In 1799 it was no small undertaking to remove with all the household gods from Königslutter to Hamburg. At that time those who moved to some little distance used to buy a van or wagon for the purpose; this Hahnemann did, and put his wife, children and movable property in it, and went out of Königslutter, as the Vicar of Wakefield left his parish, accompanied on the road for some distance by those who had received his benefactions.

No doubt Hahnemann left Königslutter with a heavy heart, for he had there begun to taste of the sweets of comfort once again, he had there put his divine discovery to the test; he had there discovered the prophylactic virtue of *Belladonna* in scarlet fever, he had there proved to his wife that his days of clogs and homespun, at the village by Leipzig, were but a, perhaps necessary, preparatory trial to a mighty future, like a run before a long leap, on the principle of *"Reculer avant de sauter."* There happened a terrible epidemic of scarlet fever at Königslutter during the last year of his stay there, and his discovery of the brilliant curative and preventive virtues of *Belladonna* in that dire disease – discovered by means of the law of similars – enabled him to save the lives of very many of the inhabitants. Hence you will not marvel that so considerable a number of them came out with him, and accompanied him some way on the road to Hamburg before bidding him "God speed."

What was the frame of mind of the gentle and genial Hahnemann as he thus wended his way towards Hamburg, with all that was near and dear to him of this world's blessings – driven away from those who loved him and thought thankfully of him for saving their lives – driven away from a certain material prosperity to strange uncertainties. This journey was destined to become memorable, for an accident happened to the wagon: it was upset going down a hill, the driver was thrown off his seat, Hahnemann and his whole family and all his goods were thrown together into once confused mass; he himself was injured, the leg of one of his daughters was fractured, his infant son mortally injured (he died shortly afterwards), and his goods were much damaged by falling into a stream at the bottom of the hill. With the help of the country folks, they were got to the next village, where he was compelled to remain for six weeks on account of his daughter's fractured limb – thus he would, of course, fritter away any little savings from Königslutter. However, he eventually did reach Hamburg.

I think a good deal of Hahnemann myself, yet I do not think he was other than a man, but he *was* every inch a man; so I can in thought put myself into his place, and methinks he may have solemnly cursed his professional persecutors as he lay at yon village with destroyed property, a bruised body, his daughter with a broken leg, and his baby son sick unto death.

Undoubtedly a change came over him after this, and he began gradually to assume a very haughty and bitter tone, and this eventuated in very strong language indeed. But not by any means too strong, in my humble judgment. Let me put it to any one of you, gentlemen, what sort of language would *you* use if you were thus drive out of house and home over and over again, and reduced to poverty, simply because you knew more, and worked harder, and cured better and more pleasantly than your neighbours? Especially if your favourite baby-boy was killed in consequence, your daughter's leg broken, and you yourself bruised and hurt?

I do not claim divine qualities for Hahnemann, and hence I not only do not blame him for his bold independence and daring, but think it right and reasonable. Even the divine Nazarene was once filled with anger. The departure from Königslutter is the starting-point of Hahnemann's freedom and considering that he was then forty-four years of age, and in mental grasp and medical knowledge vastly superior to even Hufeland, "the Nestor of German Medicine," I think the time had come for a breaking loose from the trammels whereby professional jealousy sought to reduce him to the low level of a mere medicine monger.

We once again find Hahnemann on the wander; Hamburg failed him, and he went to the neighbouring town of Altona, and not faring there any better, he removed to Möllen in Lauenburg. But here a violent longing for his fatherland came over him, and he retraced his steps back to his beloved Saxony, and planted himself at Eulenburg. Here he was again persecuted by his professional brethren through the medical officer of health for the place, and driven hence.

We find him in Dessau in 1803 writing a book against the use of coffee, that was, and is, the favourite beverage of the Germans, especially of the women and poor, as much as tea is with us. Those who are familiar with the insides of Germany hospitals know that cases of chronic poisoning with coffee are by no means rare even now; to Hahnemann's antagonism to coffee we owe the popularity of cocoa amongst the homoeopaths, the earlier homoeopaths recommending it in lieu of the forbidden coffee.

Then Hahnemann published a translation of an English work called the *Treasury of Medicines*, evidently much against the grain, and shortly afterwards wrote a German adaptation of JJ Rousseau's *"De l'Education,"* and he translated Haller's *Materia Medica* in 1806. From the time of his flight from Königslutter in 1799 till now he was maturing his discovery and fixing it.

His *Æsculapius in the Balance* is a work wherein allopathy is weighed and found wanting in such a masterly way that it would no doubt create many most implacable enemies. But this *Æsculap auf der Wagschaale* was not published till 1805, and Hahnemann's persecutions began six years previously. In this same year we have the first sketch of a *Materia Medica Pura* in Latin, under the title of *Fragmenta de viribus medicamentorum positivis*, etc., and in the following year his *Medicine of Experience*. Dr Dudgeon justly characterises this as "the most original, logical, and brilliant essay that has ever appeared on the art of Medicine."

Hereupon a whole flood of calumniators and detractors fell foul of the common enemy, Hahnemann, and no wonder, considering that human nature is what it is; and there is a good deal of this human nature in our beloved profession now as well as then. Hahnemann received for his remarkable discoveries nothing but opposition, hatred, contempt and calumny from his medical brethren. At length he could stand this no longer, and he appealed from the prejudice and injustice of his professional brethren to the public, and henceforth published his essays and papers in a magazine of general literature and science entitled *Allgemeiner Anzeiger der Deutschen*. In this journal he published a series of brilliant essays that won for homoeopathy the support of the general intelligent public, and, as Dudgeon[xxx] puts it – "The doctrines which were scornfully rejected by the scribes and Pharisees of the old school found favour with the public, and the number of his admirers and non-medical disciples increased from day to day." In 1810 he published the first edition of his great *Organon*, and then returned to Leipzig, where he soon became surrounded by a numerous crowd of patients, admirers, and followers.

It is a great wonder that the abuse and calumnies hurled against Hahnemann and homoeopathy at this time, and during the following two decades, did not drive him mad. But it did nothing of the kind, though it must have rankled in his sensitive soul. Happily, Hahnemann treated them all with silent contempt, and worked away at proving medicines and collecting pathogenetic symptoms, and in 1811 he began with the first volume of his glorious *Materia Medica Pura*, that constitutes the grandest monument ever erected to or by any physician since the world began. He no doubt said to himself, Ye poor fools, ye know not what ye do. In all Hahnemann's chequered career nothing strikes me as showing more profound wisdom than his letting his adversaries alone in their vile abuse; he might have hurled back their slanders, and defended himself and his discovery with the eloquence of a Demosthenes; but, as Celsus remarks, *Morbi non eloquentiâ sed remediis curantur*,[xxxi] and so he plodded on at his *Materia Medica*, on which much of his great glory must ever rest.

---

xxx The preceding paragraph is also nearly word for word from Dudgeon, as are likewise several others further on.

xxxi Diseases are not cured by eloquence but by remedies.

At the period at which we have now arrived, viz., 1811, Hahnemann's great idea was to establish a Leipzig *School of* Homoeo*pathy*, for the purpose of indoctrinating the rising generation of physicians with homoeopathy, both theoretically and practically, by founding a college with hospital attached. So you of the London School of Homoeopathy are strictly Hahnemannian in your efforts in this direction sixty-nine years after he tried to do the same in Leipzig.

He had, however, to content himself with giving a course of lectures on the principles and practice of homoeopathy to those medical men and medical students who wished to be instructed in the subject.

To this end he had to obtain permission from the Medical Faculty to become a Privat-Docent. This was readily granted, most probably in the hope that in defending his thesis he would show himself to be the ignorant shallow character which his detractors had announced him to be. So the day for defending his thesis arrived, and the subject thereof was *De Helleborismo Veterum*, which, as Dudgeon truly says, no one can read without confessing that Hahnemann treats the subject in a masterly way, and displays an amount of acquaintance with the writings of the Greek, Latin, Arabian, and other physicians, from Hippocrates down to his own time, that is possessed by few, and a power of philological criticism that has been rarely equalled. At this period Hahnemann was fifty-seven years old, and became at last teacher in that university in which he had been taught thirty-seven years previously. Here he lectured to medical men and students, and attached a number of these to himself, and here he built up that grand pharmacological edifice in which we reside. Hence we may truly say, as we luxuriate in our splendid *Materia Medica, Hahnemannus nobis hæc otia fecit.*

He remained at Leipzig till 1821, and was enjoying a very large practice, and making untold converts to his new system and had then attained to the age of sixty-six. But his professional brethren in Leipzig could not bear his success; they could find nothing against him; he led an exemplary life almost entirely in the bosom of his own numerous and happy family; he was almost worshipped by his patients, and he was already at the head of a considerable number of talented physicians who had declared for homoeopathy. They tell us that Hahnemann voluntarily created a schism, and thus set the profession against him. I deny this. He did every thing in his power, even at this late period, to infuse his reform into the profession itself; the profession spurned him and his better way. Is he not, at the very time of which we are treating, public lecturer on homoeopathy in the University of Leipzig? Did he not qualify himself for the post in the ordinary legal way? Did not the dean of the Faculty warmly congratulate him on his marvellous display of learning when publicly defending his thesis: *De Hellborismo Veterum?*

The medical profession expected he would come to grief in defending his thesis, and they were there to witness his downfall; he did not fall, however, but rather so staggered his opponents with his great learning that none of them any longer dared hope to hurt him on that side. Then they tried it on at his lectures in the Leipzig University, but they found in him their master, they could not impeach him for anything or even cook up a scandal against him. So they resolved to play the old game that had succeeded so well at Königslutter twenty-two years previously; they incited the guild of apothecaries against him for giving away his own medicines; this was the great crime of the noble old seer.

An injunction was obtained against him, and he was forbidden to give his own medicines under pains and penalties. He was urgently advised to defy the law and give his medicines secretly, but his noble mind revolted against such a proceeding, and his great respect for the law deterred him, moreover, from even attempting to infringe it. It was impossible for him to prescribe his medicines from his bitterest enemies the apothecaries, because some of the remedies he made use of were not kept by them, others they did not know how to prepare, and moreover, he could not trust his bitterest foes. Hence he had to quit Leipzig, and his much loved Saxon fatherland. At this time Hahnemann was the most celebrated physician of his country, and drew many from far and near to consult him. In consideration of this and in consideration of his advancing years – he was over sixty-six – one might have thought that the kind and gentle old man would have been spared by a liberal profession of which he had been so distinguished a member for forty-two years. But no; he had to leave the place that had become dear to him and find a new home once again.

We thus note that Leipzig expelled Hahnemann in 1821 because he dispensed his own remedies! There is no doubt but Hahnemann was very much distressed at this treatment. You remember that he had been a student at Leipzig, and this city was, therefore, the site of his youthful castles in the air; it was there, too, that he had got into the terrible slough of despond form which the cinchona experiment saved him; and it was there he had at last triumphantly taught where he had laboriously learned so many long years before; and it was there too that he had his first disciples whom he loved so much. *But his expulsion from Leipzig was necessary for the further development of his system.*[xxxii]

The reigning prince of Anhalt-Köthen was an ardent admirer of Hahnemann, and he offered him state rank and protection at his little capital, Köthen, which Hahnemann accepted, and thereby immortalised both the prince and his capital. At Köthen Hahnemann may be said to have entered into a haven of rest. There I take leave of him.

When I go over his wondrous life, I am profoundly impressed with his greatness as a mere man; he taught Hebrew at the age of thirteen; he knew eight languages when he went to the university at twenty; he became a doctor of medicine at twenty-four; he lived to be nearly ninety; and laboured all the time,

---

xxxii I refer to his biopathology, that is true in nature and ridiculed in books.

certainly he was a hard worker for eighty years; throughout the course of this long life I do not find one single shameful act recorded against him by real history. Of how many men can we say as much: he was indeed a great and almost a perfect man.

As a physician he stands exalted far above any the world has ever seen since the time of the divine Hippocrates. As a physician he was, indeed, incomparable; his was, and is, the truest definition of the real physician, viz., one whose sole business is that of healing the sick *citò, tutò et jucunde*.

And looking back now on the vast vista of his medical life, how can we refrain from exclaiming – *Ecce Medicus*, "Behold the physician!"

Lastly, let us look at the lessons of his life. From his boyhood, from his youth, from his manhood, and from his old age we learn industry, perseverance, love of learning, devotion to science for the direct benefit of mankind, singleness of mind, sterling irreproachable honour and probity, not having regard unto man merely, but having a firm faith in God – in a word, he dared to be wise. He sowed immortality, and deathless is his fame.

And finally, Gentlemen, if you ask me where his monument is to be found, my answer is: Look around you!

References

1 Clarke, JH. *Dictionary of Practical Materia Medica*, 2 vols., London, Homoeopathic Publishing Company, 1900-1902.
2 Burnett, JC. Obituary: *The Homoeopathic World 1843*; 199: 220-237.
3 Clarke, JH. *Life and Work of James Compton Burnett, MD*, London, Homoeopathic Publishing Company, 1904.
4 Spurling, H. *Ivy When Young. The Early Life of I Compton Burnett 1884-1919*, Chapter 4; London, Victor Gollancz, 1974.
5 Compton Burnett, J. *Ecce Medicus, or Hahnemann as a Man and as a Physician, and the Lessons of his Life, Being the first Hahnemannian Lecture, 1880*. London, Homoeopathic Publishing Company, 1881.
6 Born April 10, 1755.
7 Dudgeon, RE, *Lectures on the Theory and Practice of Homoeopathy delivered at the Hahnemann Hospital School of Homoeopathy*, London, Henry Turner, 1853.

9

HAHNEMANN AS A MEDICAL PHILOSOPHER

Introduction

Richard Hughes concentrates on Hahnemann's philosophy in this article, as he understood it from reading the different editions of the *Organon*, which he compares. He is concerned about the 'vital force', the idea of miasms, and the effects of highly diluted remedies. He challenges some of these ideas while still retaining an overall adherence to homeopathy. He is known for his adherence to the notion of 'pure' materia medica, information from provings and not from clinical experience. Having examined Hahnemann the man, and then his ideas, we now look at his therapeutics.

We can learn about Hughes from an obituary[1] and also from appreciations by RT Cooper[2] and JH Clarke.[3] The funeral took place on 10th April, the 147th anniversary of Hahnemann's birthday.

About Richard Hughes

It is with profound regret that we have to record the death of Dr Richard Hughes, which took place at Dublin on April 3rd, in the 66th year of his age. Dr Hughes was a Londoner by birth and education. He was a student of King's College and took his MRCS of England in 1857, and the LRCP of Edinburgh in 1860. In recognition of his great services to homoeopathy he received the honorary degree of MD conferred on him by the Universities of New York, Philadelphia, and St. Louis. In 1861 he became a member of the British Homoeopathic Society. He was Secretary of the Society from 1879 to 1884, Vice-President in 1885 and 1886, and in 1887 he was elected President. From 1892 to 1896 he was member of the Council, and he had edited the Society's Journal since its revival in the present form in 1892.

Early in his medical life Dr Hughes joined the late Dr Madden in practice at Brighton, and eventually succeeded Dr Madden when the latter removed to London. Dr Hughes continued to practice in Brighton until his recent retirement. During the active period of the London School of Homoeopathy, when it was revived through the efforts of Dr Bayes, Dr Hughes did consulting work in London as well; but this was afterwards relinquished and it is as "Dr Hughes of Brighton" that he has always been best known.

Dr Hughes' literary work began the year after he became a member of the British Homoeopathic Society. In 1862 he joined Drs. Drysdale and Dudgeon on the staff of the *British Journal of Homoeopathy* and continued to be one of its editors till that journal was brought to a close with its forty-second volume in 1884. In 1867 appeared the work on which the name of Dr Hughes has chiefly rested during this lifetime, his *Manual of Pharmacodynamics*, with its companion work, *A Manual of Therapeutics*. Both these works appeared first in the form of letters addressed to a supposed inquirer, and they were rapidly discovered by genuine inquirers, and were thus the means of making many converts to the new school of therapeutics. They also contained such a wealth of therapeutic matter arranged for immediate use, that they largely replaced the older authorities in the field of practice – Jahr, Boenninghausen, and the Repertories. Six editions of the *Pharmacodynamics* have appeared, though the changes in the latest of these consist of appendices devoted to additional remedies.

But no one knew better than Dr Hughes that these tractarian works of his, however popular and successful they might be, were no sufficient basis for homoeopathic practice. Hence he set himself to provide this in the way which seemed to him most desirable. The four volumes of the *Cyclopaedia of Drug Pathogenesy*, with its *Index*, are the result of this endeavour. The *Introduction* to that work full sets forth the hopes and aims of its editors, and more especially of its editor-in-chief, Dr Hughes. There will be found the rules finally adopted by the committee – rules which in our opinion are largely arbitrary and artificial, framed rather meet the views of an allopathic critic than the requirements of homoeopathic practice. However, within the limits prescribed, an immense amount of matter has been brought together describing in the order of their occurrence symptoms experienced by individual provers and in poisoning cases. This is a most desirable piece of work. But Dr Hughes expected it to be something more: he imagined it was going to replace the Schema in practice.

In point of fact Dr Hughes was more fascinated by the doctrine of homoeopathy than he was by the practice of it. His aim was to keep the doctrine – as he conceived it – pure, rather than to develop and perfect the practice.

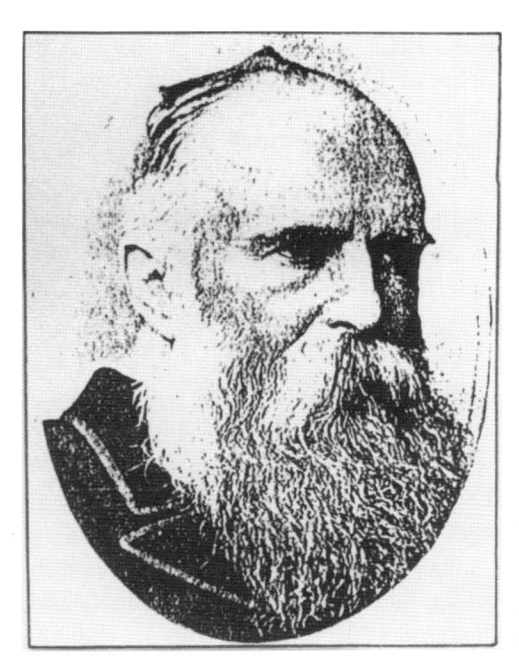

Figure 9.1 Richard Hughes (1836-1902)

Reproduced with the permission of Institute for the History of Medicine *of the Robert Bosch* Foundation

The British Homoeopathic Society, of which he had been a member forty-one years at the time of his death, was the scene of a very large part of his activities. In his time he held almost all his offices, and for many years past he has been its dominating spirit. He was rarely absent from its meetings and his voice was seldom absent from its councils.

The shock of Dr Hughes' death was so much more keenly felt in that few remembered his ever having had a day's illness. He had, however, been liable to attacks of faintness; and two years ago he had an attack of pericarditis, through which he was under the care of Dr Dudgeon. Later on he had an attack of gout. He was, however, apparently quite well at the meeting of the Society in March. Immediately preceding his death he had crossed over to Dublin with some friends on a tour of inspection of the churches of his communion. In the afternoon he complained to one of his friends staying at the hotel with him that he did not feel very well, and said he would not go out then. He sat down in a chair, and his friend left the room. On his return he found that Dr Hughes had passed away.

Hahnemann as a medical philosopher – the *Organon*[4]
Being the Second Hahnemannian Lecture, 1881
By Richard Hughes LRCP Edin. 1836–1902

Preface
The portions of this Lecture treating of Hahnemann's doctrines regarding a vital force, the psoric origin of chronic disease, and the dynamisation of medicines, were omitted in delivery for lack of time. In other respects, it stands here as its auditors heard it. Brighton, December, 1881.

Gentlemen
My predecessor in this Lectureship, Dr Burnett, conducted you through the life and work of Hahnemann up to 1821, when, in the sixty-seventh year of his age, he retired from Leipzig to Köthen. It would have been natural and fitting if I had taken up the story from this point, and showed you something of our hero during the two decades of active life yet granted to him. Circumstances, however, have otherwise determined my subject. During the last Summer Session of our School, I have been able to carry out a long-cherished project,[i] and to read with my class the Master's great exposition of his method – the *Organon of Medicine*. The study, which has been necessitated for such a task – that I might criticise, illustrate and expound aright – may well, it seems to me, be utilised for our present object. I propose, therefore, to go back somewhat upon Hahnemann's life, but to survey him in another aspect. Dr Burnett has cried *Ecce Medicus!* and has exhibited to you the man and the physician. I would ask you to consider with me the medical philosopher, as displayed in his cardinal treatise – the *Organon*.

I. The *Organon* was first published in 1810.[5] A second edition appeared in 1819;[6] a third in 1824;[7] a fourth in 1829;[8] and a fifth and last in 1833.[9] Each of these is described as 'augmented' (2nd), 'improved' (3rd), or both 'augmented and improved' (4th and 5th): and, in truth, all, save the third, show considerable changes as compared with their immediate predecessors. These editions, together with a few of the numerous translations the work has undergone, lie on the table before you.[ii] Let me say at once, that it is quite impossible to form an adequate estimate, either of the *Organon* or of its author without some knowledge of the changes it has undergone in its successive stages. Without this neither foe can criticise it nor disciple learn from it aright. For instance, the hypothesis of the origin of much chronic

---
i In my Introductory Lecture to the first Winter Session of the London School of Homoeopathy, delivered October 2nd, 1877, I said – "There ought to be a place where those interested in the matter could hear the *Organon* read and examined."

ii Materials for a sixth are said to have been left behind by the author; but the custodians of his papers have not yet received adequate temptation to publish them.

disease in psora, which not long ago was authoritatively stated to be one of the fundamental principles of homoeopathy, first appeared in the fourth edition, i.e. in 1829. The theory of the dynamisation of medicines – i.e. of the actual increase of power obtained by attenuation, when accompanied by trituration or succession – is hardly propounded until the fifth edition. On the other hand, there is the doctrine of a "vital force," as the source of all the phenomena of life, as the sphere in which disease begins and medicines act. This has been regarded by many of Hahnemann's followers, especially in France and Spain, as an essential part of his philosophy. "Voici donc," exclaims M. Léon Simon the elder,[iii] "la pensée fondamentale de Hahnemann, la pierre angulaire du système." But the earliest mention of this conception occurs in the fourth edition; and the full statement of it with which we are familiar in the fifth (§9 – 16), appears there for the first time.

II. The *Organon* is Hahnemann's exposition and vindication of his therapeutic method. It had been preceded by a number of essays in Hufeland's *Journal* – the leading medical organ of the time in Germany. Of these the most noteworthy were – *On a New Principle for ascertaining the Curative Powers of Drugs* (1792), *Are the obstacles to certainty and simplicity in Practical Medicine insurmountable?* (1797), and *The Medicine of Experience* (1806).[10] The time seemed now to have come when there should be published separately a full account of the new departure he was advocating; and hence the *Organon* of 1810.

Why did he give his treatise this name? He must, there can be little doubt, have had Aristotle in memory, whose various treatises on Logic were summed up under the common title *Organon*. Logic – the art of reasoning – is the *instrument* of research and discovery: Hahnemann designed his method as one which should be a medical logic, an instrument which the physician should use for the discovery of the best remedies for disease. But the example immediately before his mind, and through whom he was probably led to Aristotle, must have been Bacon. The second treatise of the *Instauratio Magma* of the English Chancellor is entitled *Novum Organum*: it was the setting forth of a new mode of reasoning, which in scientific research should supersede that of Aristotle, and lead to developments of knowledge hitherto unattained. That Hahnemann should aspire to do such work for medicine as was done for science in general by Bacon has been scouted by his enemies, and even deprecated by his friends, as presumption. And yet no comparison could better illustrate the real position of the man, both in its strength and in its weakness. If he erred as to special points of pathology, and even of practice, we must remember that Bacon was a doubtful acceptor of the

---

iii Hahnemann, S, *Exposition de la Doctrine Médicale Homoeopathique, par S. Hahnemann, augmentée de Commentaires par M. Léon Simon pére*. Paris: Bailliere. 1856.

Copernican astronomy and ridiculed Harvey's doctrine of the circulation, while he saw no difficulty in the transmutation of metals. But, on the other side, how truly Baconian is the whole spirit and aim of the *Organon!* Like his great exemplar, Hahnemann sought to recall men from the spinning of thought-cobwebs to the patient investigation of facts. Like him, he set up the practical - which in this case is the healing of disease - as the proper aim of medical philosophy; not seeking "in knowledge, a terrace, for a wandering and variable mind to walk up and down with a fair prospect," but rather accounting it "a rich storehouse, for the glory of the Creator, and *the relief of man's estate."* Like him, his chief strength was devoted to the exposition and perfecting of his proposed method of further progress towards this end, leaving to the future the carrying it into effect. Another Descartes may arise in medicine, whose perception of special fields of knowledge may be keener, and who may leave his mark more clearly traced on certain branches of our art. But Hahnemann, when once his method shall have won the acceptance we claim for it, will ever be reckoned the Bacon of therapeutics - the fruitful thinker who taught us what was our great aim as physicians and how we should best attain to it.

Hahnemann first called his work *Organon of the rational medical doctrine (Heilkunde)*; but from the second edition onwards the title was changed to *Organon of the healing art (Heilkunst)* - the 'rational' being here, and in all other places of its occurrence, either dropped or replaced by 'true' ('genuine,' - *wahre*). Why this alteration? The elimination of the term "rational" has been supposed to "imply that his followers were required to accept his doctrines as though they were the revelations of a new gospel, to be received as such, and not to be subjected to rational criticism".[iv] I cannot think so. To me the clue to it seems to be afforded by the coincident change from *Heilkunde* to *Heilkunst*. The name "doctrine," the epithet "rational," were in continual use for the hypothetical systems of his day. The promulgation of his views had arrayed the advocates of all these in bitter opposition against him. Hahnemann was accordingly anxious to make it clear that, in entering the lists of conflict, he came armed with quite other weapons. He was seeking, not the consistency of a theory, but the success of a practical art: to him it mattered little whether a thing commended itself or not to the speculative reason, his one concern was that it should be true[v].

III. On the title page of his first edition Hahnemann placed a motto from the poet Gellert, which has been freely rendered into English thus: "The truth an all-wise Providence intended To be a blessing to mankind, He did not bury deep,

---

iv *British Journal of Homoeopathy* 1878, 36:1 p. 63.

v Hahnemann, S, *Organon der Heilkunst*, (2nd edition). Arnold, Dresden, 1819, The preface further confirms this view.

but slightly 'fended, That any earnest search might find.'"[vi] This was replaced in subsequent editions by the words *Aude sapere*; but it continued to denote the profound conviction and motive inspiration of Hahnemann's mind. It was the same thought as that which he expressed in the *Medicine of Experience*:

IV. "As the wise and beneficent Creator has permitted those innumerable states of the human body differing from health, which we term disease, He must at the same time have revealed to us a *distinct* mode whereby we may obtain a knowledge of diseases, that shall suffice to enable us to employ the remedies of subduing them; He must have shewn to us an equally distinct mode whereby we may discover in medicines those properties that render them suitable for the cure of diseases – if he did not mean to leave his Children helpless, or to require of them what was beyond their power. This art, so indispensable to suffering humanity, cannot therefore remain concealed in the unfathomable depths of obscure speculation, or be diffused through the boundless void of conjecture; it must be accessible, *readily accessible* to us, within the sphere of vision of our external and internal perceptive facilities."

V. Hahnemann believed in the illimitable possibilities of medicine, because he believed in God. I lay more stress on this faith of Hahnemann's, from the contrast presented to it by the language of an *Address in Medicine* recently delivered,[vii] which takes homoeopathy for its theme and the *Organon* for its text. The able and candid physician to whom we owe this utterance asks in it – "What grounds of reason or experience have we to justify the belief that for every disease an antidote or cure will sooner or later be discovered?" and, going farther still, declares it to be in his judgment "Utopian to expect that diseases generally shall become curable by therapeutical or any other treatment." That this melancholy Pyrrhonism is of extensive prevalence appears also from the fact, witnessed to by the leading medical journal,[viii] that at the recent International Congress in London "therapy" was conspicuous by its absence. It was not so at the Homoeopathic Convention which preceded it; and this just stamps the difference between the two attitudes of mind. I cannot prove – at any rate here – that the faith of the founder of homoeopathy was sound, and the scepticism of its critics otherwise; but it is evident which is the more fruitful. As a lover of my kind, and not a mere man of science, I can say, "*Malo cum Hahnemanno errare quam cum*" – well, it would be personal, not to say difficult, to Latinise the rest, but my hearers will supply it.

---

vi *British Journal of Homoeopathy*, 1882, 35:4, p. 366.

vii The *Address in Medicine*, delivered before the British Medical Association in 1881, by John Syer Bristowe, *British Medical Journal*, 1881, 41:13th August.

viii *The Lancet* 1881, 58: 27th August.

VI. Hahnemann, whose heart was indeed bubbling up with his good matter, and whose tongue was certainly the pen of a ready writer, has written a separate preface for each edition of his work. I cannot give any account of them here; but they are all well worth reading. The second especially deserves notice as a full statement in brief of Hahnemann's view of the existing state of medicine; and nowhere does Bacon speak more clearly through him than in his emphatic statements here regarding the relation of reason to experience in the study of medicine.

VII. I come now to the Introduction, which in every edition forms a considerable proportion of the whole volume. It has altered very much, however, between its earliest and latest appearance. In the first three editions, it consists of a series of unintentional homoeopathic cures (so considered) taken from medical literature, with a few prefatory and concluding remarks. But in the second and third Hahnemann had introduced into the body of the work a long section of destructive criticism on existing theories and modes of treatment; and this, when he issued the fourth, seemed to him to find a more appropriate place in the Introduction. Thither, accordingly, it was transferred, forming – under the title *Survey of the Allopathy*[ix] *of the hitherto-prevailing School of Medicine* – a first part; while the "Instances of involuntary homoeopathic cures" took place as a second. In the fifth edition, these last disappeared altogether, being merely referred to in a note; and the Introduction became a continuous essay, its subject being the medicine of the author's contemporaries and predecessors.

VIII. I think that no one who is acquainted with the state of medical thought and practice in Hahnemann's day will question the general justice of the strictures he here makes upon it. The recent critic to whom I have referred admits "the chaotic state of therapeutical theory and practice at that time prevalent;" but he hardly appreciates Hahnemann's merit in proscribing and stigmatising it as he did. Chaos itself, to the habitual dwellers in it, seems to be cosmos: it can only be apprehended for what it is by those who have the cosmos in their souls. This was Hahnemann's case. He saw all around him the two things which he cites Gregory the Great as pronouncing ἀτελές - ἄλογος πραξις and λογος ἄπρακτος.[11] On the one side were the men of note – the Stahls and Hoffmanns and Cullens – building up their ingenious and ambitious systems on hypothetical data: on the other were the mass of practitioners, quite unable to utilise these imaginings, and treating disease according to

---

ix So written in the fourth edition of the original, but in the fifth more correctly given as 'allœopathy,' which the translators should have reproduced. Ἀλλοίου πάθος, not ἄλλου, is Hahnemann's antithesis to ἄμοιυ πάθος; and as the latter forms homoeopathy, the former should be allœopathy.

empirical maxims or the directions of the prescription book.¹² The physician's art was the butt of every satirist, the dread of all who fell ill, the despair of the minds that formed a nobler ideal of it. Hahnemann himself, as Dr Burnett has told you, for a time gave himself up to such despair; till his experiment with cinchona bark proved Newton's apple, the clue of *Ariadne*, which suggested the true law of the phenomena and led the way to better things.

If we were going thought the Introduction in detail, there would be many points on which criticism and correction would be necessary; but the general soundness of its attitude must be sufficient for us to-day. It bears to the body of work the same relation as Bacon's *De Augmentis* to his *Novum Organum*, and the treatise on *Ancient Medicine* to the *Aphorisms* of Hippocrates. Before leaving it, I must say a few words about the instances of cure, which, though dropped by himself, have been inserted form the fourth edition in the translation Dr Dudgeon has given us, and are therefore familiar to all.ˣ His critic has singled out the first and last of these, and has had no difficulty in disposing of them as without bearing on the point to be proved. But a more thorough examination would show that *e duo discere omnes* was hardly a safe mode of proceeding. Of the forty-five references made, six are indeed quite worthless, and fifteen more dubious but the remaining twenty-four will stand the most searching examination. The cures were reported by the best observers of their time; the remedies employed were undoubtedly homoeopathic to the disorders present, and have no other mode of action to which their benefits could with any plausibility be traced. We could multiply, and perhaps improve upon them, now; but, such as they are, they do speak the language as utterers of which Hahnemann cited them.

IX. We come now to the *Organon* proper. It consists of a series of aphorisms – in its latest form 294 in number, to which are appended numerous and often lengthy notes. This is a form of composition eminently suggestive and stimulating. It is endeared to many of us by Coleridge's *Aids to Reflection*; but Hahnemann must have taken it from the *Novum Organum*, perhaps also with a recollection of the work of the Father of medicine which derives its name therefrom.

While each aphorism is complete in itself, and might be made the text of a medical discourse, the work they collectively constitute has a definite outline and structure, which remains unchanged through the successive editions, and is as evident in the first as in the last. This outline is given in the third aphorism, which – with the exception of 'rational' for 'true' practitioner in the first – is identical in all editions:

---

x Dr Dudgeon, not having the original of the fourth edition at hand, transferred them from Devrient's translation; and there are several errors accordingly.

X. "If the physician clearly perceives what is to be cured in diseases, that is to say, in every individual case of disease; if he clearly perceives what is curative in medicines, that is to say, in each individual medicine; and if he knows how to apply, according to clearly-defined principles, what is curative in medicines to what he has discovered to be undoubtedly morbid in the patient, so that recovery must ensue – to apply it, as well in respect to the suitableness of the medicine which from its kind of action is most adapted to the case, as also in respect to the exact mode of preparation and quantity of it required, and to the proper period for repeating the dose; if, finally, he knows the obstacles to recovery in each case, and is aware how to remove them, so that the restoration may be permanent – then he understands how to treat judiciously and reasonably, and is a true practitioner of the healing art."

XI. The three desiderata, then, are –

XII. 1st. The knowledge of the disease – which supplies the indication:

XIII. 2nd. The knowledge of medicinal powers – which gives the instrument:

XIV. 3rd. The knowledge how to choose and administer the remedy – which is the thing indicated.

The first part of the *Organon* (down to §70) treats of these points doctrinally, by way of argument:[xi] the second practically, in the form of precept. The summing up of the doctrinal portion is contained in §70, in these words: –

"From what has been already adduced, we cannot fail to draw the following inferences: –

"That everything of a truly morbid character, and which is to be cured, that the physician can discover in diseases consists solely in the sufferings of the patient and the sensible alterations in his health, in a word, solely in the sum total of the symptoms, by means of which the disease demands the medicines adapted for its relief; whilst, on the other hand, every internal cause assigned to it, every occult quality or imaginary *materies morbi*, is but an empty dream:

"That this derangement of the health, which we term disease, can only be restored to soundness through another revolution in the health by means of medicines, whose sole curative power consequently, can only consist in deranging man's health, that is, in an excitation of morbid symptoms peculiar to each, and this is learned with most distinctness and purity by proving them on healthy individuals:

"That, according to all experience, a natural disease can never be cured by medicines that possess the power of producing in the healthy individual

---

xi § 5 – 18 discuss knowledge of disease; 19 – 21 knowledge of medicines; 22 – 27 knowledge of application of one to the other; 28 – 69 are an explanation and defence of the mode of application by similarity.

an alien morbid state (dissimilar morbid symptoms) differing from that of the disease to be cured (never, therefore, by an allœopathic mode of treatment), and that even in nature no cure ever takes place, in which an inherent disease is removed, annihilated and cured by the accession of another disease dissimilar to it, be the new one ever so strong:

"That, moreover, all experience proves that by means of medicines which have a tendency to produce in the healthy individual an artificial morbid symptom antagonistic to the single symptom of disease sought to be cured, the cure of a long standing affection will never be effected, but merely a very transient alleviation, always followed by aggravation; and that, in a word, this antipathic and merely palliative mode of treatment is, in long standing diseases of a serious character, quite incapable of effecting the desired object:

"That, however, the third and only other possible mode of treatment (the homoeopathic), in which there is employed against the totality of the symptoms of the natural disease a medicine (in a suitable dose) capable of producing the most similar symptoms possible in the healthy individual, is the only efficacious method of treatment, whereby diseases, as mere dynamic derangements of the vital force, are overpowered, and being thus easily, perfectly and permanently extinguished, must necessarily cease to exist – and for this mode of procedure we have the example of unfettered nature herself, when to an old disease there is added a new one similar to the first, whereby the old one is rapidly and for ever annihilated and cured."

Then, in §71, Hahnemann propounds the practical questions which in the remainder of the treatise he seeks to answer, thus: –

"I. How is the physician to ascertain what is necessary to be known in order to cure the disease?

"II. How is he to gain a knowledge of the instruments adapted for the cure of the natural disease – the pathogenetic powers of medicines?

"III. How is he to employ most appropriately these artificial morbific potencies (medicines) for the cure of diseases?"

In reply to the first, he gives rules for the examination of the patient; to the second, for the proving of medicines on the healthy; to the third, for the determination of similarity, the choice and repetition of the dose, the preparation of drugs, the diet and regimen to be observed, and so forth.

This is, in the authors own words, the ground-plan of the *Organon*. Of course each position taken up needs justification on its own merits; and this we shall enquire immediately how far we can award. But I would first call your attention to the simplicity of Hahnemann's conception, to its entire freedom of hypothesis and completeness within itself. All other medical systems had been based upon certain doctrines of life and disease: Hahnemann's method was utterly independent of them. His whole argument might be conducted, as it is indeed in the first three editions of his work, without any discussion of physiological and pathological questions. I would impress this fact upon such of his disciples as represent homoeopathy to be complete scheme of medical philosophy; who would make the dynamic origin of all maladies a plank of the platform on which we must stand, and call the psora-hypothesis "the homoeopathic doctrine of chronic disease." This is an entire mistake. There are certain views in physiology and pathology which seem more harmonious than others with homoeopathic practice: Hahnemann thus came to hold them, and most of us tend in the same direction. But they might all be disproved and abandoned, and homoeopathy would still remain the same: we should still examine patients and prove drugs and administer remedies on the same principles, and with the same success.

But I would commend this consideration also to Hahnemann's critics. He has had critics from the first, though nothing is wider of the mark than to speak of "the contempt which experienced physicians felt and freely expressed for him and his whimsical doctrines." Not thus did Hufeland and Brera and Trousseau and Forbes write of the new method and its author. But the first-named of these made a remark which is full of significance: he said that if homoeopathy succeeded in becoming the general medical practice, it would prove "the grave of science." Now this I make bold to claim as an unintentional compliment: for it describes our system as being true medicine, which is not science, but art. This is a truth very much forgotten now-a-days. Hahnemann, in the opening paragraph of *Organon*, proclaims that "the physician's high and sole mission is to restore the sick to health – to cure, as it is termed." It is with this direct aim that he is to study disease and drug-action, and the relation between the two. He is not, primarily, a cultivator of science: he is a craftsman, the practiser of an art, and skill rather than knowledge is his qualification. His art, indeed, like all others, has its associated sciences. Physiology and pathology are to it what chemistry is to agriculture, and astronomy to navigation. So far as they bring real knowledge, the more versed the physician is in them the better for himself and for those in whose aid he works. But he was before they had being, and his art should have a life of its own independent of the nourishment they bring. They must, being progressive, consist largely of uncertainties – working hypotheses and imperfect generalisations, destined ere long to be superseded by more authentic conceptions. Medicine should not vary with their fluctuations, or hold its maxims at the mercy of their support. While grateful for the aid they bring, it should go on its own separate way and fulfil its distinctive mission.

One great value of the method of Hahnemann is, that it dwells in this sphere of art. It *is* "the grave of science;" for science, as such, has no existence here – it dies and is buried. But its corpse enriches the ground which covers it, and thereon grass springs up and fruits ripen for practical use. On the other hand, the great weakness of the general medicine of to-day is that, so far as it is more than blind empiricism, it is an applied science rather than an art. It shifts from heroism to expectancy, from spoliation to stimulation, with the prevailing conceptions of the day as to life and disease. Maladies are studied with the eye of the naturalist rather than of the artist; and the student is turned out thoroughly equipped for their diagnosis, but helpless in their treatment. Hence the nihilism of so much of modern teaching: hence, at the late Congress, the miserable halfpenny-worth of therapeutic bread to the gallons of scientific sack. It would be well for its three thousand members if they would go home to meditate the words of the man they despise – "the physician's high and sole mission is to restore the sick to health;" if they would recognise medicine as the art of healing, and cultivate it accordingly.

Let us now consider the three positions Hahnemann takes up: – his attitude (1) towards disease, (2) towards drug-action, and (3) towards the selection and administration of remedies.

1. In the resume of his conclusions which I have quoted (§70), Hahnemann speaks of the sum total of the symptoms of a patient as the only curative indication which the physician can discover. In this he hardly does himself justice; for in §5 he has pointed to the knowledge of the *causes* of the malady as important, and in §7 and its note has assumed as obvious that an exciting or maintaining cause which is discoverable and reachable shall be removed. He has further reminded us, in §3 and 4, that both to prevent disease, and to make his curative treatment unobstructed and permanent, the physician must also be a hygienist. It would hardly be necessary to mention such points, but that we have lately heard it said that "for him, preventive medicine, which deals specially with the causes of disease, and has been successful only in proportion to its knowledge of them, would have been a mockery and a snare."[xii]

2. With these qualifications, however, Hahnemann's doctrine is that the totality of the symptoms – the sum of the sufferings the patient feels and the phenomenon he exhibits – constitutes, *for all practical purposes*, the disease. He does not say that they alone *are* the disease. On the contrary, he constantly speaks of them as the "outwardly reflected picture," the "sensible and manifest representation" of what the essential alteration is. His point is, that at this last you cannot get, and – to cure your patient – need not get. If you can find means for removing the sum total of his symptoms, he will be well, though you may know as little as he wherein, essentially, he was ill (§6 – 18).

3. Now what objection can be taken to this thesis? If any one should seriously maintain that symptoms and morbid changes are not correlative; that there is any way of inferring the latter except from the former – as a whole – except by

---

[xii] Bristowe, op cit.

righting the latter – their proximate cause, I will refer him to the Introductory Lecture delivered here in 1878 by Dr Dyce Brown,[xiii] in which the point is thoroughly discussed and settled. Our recent critic is too acute to say much of this kind. His main charge against Hahnemann's view of disease is that it ignores pathology and more especially morbid anatomy, so that the "laborious investigations conducted in our dead-houses, which we fondly imagine to add to our knowledge of diseases" would be "looked upon by him with contempt." But in so speaking he forgets Hahnemann's aim. He is laying down what are the *curative indications* in disease, what the physician can and should know of it in order to remove it. Do the investigations of the dead-house help us here? The changes they discover are the *results* – generally the ultimate results – of morbid action; but in this stage of the process such action is no longer amenable to remedies. If it is to be cured, it must be taken at an earlier period, before there has occurred that "serious disorganisation of important viscera" which Hahnemann speaks of as an "insuperable obstacle to recovery."[13] And how shall it then be recognised, except by its symptoms? No microscope can see the beginnings of cirrhosis of the liver or of sclerosis in the brain and cord. But the patient can feel them, and my even exhibit them. Some slight hepatic uneasiness, some dart of pain or altered temper or gait, may and often do supervene long before the pathognomonic physical signs of such maladies appear. It is impossible to say how much suitable remedies at this time applied may not do – may not have done – to arrest the morbid process then and there. The Hahnemannic pathology is a living one, because it seeks to be a helpful one. It was wisely pointed out by the late Clotar Müller that the contemplation of disease mainly in the light of its ultimate organic results had a discouraging effect; whereas, if we would just apply our method fully to each *tout ensemble* of disorder as it came before us, our possibilities were boundless.[xiv]

4. But Hahnemann has been accused of ignoring pathology in another way, viz.: by "objecting to all attempts on the part of systematic writers and practical physicians to distinguish and classify diseases." He is supposed to have been – and the utterances of some of his own disciples lend colour to the charge – a mere individualiser, regarding the maladies which affect mankind as, "with a few exceptions, simply groups of symptoms, mosaics of which the component pieces admitted of endless re-arrangement." But his, again, is a great mistake, as I have endeavoured to prove in a paper on "Generalisation and Individualisation" which I submitted to our late Convention, and which you may see in its *Transactions*. I there showed, by numerous quotations, that

---

xiii To be had of the Secretary to the School.
xiv See also essay on the *Relation of Pathology to Therapeutics* in Dunham, C, *Homoeopathy, the Science of Therapeutics*, FE Boericke – Hahnemann Publishing House, Philadelphia, 1877, p. 99.

Hahnemann recognised as freely as any other physician the existence of definite types of disease, of fixed character because resulting from an unvarying cause, to which distinctive appellations might be given and specific remedies (or groups of remedies) allotted. He varied from time to time, as pathology itself has varied, in the list of those to which he would assign such place; but at the lowest estimate they cannot fairly be described as "a few exceptions." They embrace the whole field of "specific" disease - acute and chronic. Take the instance of intermittent fever, which has been cited. Hahnemann is supposed to have declared these fevers innumerable, and each instance of them that came before him an independent disease. But read the section of the *Organon* expressly devoted to the subject (§235 - 244). You will see there that it is only sporadic intermittents occurring in non-malarious districts that he thus describes. The true endemic marsh-ague he recognises as a disorder of fixed type, always curable by bark if the patient is not otherwise unhealthy; while the epidemic intermittents, though distinct among themselves, have each a specific character, so as to be amendable to one common remedy. It is in these (and the sporadic cases) only that he reprobates the blind cinchona-giving practised in his day.

5. Here also, then, Hahnemann must be vindicated from the charge of ignoring any real pathology, however little he valued the speculations of his own time which laid claim to that title. It is in the first part of the second division of the *Organon* (§72 - 82) that his views on this subject are expressed; and, allowing for the fact that they are fifty years old, and therefore to some degree antiquated, there is nothing in them unworthy of a learned and sagacious physician. I reserve his theory about "psora," intercalated in the fourth and fifth editions, which must subsequently receive a few words on its own merits.

6. Hahnemann concludes this portion of his subject with some suggestions as to the examination of patients (§83 - 104), of which all that need be said is that they are, as becomes their object, thorough. The homoeopathic physician does not listen and enquire merely to find out to what class of maladies his patient's troubles are to be relegated. For this end but few symptoms are necessary, and the rest can be left. He has to get at their totality, that he may "cover" them with a medicine capable of producing them on the healthy subject; and in pursuit of this aim he must not account any detail superfluous. It has been objected that we should come off badly upon such a method with Mrs. Nickleby for a patient. But happily all patients are not Mrs. Nicklebys; and when we do meet them common sense must deal with them accordingly. Of course, proportion must be observed; and anything we *know* to be merely incidental may be omitted. Our colours must be mixed, like Opie's, "with brains, Sir." But if we only *think* a detail unimportant, our wisdom will be to give the patient the benefit of the doubt, and insert it in our picture.

7. Such is Hahnemann's attitude towards disease; and I think it comes out from examination proof against every objection, and fitted at all points for its object. Still more incontrovertibly can this be said of the position he takes up with reference to drug-action (§19 - 22). His one insistence is that this can only be ascertained by experiment on the healthy human body. Few now-a-days question the value of this proceeding, and many adopt it; but Hahnemann has hardly yet been awarded the merit which belongs to him as its pioneer. Haller had indeed preceded him in affirming its necessity, and Alexander and a few others had essayed tentatively - very tentatively - to carry it out; but Hahnemann developed Haller's thought into a doctrine, and multiplied a hundred-fold Alexander's attempts at proving. When the profession comes to know him in his true worth, he will be recognised by all as the Father of Experimental Pharmacology.

    The great value of choosing the human subject for our provings of drugs is, that thereby their subjective symptoms - the sufferings as well as the phenomena they cause - can be ascertained. There is of course the inevitable shadow here - the counter-peril that a number of sensations of no moment shall be reported by the experimenters, and cumber our pathogeneses. This is inevitable; but Hahnemann at least saw the inconvenience, and did his best to avoid it. Let his rules for proving in the *Organon* (§105 - 145) be read, and the information we have elsewhere as to his manner of proceeding be considered, and it will be seen that he did all that his lights suggested to make experimentation of this kind pure and trustworthy.

8. We pass now to the third division of the "vocation of the true physician," as conceived by Hahnemann. How is he to use his knowledge of drug-action in the treatment of disease? How wield the potencies the former gives him for the favourable modification of the latter?

9. To the answer to these questions are devoted forty-eight aphorisms (§22 - 69) of the first and a hundred-and-forty seven (§146 - 292) of the second division of the *Organon*. Hahnemann argues that there are only three conceivable relations between the physiological effects of a drug and the symptoms of disease, and therefore only three possible ways of applying the one to the other. The two may be altogether diverse and heterogeneous, as the action of a purgative and a congestive headache; and if you use the former to relieve the latter, you are employing a foreign remedy - you are practising *alloeopathy* - (ἀλλοίου πάθος). Or they may be directly opposite, as the influence of a bromide and the sleeplessness of mental excitement: then, to give bromide of potassium to induce slumber is to act upon the enantiopathic or antipathic principle (ἐυαυίου, ἀυτί, πάθος). Or, thirdly, they may be similar, as strychnine-poisoning to tetanus or that or corrosive sublimate to dysentery. If such drugs are used for their corresponding disorders, you are evidently

homoeopathising (ὁμοίου πάθος). Now, of these, alloeopathic medication must be condemned, both on the ground of its uncertainty, and on that of the positive injury it does by disordering healthy parts and by flooding the system with the large doses of drugs necessary to produce the desired effects. Antipathic treatment is certainly and rapidly palliative; but the inevitable reaction which follows leads to a return of the evil, often in greater force. It can rarely, moreover, deal with more than a single symptom at a time; and even then its capabilities are limited by the very few really opposite states which exist between natural disease and drug-action. Antipathy may do tolerably well for immediate needs and temporary troubles; but it is not competent to deal with complex, persistent, or recurrent maladies. For these we are shut up to the homoeopathic method, if we are to use drugs in disease at all. This operates "without injury to another part and without weakening the patient." It is of inexhaustible fertility for the analogies between natural and medicinal disorder are endless. It is complete, for the one order of things may cover the other in its totality. It is gentle, for no large and perturbing dosage is required for its carrying out. It is, lastly, permanent; for the law of action and re-action which makes the secondary effects of antipathic palliatives injurious here operates beneficially. The primary influence of the drug being in the same direction as the morbid process, the secondary and more lasting recoil will – after (it may be) a slight aggravation – directly oppose and extinguish it. It is thus that Hahnemann explains the benefit wrought by homoeopathic remedies: thus, and also by the theory (§28 - 52) of a substitution of the medicinal for the actual disease, for which he cites parallels in nature.

10. Here again we pause to ask what objections have been taken to Hahnemann's position. His doctrine of the three relations between drug-action and disease seems too simple for certain minds. One (Anstie) calls it metaphysical; another (Ross) geometrical; a third exclaims, "how curious, how ingenious, how interesting!" and imagines that in so designating it he excludes the possibility of its conformity to nature. But why should it not have these features and yet be true? What other alternative is possible? What fourth term of comparison can be found between (be it remembered) the effects of drugs on the healthy and the symptoms of disease? If you use the one for the other, you must do so allœopathically, antipathically, or homoeopathically. Medical men seem very fond now-a-days of disclaiming any system in their practice, and announcing themselves as altogether lawless and empirical. But they can no more help practising upon one or other of these principles than M. Jourdain could help speaking prose unless he launched into verse. If they would only analyse their own thoughts, they would see that directly they learn the physiological action of a drug they consider what morbid states it can indirectly modify or directly oppose. These are two of the members of Hahnemann's

triad; and the difference between us and them is that our first thought is as to what disorders the drug phenomena most resemble. We would not neglect the two other directions in which the medicine might be utilised, if we had reason to think it advantageous to follow them; and our complaint is that the profession at large do neglect and ignore the third, to the great loss of their patients.

Why should they do so? Some have answered that the method is rarely practicable, that real parallels between disease and drug-action are rare. To speak thus, however, implies a very deficient knowledge of pharmacodynamics. Others have expressed a more general and natural objection when they have argued that medicines which are truly similars must aggravate rather than benefit, if they act at all. It would seem so; and it is not surprising that in the older works on Materia Medica morbid states analogous to the action of drugs are set down as contra-indicating their employment. But this difficulty *solvitur ambulando*. Let any one take an obvious instance of such a contra-indicating condition – a sick stomach for *Ipecacuanha*, a congested brain for *Opium*, a dry febrile tongue for *Belladonna*. If he gives a quantity capable of exciting such states in the healthy, he may undoubtedly aggravate. But let him reduce his dose somewhat below this point, and he will get nothing but benefit. This has been tested over and over again, and no one has reported adversely to it: on the contrary, uses of medicines derived from the method are now becoming as popular in general practice as they have long been in ours. Why should this benefit result? We have heard Hahnemann's explanation, that such remedies work by substitution and by exciting reaction. It is one in which it is not difficult to pick holes, and he himself says, in propounding it, that he does not attach much importance to it (§28). Any discredit, however, resulting from its disproval must attach equally, as regards substitution, to Bretonneau and Trousseau, as regards re-action, to more than one ingenious thinker of our own country (Fletcher, Ross, Rabagliati). More recently, the hypothesis has been advanced that medicines have an opposite action in large and small quantities, so that the reduction of dose necessary to avoid aggravation gives you a remedy acting in a direction contrary to the disorder, while its choice by similarity secures practicability and complete embracement. It myself feel great difficulty acceding to this theory as a general account of homoeopathic cure; but there is no justification for representing its adoption as an abandonment of the homoeopathic position. It is an attempt at explanation, that is all: the fact that likes are cured by likes is the all-important thing, account for it how we may. So Hahnemann said, and so all homoeopathists believe.

The side of Hahnemann's position on which he is most vulnerable is its exclusiveness, in which he maintains his method to be applicable to all non-surgical disease, and to render all other ways of employing medicines superfluous and hurtful. This led him, as has been fairly urged, to regard intestinal worms as products of the organism, and to ignore the acarus as the exciting cause of scabies; it has resulted among his followers in a denial of palliatives to their patients by which much suffering might have been spared. In the first matter, however, he erred in common with most of his contemporaries; and in the second he is not responsible for the excesses of disciples who are often more Wilkesite than Wilkes himself. The rational homoeopathist recognises, indeed, the inferior value and limited scope of antipathic palliation. He knows that it is only properly applicable to temporary troubles. But in these he makes full use of it. He does not allow his patient to endure the agonies of angina pectoris, when he knows that amyl nitrate will relieve them; he does not refuse chloroform during the passage of calculus any more than during that of a foetus. Hahnemann's exclusiveness is not to be justified; but it may fairly claim excuse as the enthusiasm of a discoverer, full of the sense of the power of his new method, and naturally led to apply it everywhere and to esteem it without rival.

The treatment of this subject in the second part of the *Organon* is purely practical. It gives instructions for the selection for remedies upon the homoeopathic principle, and for their judicious employment when selected. It enquires what should be done when only imperfect similarity can be obtained, when more than one medicine seems indicated and when the symptoms are too few to guide to a satisfactory choice. He considers the treatment on the new method of local diseases (so-called), of mental disorders, and of the great class of intermittent affections. He gives directions for diet and regimen; for the preparation of medicines; for the repetition of doses, and for their size.

It is on the last of these points only that I can touch here: for the rest I must refer to the work itself. Hahnemann's treatment of the subject of dose has not had justice done to it, in consequence of our only knowing the fifth edition of the *Organon*. In the year 1829, after the publication of the fourth edition, he unfortunately determined to secure uniformity in homoeopathic usage by having one dilution for all medicines, and this the decillionth – the 30th of the centesimal scale. Our present *Organon* represents this view; but the first four editions make no such determination, and are entirely moderate and reasonable in the principles of posology they lay down. The dose of a homoeopathically selected remedy, they say, must obviously be smaller than that of one intended to act antipathically or allœopathically. If too large, it will excite needless aggravation and collateral suffering. It should be so far reduced that its primary aggravation (which Hahnemann supposed a necessary result) should be hardly perceptible and very short. How far this must be varies with the medicine used; and for suggestions on this point he refers to his *Reine Arzneimittellehre* where the dosage recommended ranges from the mother tincture to the 30th – the latter, however, being of exceptional height. He alleges experience alone as having led him to attenuate so far; but argues the reasonableness of so doing from the increased sensitiveness of the diseased body, pointing out also that dilution does not diminish the power of a substance in proportion to the reduction of its bulk. Excluding the specific doses mentioned in the other treatise referred to, which are simply questions of fact and experience, there is nothing in this part of the *Organon* - in its essential structure - to which fair exception could be taken.

I wish I could have stopped here; that there had been in the volume I am now expounding nothing more difficult to defend than what has gone before. In its first three editions - i.e., up to 1824 - there is not. Almost everything in Hahnemann's work during the first quarter of this century is of enduring worth; it is positive, experimental, sound. But from this time onwards we see a change. The active and public life he led at Leipzig, with the free breath of the world blowing through his thoughts, had been exchanged, since his exile to Köthen in 1821, for solitude, isolation, narrowness. The reign of hypothesis began in his mind - hypothesis physiological, pathological, pharmacological. The theories he was led to form in all these branches of thought found their way into the later editions of the *Organon* and so demand some consideration from us here. But let it be remembered throughout that they are not of the essence of its argument; that its structure and substance were complete before they appeared, and - in the judgment of many of us - are rather injured by their interpolation. Without them, all is inductive reasoning or avowedly tentative explanation; they, dogmatically asserted but all unproven, introduce a new and questionable element, they constitute what Drs. Jousset and Gaillard have well called "the romance of homoeopathy."

The first of his hypotheses is that of a *vital force*, as being the source of all the phenomena of life, and the sphere in which disease begins and medicines act. Hahnemann would probably at all time have called himself a vitalist, in distinction alike from the *animism* of Stahl (which made the immortal soul the principle of life), and form the views of those who would bring all vital phenomena under the laws of physics and chemistry. He early, moreover, employed the term *dynamic* to denote also the sphere in which true disease took its origin, and those effects of drugs which require vitality for their production. Disease has its *materies morbid* and organic changes; but all these may be - Hahnemann would have it always are - secondary products and effects, the primary derangement being invisible and intangible, manifest only in altered sensations and functions. Drugs, again, produce - many of them - chemical and mechanical effects; but these might occur in the dead as in the living body. The exclusively vital reactions they set up in the crucible of the organism belong to another sphere: they correspond with the beginnings of disease, like them are revealed by altered sensations and functions, like them are to be characterised as "dynamic."

Had he gone no farther that this all would have been well. It is easy to read into his language the present protoplasmic doctrine of life; while the frequent commencement of disease in molecular rather than molar changes,[xv] and the dynamic – as distinct from the mechanical and chemical – action of drugs, are recognised by all. But in his later years Hahnemann advanced from this thoroughly tenable position into one far less easy to maintain. He adopted the view that vitality was a "force," analogous to the physical agencies so called, without which the material organism would be without sensation and functional activity, which animates and energises it during life and leaves it at death. It is this 'vital force' (*Lebenskraft*) which is primarily deranged in illness, and on which morbid potencies – both natural and medicinal – act through the sensory nerves. Its behaviour under medicinal influence is ingeniously imagined and elaborately designed (§127); and in the fifth edition of the *Organon* it is frequently mentioned as the actor or sufferer where previously the author had been content to speak of the organism (as in §148).

Now Hahnemann can hardly be thought the worse of for entertaining this view, since, in some form or other, it was almost universally prevalent in his day. If the advice of the present Pope is taken it will continue to be the teaching of all Catholic colleges; for it is simply the Thomist doctrine – itself derived from Aristotle – under another name. But the tendency of recent science is to regard the organism as no monarchy, wherein some 'archæus' lives and rules, but as a republic in which every part is equally alive and independently active, the unity of the whole being secured only by the common circulation and the universal telegraphic system of nerves. It unfortunate, therefore, that Hahnemann should have committed himself and his work to another conception. Either or neither may be wholly true; but one would have been glad if the *Organon* had kept itself wholly clear of such questions, and had occupied only the solid ground of observation and experiment.

And now of the *psora theory*. This is far too large a subject for justice to be done to it here. It has been fully handled elsewhere;[xvi] and any one who would desire to deal fairly with Hahnemann on the point has abundant material for so doing. I can only say a few words as to what it purports to be and what it really is.

It is sometimes averred by Hahnemann's critics that he made all chronic disease – or at least seven-eights of it – originate in itch. But this is a misconception. He

---

xv Hahnemann himself would have allowed this "frequent" to be more correct than "invariable"; for he considered cholera due to the invasion of a cloud of minute organisms, and on this ground advised camphor to be used so freely for it (see *Lesser Writings*, op cit, p. 851 & p. 854). He is thus granting, in principle, the germ theory of infectious diseases, and the propriety of parasiticide treatment in them.

xvi See Dudgeon, RE, *Lectures on the Theory and Practice of Homœopathy delivered at the Hahnemann Hospital School of Homœopathy*, Henry Turner, London, 1853, chapters IX and X; and my own: Hughes, R, *Manual of Pharmacodynamics* (4th edition), Leath & Ross, London, 1880, pp 87, 90 & 839.

begins by excluding from the category of true chronic maladies those which arise from unhealthy surroundings, noxious habits, and depressing influences (§77); for these, he says, disappear spontaneously when the lædentia are removed. Neither will he allow the name to the medicinal affections which the heroic treatment of his day made so common (§74 - 6), and which he regards as incurable by art. True chronic disease consists of such profound disorders as asthma, phthisis, diabetes, hypochondriasis, and the life - disorders insusceptible of cure by hygiene, and tending to permanent stay and even increase. A certain proportion of the affections so characterised were traceable to specific infection; and it seemed to him that the remaining seven-eighths (it is here that these figures come in) must have some analogous 'miasmatic' origin. In the medical literature of his day he found numerous observations (he cites ninety-seven of them) of the supervention of such diseases upon the suppression of cutaneous eruptions, among which scabies - then very prevalent - took a prominent place. In this last he thought he had found the 'miasm' he wanted. It resembled syphilis in its communication by contact, its stage of incubation, and its local development, while it was far more general. He thereupon propounded it as - together with the other contagious skin affections, which he regarded as varieties of it - the source of the nonspecific chronic diseases, understood as defined.

Now it is easy for us, knowing what we know (or suppose we know) about itch, to make merry over this theory of Hahnemann's. But to condemn or ridicule him for it is a gross anachronism. We forget that the modern doctrine of scabies dates only from Hebra's writings on the subject in 1844. Before that men like Rayer and Beitt could deny the existence of the acarus; and it was quite reasonable to regard it as only the product of the disease. Hahnemann, who was one of the most learned physicians of his time, knew all about it, and had, in 1792, written upon it.[xvii] He nevertheless, in 1816, described scabies as a specific miasmatic disorder, forming itself in the organism after contagion (as syphilis does), and announcing by the itch-vesicle its complete development within. It was thus regarded that he propounded it as the origin of much chronic disease. We, understanding it better, must refuse it such a place. But when we look beneath the surface of his doctrine, we find it far from being bound up with his view of scabies. It rests upon the broader ground of morbid diathesis, and especially upon that form of it associated with cutaneous disorder which has led the French pathologists to speak of a *diathése herpetique* or *dartreuse*. Translate Hahnemann's 'psoric,' now into these terms, now into *scrofulous,* and you have the substance of his thought, which is absolutely true and of the utmost importance. It was for therapeutic purposes that he arrived at it, and these it has subserved in no common degree, giving us a wealth of new remedies, of long and deep action, which are our most valued means

---

xvii Hahnemann, S, Hahnemann on the Itch Insect, *British Journal of Homoeopathy*, 1868, 21:4, p. 670.

in chronic disorders. Compare, for instance, our use of *Sulphur* with that which generally obtains – with that even which obtained in our own school before the psora doctrine was enunciated, and you will see what we have gained by it.

Here again, then, we cannot allow Hahnemann to be depreciated on account of his hypothesis, strange as it may seem to us. But we must regret that he incorporated it in his *Organon*. Neither it nor its practical consequences form any part of his method, as such; and pathological theory is out of place in the exposition of a mode of proceeding which is wholly independent thereof. In reading the *Organon*, let us determine to ignore it, or to translate its language in the way I have suggested: we shall then do greater justice to the main argument of the treatise.

And now a few words upon the theory of *dynamisation*, which is a subject quite distinct from that of infinitesimal dosage. We have see that Hahnemann was led to adopt and defend the latter on grounds whose legitimacy all must admit, whatever they may think of their validity. For the first quarter of a century of his practice in this way (he began it in 1799) he thus regarded and justified it. He maintained, as I have said, that by the multiplication of points of contact obtained, dilution does not weaken in proportion to the reduction of bulk; but, in so speaking, he admitted that it did weaken. He even attempted to fix the ratio of the two processes, estimating that each quadratic diminution of quantity involved loss of strength by only one half; and this calculation remains unaltered in all editions of the *Organon* (note to §284). In the third edition, however – *i.e.*, in 1824 – there appears for the first time the note we now read as appended to §287. He here speaks of the unfolding of the spirit of a medicine as effected by the pharmaceutic processes of trituration and succussion, and in proportion to the duration of the one and the repetition of the other. By regulating these, accordingly, we can secure either moderation of excessive crude power or development of finer and more penetrating medical energy. In publications of 1825 and 1827 he carries yet farther this new thought. At first he had ascribed the increase of power to the more intimate mixture effected by his processes; but now he declares it to be something over and above this – a change, a liberation of the dynamic, a development of the spiritual, powers of the drugs, analogous to the production of heat by friction. Treated in this way, he affirms, "medicines do not become by their greater and greater attenuation weaker in power, but always more potent and penetrating;" there is "an actual exaltation of the medicinal power, and real spiritualisation of the dynamic property, a true, astonishing, unveiling and vivifying of the medicinal spirit."

These views were so little in accordance with those expressed in the *Organon* that we find scant further trace of them in the edition of 1829. In the note before mentioned 'refined' (*verfeinert*) becomes 'potentised,' as we have it now; and in the directions for proving medicines a note is added to §129, saying that recent observation pointed to greater attenuation and potentisation rather than larger quantity as best giving the strength required for the purpose. This is all. In 1833, however, the pharmaceutical portion of the treatise has two new aphorisms (269, 270) embodying them. Its posological section remains unchanged, save in §276. here Hahnemann had said, in former editions, "a medicine, even though it may be homoeopathically suited to the cure of disease, does harm in every dose that is too large, the more harm the larger the dose, and by the magnitude of the dose it does more harm the greater its homoeopath city." In the fifth edition he adds – "and the higher the potency selected," which obviously changes the whole meaning of what has gone before, and makes a dose a mere question of number of drops or globules. I mention all this to show how entirely the doctrine of dynamisation was an after-thought, and how little the *Organon* proper (with which we are immediately concerned) has to do with it.

But what shall we say of the theory itself, in its bearing on Hahnemann as a medical philosopher? This must depend very much upon the stand-point from which we regard it. Was it a gratuitous hypothesis, at best a mere logical consequence of the other views of the originator? or was it an attempt to account for facts – these being in themselves genuine? Hostile critics of homoeopathy assume the former position, and judge accordingly. We, however, cannot do this. Whatever our own preferences in the matter of dosage, it is impossible to read the history of homoeopathy – still more to be acquainted with its periodical literature, without recognising that highly attenuated medicines have an energy *sui generis*. They show this in provings on the healthy as well as in the treatment of the sick; and not here and there only, but in such multitudinous instances as to make coincidence and imagination utterly inadequate as accounts of the phenomena. The Hahnemannic processes certainly do develop virtues in drugs which in their crude state are altogether latent. Brimstone, oyster-shell, flint, charcoal, common salt – these substances in mass have a very limited range of usefulness: but what cannot homoeopathy do – what has it not done – with *Sulphur, Carbo vegetabilis* and *Natrum muriaticum*, in the dilutions from the 6th to the 30th? In this form they are in our hands as well-tried agents as any on which ordinary medicine depends. Their potency is a fact to us: how are we to account for it? Hahnemann's dynamisation, in the light of later science, must be held untenable; but to this day we have nothing to put in its place. And, even if we had, we should not the less honour the philosopher who perceived the necessity of the explanation; who brought to light the hitherto unknown phenomena, and set us to work at giving a scientific account of them.

My task is now complete. I have strictly confined myself to the announced subject of my lecture – the exhibition of Hahnemann as a medical philosopher by means of his *Organon*. But we are accustomed now-a-days to require more of philosophy than that it shall be sound in method: it must also show its power in bearing fruit. Hahnemann's need not fear the challenge. There is a fine passage in Macaulay's essay on Bacon, in which he recounts the numerous gains to mankind which the science of the last two hundred years has contributed. If the writer of the *Novum Organon* could have looked forward, he says, he might well have rejoiced at the rich harvest which was to spring up from the seed he had sown. In like manner has even the immediate future responded to the impulse given by our Organist. Could he have foreseen the medicine of to-day, how much there would have been to gladden his heart. He lived in a time when heroic antiphlogisticism was in full force; when physicians "slew," as in Addison's day, "some in chariots and some on foot;" when every sufferer from acute disease was drained of his life-blood, poisoned with mercurials, lowered with antimonials, and raked by purgatives. He denounced all this as irrational, needless, injurious; and it has fallen – never, we trust, to resume its sway. The change thus wrought even in the practice of the old school would be a matter for great thankfulness on his part; but how his spirit would have bounded when he looked upon the band of his own followers! The few disciples made during his life-time have swelled into a company of some ten thousand practitioners, who daily, among the millions of their *clientéle*, in their scores of hospitals and dispensaries and charitable homes, carry out his beneficent reform, making the treatment of disease the simple administration of a few (mostly) tasteless and odourless doses, and yet therewith so reducing its mortality that their patients' lives can be assured at lower rates. He would see the *Aconite* and *Belladonna*, the *Bryonia* and *Rhus*, the *Nux vomica* and *Pulsatilla*, the *Calcareas*, *Silica*, *Sulphur*, which he created as medicines, playing their glorious parts on an extensive scale, robbing acute disease of its terrors and chronic disease of its hopelessness. He would see his method ever developing new remedies and winning new victories – evoking *Lachesis* and *Apis*, *Kali bichromicum*, *Gelsemium* – winning laurels in yellow fever as green as those which crowned it in the visitations of cholera. He would see his principles gaining access one by one to the minds of physicians at large – the proving of medicines, the single remedy, the fractional dose already accepted, and selection by similarity half adopted under other explanations and names. He might well feel, like Bacon, about the *Philosophia Secunda* which should er d his *Instauratio Magna*. He had given its *Prodromi sive Anticipationes*: "the destinies of the human race must complete it – in such a manner, perhaps, as men, looking only at the present, would not readily conceive." The destinies of the human race, in respect of disease and its cure, are completing it; and will be yet more profoundly modified for the better as that completion goes on.

With these thoughts I commit the fame of Hahnemann as a medical philosopher to the impartial judgement of the great profession he has adorned.

References

1. Obituary: Richard Hughes MD, *The Homoeopathic World* 1902, 1 May, 231–233.
2. Cooper, RT. Dr Richard Hughes, a study, *The Homoeopathic World* 1902, 1 May, 200–202.
3. Clarke, JH, Editorial: Hughes, *The Homoeopathic World*, 1902, 1 May, 193–197.
4. Hughes, R. *Hahnemann as a Medical Philosopher – The Organon, Being the Second Hahnemannian Lecture,* 1881. London, E Gould & Son, 1881.
5. Hahnemann, S, *Organon der rationelle Heilkunde,* Dresden & Leipzig, Arnold, 1810.
6. Hahnemann, S, *Organon der Heilkunst,* Dresden & Leipzig, Arnold, 1819.
7. Hahnemann, S, *Organon der Heilkunst,* Dresden & Leipzig, Arnold, 1824.
8. Hahnemann, S, *Organon der Heilkunst,* Dresden & Leipzig, Arnold, 1829.
9. Hahnemann, S, *Organon der Heilkunst,* Dresden & Leipzig, Arnold, 1833.
10. Hahneman, S, *Lesser Writings,* (trans Dudgeon RE). London, W.Headland, 1851. (All three essays are translated and reprinted in this book).
11. *ibid*; p 501.
12. Hahnemann, S, *Organon der Heilkunst* (2nd Edition). Dresden & Leipzig, Arnold, 1819. (See Preface)
13. Hahnemann, S. *Lesser Writings* (trans Dudgeon RE). London, W. Headland, 1851. p 561.

10

HAHNEMANN AS A SCIENTIST, BY HIS CHIEF TRANSLATOR

Introduction

It is rare that creative the voice of Robert Ellis Dudgeon is heard in his own right in modern homeopathy, yet we rely on his version of Hahnemann for much our interpretation and understanding, No analysis of the linguistics has appeared, no comparison of the translations of Dudgeon.[1,2,3] with those of Charles Hempel[4,5] or Louis Tafel[6] for example. Here Dudgeon uses great erudition to explain the development of Hahnemann's thought in a context of the history of medicine. We learn that the dawning of the new principles of homeopathy may have been sparked by one experiment but were verified many times before publication.

About Robert Ellis Dudgeon[7,8]

Born at Leith (the port of Edinburgh) on March 17, 1820, Robert Ellis Dudgeon was a younger son of a wealthy timber merchant and ship-owner of that town, trading principally with Sweden and Norway. The name of the firm was "Dudgeon and Dickson," and for business purposes the Dickson of the firm took up his residence in Sweden, permanently as it turned out. The late Baron Oscar Dickson, of Sweden, was his son.

At an early age Robert was sent to a boarding school, of which he used to give an amusing description – it was a school of the "Dotheboys Hall" type, though his fond parents were in blissful ignorance of this fact. But whatever the opportunities for instruction might or might not be, nothing could prevent young Robert taking in learning. When still a boy, he passed on to Edinburgh University, and by the age of nineteen he had passed all his examinations for the MD degree, and had received the qualification of the Royal College of Surgery of Edinburgh. Although he had passed all his examinations, his MD degree could not be conferred until he was of age, so he spent the two intervening years in further studies in the medical schools of Paris and Vienna. To his residence in these capitals is probably due his

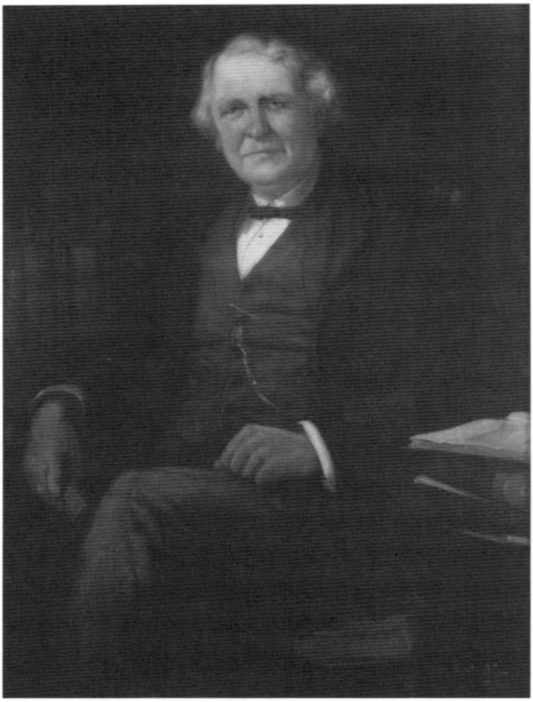

Figure 10.1 Robert Ellis Dudgeon (1820-1904)

Reproduced with the permission of CAMLIS, Royal London Homoeopathic Hospital.

familiarity with the French and German languages, which proved of such service in after years.

Contemporaries of his, and fellow sons of Midlothian, were John Drysdale, Rutherford Russell, and Francis Black. When at Vienna, Dudgeon met his old friends, Drysdale and Russell, who had come to study homeopathy at Fleischmann's hospital. But Dudgeon was engaged in other studies, and could not be induced to look into the new cult. It was after all had returned home that Dudgeon became interested, and in this way: Drysdale and Russell asked Dudgeon to help them with some translations they were making from the German. Dudgeon, then as always ready to help his friends, undertook a share of the work. He then became interested indeed; so much so that he made another journey to Vienna to study homeopathy for himself. From that time to his death – for over sixty years – his life has been spent in the service of the homeopathic cause.

Literary Works

The *British Journal of Homoeopathy* was started on its long and honourable career in the year 1842, under the editorship of J Rutherford

Russell and JJ Drysdale. Three years later Dudgeon joined the staff, and continued to be one of its editors until it ceased to appear, and was its editor-in-chief for the greater part of its existence. The *British Journal of Homoeopathy* was a quarterly journal, whose solid contributions an extremely practical part of the foundation of the practice of today.

Gifted in an eminent degree with the literary faculty, Dr Dudgeon's writing was by no means confined to journalistic work. Homeopathy has never wanted representatives who have the power of expressing themselves clearly in direct and vigorous language, and to this faculty it owes many of its treasures. Of literary homeopaths Dr Dudgeon must always occupy an honoured place in the very first rank. His translations of Hahnemann's works into English are as immortal as those works themselves, and are destined to be even better known, and more widely read than the originals, by reason of the great prevalence of the English language over the German. Hahnemann himself had great literary powers and, like Dr Dudgeon, he was a great linguist and translator. It was Hahnemann's translating work, which led him to discover the homeopathic law, as it was Dr Dudgeon's translating work which made him a homoeopath.

In the year 1886 the Homoeopathic League came into existence, and Dr Dudgeon's unrivalled knowledge of homeopathic controversy again came into action. The League work crystallised itself into the issue of a series of tracts. These tracts were for the most part written by Dr Dudgeon himself, and those that he did not write he edited, and he indexed the whole. Thus the three volumes of *Homoeopathic League Tracts* may be put down to his credit as practically one of his own original works.

Inventions and works on optics

Dr Dudgeon wrote and translated several books and articles on the subject of the human eye – e.g., *The Human Eye, its Optical Construction* (1878); a translation of Fuch's *Causes and Prevention of Blindness* (1885); of François Sacey's *Mind Your Eyes* (1886). These were books. His articles were, "Cure of Pannus by Inoculation" (*London and Edinburgh Journal of Medical Science*, 1844); "On Subaqueous Vision" (*Philosophical Magazine*, 1871).

The last work dealt with one of Dr Dudgeon's inventions – spectacles for seeing under water. The human eye is constructed for aerial vision, as the eye of fish is for subaqueous vision. The consequence is that to the human eye when under water the refraction is so great that objects cannot be seen in their true positions. Dr Dudgeon invented spectacles that enabled him to do this. The invention consisted in making a lens of air hermetically enclosed between two concave glasses. The curves of the glasses were so arranged as to correct the refraction of the water. In his work on the human eye, Dr Dudgeon gave an account of these, and also interesting illustrations of how objects appear under water, and above the surface of the water when looking through the glasses from beneath.

In 1882 Dr Dudgeon's work *The Sphygmograph* appeared. This contained a description of his new pocket Sphygmograph, now so well known, but then recently perfected by him. The original sphygmograph was that of Marey invented some years before. Singularly enough, Marey's death occurred, at a great age, only a few months before that of Dr Dudgeon. Marey's sphygmograph was a clumsy affair compared with that of Dr Dudgeon, and was quite out of the question as an instrument for use in general practice. Dr Dudgeon made it possible for any one who so desired to take sphygmograms almost as easily as to feel the pulse.

Hahnemann, the founder of scientific therapeutics[9]
By Robert Ellis Dudgeon MD

"Man, as the minister and interpreter of nature, does and understands as much as his observations on the order of nature, either with regard to things or the mind, permit him, and neither knows nor is capable of more." – *Nov. Org.*, aph. I.

Nec fas est propius mortali attingere dirum.

In Memoriam
The London School of Homoeopathy may almost be said to owe its existence to Dr William Bayes. As its first honorary Secretary, he worked zealously and unremittingly to place it on a sound financial basis. In this he succeeded beyond expectation. His earnestness and the charm of his manner won over to the cause of this School a large number of supporters, both lay and medical, and his preeminent administrative faculty moulded it into its present form. The project of an annual Hahnemannian lecture, and its publication for distribution among the Governors of the School, was eagerly adopted by him. While these pages are passing through the press, the sad news of his untimely death reaches me. I may be permitted to dedicate this lecture to his memory, and to the remembrance of a friendship of many years' standing, which was never interrupted by any differences of opinion we may have had respecting the best measures for promoting the usefulness of the School. December, 1882.

Gentlemen,

Hahnemann has been dead nearly forty years. He now belongs to history. We occupy the position of posterity in relation to him. We can view him in perspective, and can estimate him in comparison with the great medical personages of the past. We are now able to fix accurately his place in the history of medicine. In this lecture I shall endeavour to show what that place is. To this end I must cast a retrospective glance over the past.

As a preliminary, I will ask, what is the aim and object of medicine? It is the cure of disease. As Hahnemann expresses it in the first aphorism of his *Organon*, "The high and only mission of the physician is to restore the sick to health." It is necessary to remember this, for it has often been forgotten by some of the most illustrious names in the history of medicine. Anatomy, physiology, pathology, botany, chemistry and all the other so-called collateral branches of medical science, are but the means to an end – that end being the cure of disease. But the means have often been cultivated as though they were the end; and the cultivators are wont to look down on the therapeutist, as though the cure of disease was but a poor thing in comparison with the study of disease as branch of natural history, or with physiological or anatomical research.

It is impossible to say when or to whom the idea first occurred that diseases could be cured by drugs. In the first edition of the *Organon*, §7, Hahnemann says:

"There must be in medicine a healing principle; common sense tells us this."

But to the common sense of many there is no "must" about the matter. Unless we had been told that medicines have a "healing principle," we should scarcely have suspected it. On the contrary, seeing their uncomfortable effects when we swallow them, we might easily come to consider them, and class them among disease-producers rather than disease-removers. That, however, medicines were believed to possess a healing principle from a very early age is sufficiently obvious. We may suppose the belief to have originated in this way: Primitive man seeing animals eating the herbs that grew about, would imitate these creatures. Some herbs he would find nourishing and good; others, he would observe, made him more or less uncomfortable and ill. These he would note and set aside. When attacked by disease, which he would endow with a personality or entity, as he did all the forces of nature, the idea might occur to him, that as those herbs gave him a good scouring out, he might, when sick, eject his troublesome disease by taking what would make him vomit, or purge him, or give him a thorough shaking, and if his disease left him *post hoc*, he would ascribe it *propter hoc*, and recommend it to all his similarly affected friends. The earliest historical records we possess are probably the votive tablets preserved in the temples of Æsculapius. Pious persons who had been cured, or thought they had been cured of diseases, used to hang up tablets in their temples, recording their name, their disease, and the treatment they imagined had cured them. In this way medical facts were accumulated, and patients visiting these temples might, from a study of these votive tablets, he enabled to cure their own diseases by the same means. "Ομοιον πάθος, ομοιον φάρμακον", as they used to say, i.e., for a like disease a like remedy, and thus an empirical therapeia was gradually formed. But it could hardly have led to much, there were so many chances against accuracy. The pious votary might have wrongly named his disease, or he might have been mistaken in his opinion as to what had cured him, or the patient who sought to profit by his experience might err in thinking he had the same disease, or might misapply the remedy. It is true the priests of Æsculapius were there to direct him, guided by the records of the tablets, but they would be just as liable to err. So, on the whole, the gain to therapeutics from this system would be but small, and this method gradually fell into discredit, though its still survives among the learned under the name of *usus in morbis*, and, with modifications, occupies the chief place in the domestic medicine of the people.

When medicine came to be cultivated as a special profession, the primitive empiricism of the Æsculapian priests was scorned by the race of learned physicians, and hypothesis and speculation were employed to determine the nature of diseases and the virtues of medicines. Diseases were classified as dry and moist, hot and cold, and medicines were arranged in similar classes. Dry diseases were treated with moist remedies, hot diseases with cold remedies, and *vice versa*. But this classification was purely arbitrary and fanciful, and had no foundation in nature; and yet it lasted through many ages, and was not extinct in the end of the eighteenth century, when Hahnemann commenced his researches. With the increase of scholastic learning the simplicity of the ruder ages of medicine gave place to scientific complexity. No prescription was considered complete or *secundum artem* that did not contain at least a base, an adjuvant, a corrigent, and an excipient, and the greater the number of ingredients that could be introduced into the composite remedy, the better satisfied was the prescriber. As pathological theories changed so did prescriptions. But it mattered little what pathological theory was in the ascendant, prescriptions remained as complex and irrational under one regime as under another. The vitalist and the humoralist found reasons equally plausible for bleeding, purging, and blistering, and for writing long prescriptions containing often several dozens of medicines more or less powerful, which only failed to poison the patient because the ingredients were mutually antagonistic, or because the prescription contained some powerful emetic or purgative that quickly swept aside the whole of the poisonous rubbish out of his system before it had time to do much harm. It is astonishing that the faith in drugs lasted so long among physicians as it did. Up to the date of Hahnemann's discovery, and, indeed, long afterwards, we find the foremost representatives of medicine gravely prescribing these wonderful compounds, and repeating without hesitation the hypothetical fictions regarding the virtues of drugs that had been current since the days of Dioscorides.

The prescriber's art seems to have attained the climax of complex absurdity shortly before Hahnemann's days. A work published in 1683 - i.e., at a time not more distant from the initiation of Hahnemann's reform than the latter is from our day - gives us a detailed account of the therapeutics of that time. It is entitled *Doron Medicum, or a supplement to the New London Dispensatory*, its author is William Salmon, Professor of Physik. We there find long lists of primary and secondary alteratives; purgatives, divided into choler purges, phlegmagogues, melanagogues, hydragogues, and holagogues. Then medicines are classified by their temperaments. "All medicines," we are told, "simply considered in themselves, are either hot, cold, moist, dry, or temperate." Then follow lists of medicines: temperate; hot in the first degree, hot in the second degree, hot in the third degree, hot in the fourth degree; cold in the first degree, &c.; dry in the first degree, &c.; moist in the first, second, third and fourth degrees. Next, medicines are classified according to their "appropriation," as cephalicks, pectorals, cordials, stomachicals, hepaticals, nephriticks, spleneticals, hystericals, arthriticals. Then hot medicines are arranged into those heating the head, the breast, the stomach, the heart, the liver, spleen, bowels, veins, womb, joints. Cold medicaments are arranged into those cooling the same organs. Again, medicines are classified according to their properties, as emollients, relaxers, rarifiers, aperitives, attenuaters, astringents, attractives, repercussives, discussives, cleansers, anodyns, narcoticks, carminatives, diaphoreticks, alexipharmicks, pyroticks, suppuratives, sarcoticks, glutinatives, epiloticks, diureticks, emmengogicks, traumaticks, cosmeticks. Purging medicaments are: catharticks, emeticks, diureticks, sudorificks, ptermicks, salivaticks. They are further divided into medicines purging choler, flegm, melancholia, water, all humours; by vomit, by urine, by sweat, by the nose, by the palate.[i]

The following are some of the queer remedies physicians prescribed and their patients swallowed in all faith:

Quinta Essentia Bufonum Fabri, (Faber's Quintessence of Toads) - R.
Toads are in great numbers in the month of June. Hang them up and dry them in the sun, then calcine till the ashes are white, from which, with *Carduus* or *Scabious* water, or water of Limon-Peels, extract a salt to the highest whightness: mix, and keep this Salt with Treacle water. There are some which order this Quintessence to be made with the distillation of live Toads; but Faber affirms that water to be the highest poison, and, from its Volatile Spirit, to kill by its odour. This salt is one of the chiefest Antidotes against Poison, resisting all Venom to a wonder."

---

i The spelling of the original is retained.

Quinta Essentia Ossium Humanum Fabri. Quintessence of Man's Bones. – R.
Mans bones in gross powder (and infused in generous wine for 8 days) of which make an Oyl per descensum, which rectify by a seavenfold distillation in a Retort. The faeces or Caput Mortuum calcine in a strong fire, from which Calx, with boyling water, extract a Salt, which purify and make white; then conjoin it with its afore-prepared Oyl, and digest, that they may be perfectly incorporated. This will be best and most efficaciously done, at Sol his entrance into Aries, which is about the tenth day of March every Year. The same ought to be observed in making the Salt of Mans skull, with sweet Spirit of Vitriol. There is nothing in Rerum Natura more powerful than this Balsam in curing and taking away all manner of arthritick pains and torments. It speedily takes away all kinds of rottenness, and corrects every other vice of the Bones. Let it be applied warm in manner of a Balsam, with Lint, to the part affected. The Potestates Cranii Humani is a similar preparation employed chiefly for the cure of Epilepsia or Falling Sickness."

I need not waste time by giving the details for the preparation of Pulvis Viperinus or Powder of Vipers, a specifick against Scabs, Itch, Morphew, Breakings out, Erysipelas and Leprosies, and many other diseases, nor those for making the Balsamum ad Cancrum, containing amongst other choice ingredients, Mummy, Powder of Dryed Toads, and Oyl of Soot.

I shall pass on to –

Unguentum Sympatheticum, the Sympathetic Oyntment. – R.
Bears Grease, the Brains of a Boar, Powder of washed Earthworms, red Sanders, Mummy, Bloodstone, ana, 3i; Moss of a dead Mans Skull, not buried, 3j; make an oyntment according to Art. or thus according to Barbet (which he affirms to be the best description): R. Oyl of Roses, fine Bole, ana, 3j, Oyl of Linseed 3ij, Moss of a Dead Mans Skull, Mans Fat, ana, 3ij, Mummy, Mans Blood, ana, 3ss. Mix and make an Oyntment. All wounds are cured by this Oyntment (provided the Nerves and Arteries, or some of the principal Members be not hurt) thus: Anoint the Weapon that made the Wound daily once, if there be need and the Wound be great, otherwise it will be sufficient to anoint it every other day. When note, 1. That the Weapon be kept in clean Linnen, and in a temperate heat; for if the dust fall, or Wind blow upon it, or it be cold, the Sick will be much tormented; so also if it be kept too hot. 2. That if it be a stab, the Weapon must be anointed towards the point descending. 3. That if you want the Weapon, take Blood from the Wound upon a stick, and use it as if it were the Weapon. Thus the Tooth-ache is cured by pricking the Gums and anointing the Instrument."

Many other medicines of a too disgusting character to be named to ears polite are described in this book, and the most marvelous healing virtues attributed to them.[ii] Directions are given for preparing amulets to protect the wearer from the

---

ii As this lecture was delivered to an audience presumably consisting of medical persons and students, whose minds are case-hardened by their studies to all nastiness, I made no concealment as to the nature of these revolting remedies. But a valued friend and colleague has reminded me that the lecture, in its printed form, is for general distribution among the Governors of the School, who are not all medical men, nor yet all men, but the reverse; and that, therefore, it might be as well not

plague and other malignant diseases, and full particulars are given for making the *Universal Medicine*, which ought to have rendered all others superfluous.

The book in which these ridiculous and often loathsome remedies are gravely described and seriously recommended was published thirty-seven years after the death of Bacon, twenty-five years after the death of Harvey, during the life of Sydenham and Boerhaave, and only twenty-five years before the birth of Cullen.

It may perhaps be thought that the work I have been quoting from contains the vagaries of an eccentric, and that such filthy medicines as he describes were peculiar to himself. But this is not so. The writer was a learned physician, the author of many other works on medicine, chemistry, botany and astrology. We find, besides, that most all the objectionable ingredients of his prescriptions have formed the subjects of learned essays and dissertations by his contemporaries and successors far into the eighteenth century. Those curious in these matters will find in the great *Dictionary of Materia Medica* of Merat and De Lens, numerous references to works published in all countries of Europe extolling the medicinal virtues of the most repulsive substances.

I do not suppose that these loathly and grotesque remedies were patronised by Stahl, Hoffmann, Boerhaave, Haller and Cullen, the great medical authorities of the eighteenth century, to which Hahnemann belonged; but medicine has never been practised solely by great men, and it was long before their half-hearted teachings of an unprincipled therapeia exercised much influence on the practice of the rank and file of the medical profession, as they could give no more reason *for* the remedies they proposed than *against* those they denounced. Down to a very recent period some of the most repulsive remedies were employed by physicians of high standing, and though most of the filthy compounds I have alluded to without naming (for fear of shocking my readers) were eliminated form the published works on *Materia Medica,* some of them still retained their reputation among individual practitioners, even to our times. From want of a guiding principle for ascertaining the curative properties of medicines, therapeutics had degenerated into a senseless farrago of uncleanness and absurdity, a *caput mortuum* of inert rubbish, a cesspool of filthy abominations, and a torture chamber of painful and noxious appliances. But though some of the grosser elements were discarded by the contemporaries of Hahnemann, the therapeutics of his time and for many years afterwards remained as irrational as ever.

When, in 1796, he first tentatively put forward the idea that, in the treatment of chronic diseases, medicines might be given on the *similia similibus* principle, and when he launched his system perfectly excogitated, in his *Organon,* in 1810, no sign had been given by the chiefs of the medical schools that they thought that

---

to call a spade a spade, but to employ some such euphemistic paraphrase as "horticultural implement." On the whole, I think it best to omit the description of the spade altogether, for fear it might be thought to bear to great a likeness to a *graip*.

complex prescriptions were irrational, that inflammations were not best treated by blood-letting, that frequent purgation was not eminently conducive to health, in spite of the wise saying of Sauvages "*nil magis nocet quam repetita evacuantia*," that alteratives – meaning thereby, generally, mercury pushed to salivation – were not scientific remedies, or that painful processes under the theoretical name of "counter-irritants" were not indispensable curative agents. Homoeopathy was not "in the air" when Hahnemann wrote about it, nor, I may say, for some years after the *Organon* appeared. Thirteen years after the publication of the *Organon*, a new medical periodical was set up in London, and it took the title *The Lancet*, as though blood-letting was the chief of remedies. The earlier editions of Sir Thomas Watson's great work on the *Practice of Physic* recommended blood-letting for everything inflammatory without a doubt as to its excellence. Even in 1858 he says about peritonitis, "It is of great importance that blood-letting should be performed early. After a full bleeding from the arm, such as has produced some sensible impression upon the circulation and brought the patient to the verge of syncope, the surface of the belly should be covered with leeches – from 20 to 40 may be applied at once." But in the same edition he makes an exception in the case of pneumonia: "Years have passed by since I have met with any instance of that disease which has required blood-letting. I may say the same of inflammatory diseases in general. They have all become less tolerant of blood-letting since the cholera swept over us in 1832." It is not easy to understand how the sweeping over us of cholera should render pneumonia and inflammatory diseases less tolerant of blood-letting; but, as the celebrated article by Sir Daniel Sandford on "Homoeopathie" appeared in the *Edinburgh Review* in 1830, and as, about the same period, the practice of homoeopathy was introduced into Britain, and began to be much talked about, it is more likely that the "sweeping over us" of homoeopathic knowledge, rather than of the cholera, made *patients* less tolerant of blood-letting, and so doctors had to give it up; and as they found that diseases did better without it, they had to alter the teachings of their text books accordingly, and they had to invent some other reason for their altered practice, and the "sweeping over us of cholera," or the "change of type of disease" served to save their dignity and excuse their change of front. But that was not till many years after the publication of the *Organon*.

Hahnemann gradually led up to his finished method by a careful examination of all the systems of therapeutics that had previously been advocated. I say, "all" the systems, but indeed, they were only two in number, viz., the treatment of disease by medicines having action *contrary* to the disease, and that by medicines have an action *different* to the disease. He showed that these were irrational, futile, and when not useless, pernicious. He demonstrated by reasoning and experimental proof that the true rule of drug selection, was to employ in a disease a medicine whose pure effects on the healthy body were similar to the phenomena of the disease to be cured. This was not a theory but a logical deduction from observed facts arrived at in the true experimental way. Thus: certain diseases were known to be curable by certain medicines. These medicines he tested on himself and others, and found that they caused morbid states, closely resembling the diseases they were known to cure. He did not jump to this conclusion form his one experiment with cinchona bark. That experiment set him thinking and led him to other experiments with other drugs. After six years of patient reflection and experiment he suggested that the administration of medicines according to the rule *similia similibus curentur* might be the best method of treating chronic diseases – acute diseases might still be best treated by the contrary or palliative method. His suggestion fell unheeded by the great and the small men of the day. They were quite content with their old and traditional methods, their bleeding, blistering, purging, salivation and complex prescriptions. Hahnemann, nothing daunted, went on with his experiments, and nine years later published a work in Latin *On the Positive Effects of Medicines*, partly ascertained by experiment on himself and the members of his own family – for as yet he had no disciples – partly culled from the records of poisoning and observations of the effects of drugs in the writings of medical authors. At the same time he published that remarkable work *The Medicine of Experience*. Fortified by his nine years of diligent experimentation with medicines, in order to ascertain their pathogenetic powers, and his equally long trials of the curative powers of medicines given on the *similia similibus* principle, he felt himself justified in declaring this therapeutic rule to be of general application, and the use of palliatives to be limited to tiding over temporary difficulties, such as apparent death from freezing or asphyxia, and hysterical convulsions. He was practising at Torgau, a small town on the Elbe, at this time. Five years more of reflection and experiment enabled him to perfect his system to such a degree, that he published his great work, to which he gave the title *of Organon of Rational Medicine, according to Homoeopathic Laws (Organon der rationellen Heilkunde, nach Homöopathischen Gesetzen)*. Simultaneously with the appearance of this work he came to Leipzig, and the following year he published the first volume of the *Materia Medica Pura*. The actual provings in this volume were made by himself alone, probably assisted by some of the members of his family. But he was now in a famous university town, where there were many medical students, some of whom he might hope to get to assist him in his gigantic undertaking, the construction, namely, of a materia medica which should contain nothing but the experimentally ascertained positive effects on the healthy human body of the medicines treated of. Such a thing had never before been attempted, nor even suggested – unless we are to consider the oft-repeated quotation from Haller as a suggestion. Hahnemann felt that his own unaided provings would not suffice to furnish the ideal materia medica his therapeutic system required. The art was too long and his single life too short for such a task. He must have the assistance of intelligent co-operators, who were convinced of the truth or at least of the reasonableness of his therapeutic rule. How to get these zealous co-operators was the problem. If he could become a teacher of medicine as he understood it, he might succeed in convincing a class of students of the truth of his rational therapeutics, and enlist them in his work. He applied to the authorities of the Faculty of Medicine of the University for permission to teach medicine. He was informed that he would only be allowed to do this by passing an examination and defending a thesis before the Faculty of Medicine. He willingly complied with these conditions. He wrote a thesis on the *Helleborism of the Ancients*, which was so excellent, that when he came to defend it before the Faculty, his examiners could find no fault with it, and were forced to acknowledge its superlative merits. Having thus obtained the licence to teach, he soon collected around him a class of enthusiastic young men, who entered heart and soul into his scheme, and aided him so effectually in his work of proving medicines that, between 1816 and 1821 he was enabled to publish five more volumes of his pure materia medica. The six volumes of this colossal work contain the positive effects of sixty-four medicines. It constitutes a real treasury of materia medica, displaying the accurately observed effects of medicines on the human body, without any alloy of hypothesis or conjecture. Such a materia medica had never been offered to the medical world since medicine had been cultivated as an art. It upset and rendered useless all the treatises and text books on materia medica that had hitherto passed current in medicine. These contained mere hypothetical or traditional accounts of the supposed virtues of medicines. Hahnemann's materia medica, excluding hypothesis, recorded only the well-ascertained effects of medicines on the human body. Hahnemann's provings were the necessary corollary to his therapeutic rule. Previous to his time a distinction had been made between poisons and medicines. All drugs which were so powerful that they could not be given in ordinary doses without danger, were banished from the materia medica, and those only that could be given in considerable quantities without much risk were allowed to be medicines. Hahnemann abolished this distinction. He said with Shakespeare, "in poison there is physic," and he might have said "the stronger the poison the greater the physic."

It will be observed that, during his say in Leipzig, Hahnemann had no thought of separating himself from the established medical school. He qualified himself to be a teacher in that school in the usual manner. He gave lectures and formed a class of students in connexion with the existing Faculty of Medicine, and though the doctrines he taught were novel and original, he was quite within his legal right in teaching medicine as he understood it, and any medical teacher would do the same. During all this period he broached no theory either as to the nature of the disease or the mode in which the cure was effected. He proved his medicines in substantial doses, and he reduced the dose of the medicine he administered for the treatment of disease, expressly in order to avoid the too violent effects of large doses. He varied his doses according to the nature of the medicine and of the disease. When I say he broached no theory as to the curative action of medicines, I may be reminded that he held that medicines cured diseases by substituting a more powerful medicinal artificial disease for the weaker natural disease; but this, though apparently a hypothesis, was in fact a deduction from what he believed he observed in every case in which a medicine acted curatively, viz: that it caused an apparent aggravation of the natural disease. We may believe he was mistaken in this, and probably he may have got the idea from a statement of John Hunter, as Dr Fredault supposes; still it was a legitimate deduction from what he believed to be facts – but which we now think we have found not to be facts – a logical inference from the premises, only we now hold these premises to have been unsound. However, this is a matter of quite secondary importance.

The great central truths of Hahnemann's teaching up to the time when he was driven from Leipzig by the hostility of his colleagues, were these: the demonstration by reasoning and proof of the truth of the therapeutic rule *similia similibus curantur* – let likes be treated by likes; the necessity for ascertaining the effects of medicines on the healthy human body; the administration of medicines in disease singly and alone, and in the precise form in which they had been proved; the diminution of the dose for the purpose of avoiding its too violent action. There is nothing theoretical here, all these maxims are derived from observation and experience; conjecture and speculation have no part in them.

No theory of disease or of medicinal action is involved in the therapeutic rule; the reasoning employed in its discovery is strictly logical. Certain medicines are known to cure certain diseases, these medicines, when tested on the healthy human being, are found to cause morbid states similar to the diseases they cure. This is found to be the case with all medicines that have been subjected to trial; it is, therefore, so far as can be judged, a general rule that medicines that can cure diseases can produce on the healthy morbid states resembling those diseases; and, conversely, medicines that can produce on the healthy certain morbid states can cure diseases resembling those morbid states. Hence the therapeutic rule: in order to cure any disease select a medicine that can produce a similar morbid condition on the healthy – *similia similibus curantur* – let likes be treated by likes. This is a practical rule deduced from experience. Hahnemann first called his system the "Medicine of Experience." The, as if to show its logical character, he called it "Rational Medicine," and later on simply "Medicine," or "the Healing Art," as though there were none other that deserved the name.

To render it possible to apply this rule some one must undertake the heavy task of ascertaining the effects of medicines on the healthy human body. Hahnemann did not shrink from this herculean labour. For years and years he worked away silently and solitarily at the task of rendering the rule he had discovered of practical use. It was only after he came to Leipzig that he received any help from others. It was fortunate, indeed, for homoeopathy that he came to Leipzig, for had he lingered on in the paltry little town of Torgau, he could never have attracted disciples around him able and willing to assist him, and homoeopathy might have remained in its initial stage – the revelation of the true rule for treatment, but incapable of being applied for lack of proper instruments.

The single remedy was a necessity, for if medicines cured by virtue of their power to produce certain morbid states on the healthy, they must be given in the same shape in which they had been proved to produce these morbid states. If given in combination with other medicines having different effects, or if given deprived of any of the constituents they possessed when they produced these morbid states, we could have no warranty that they would possess the power, under this new form or combination, of acting as they had acted when given singly and simply. If a chemist tells us that, according to the laws of chemistry, if we wish to produce a certain effect on a solution of carbonate of soda we must add a certain substance called tartaric acid, we would never be so foolish as to expect to obtain the same effect if we gave the tartaric acid in combination with other things, say potash, magnesia, and nitre, even though we should learnedly bestow on our additions the titles of adjuvant, corrigent and excipient, nor if we gave the carbonic acid alone, or the soda alone.

The small dose was also a deduction from experience, which taught that the ordinary large doses act too violently. Experience taught that diseased parts of the human organism are more sensitive to the action of medicines having a particular affinity to them as evidenced by their causing effects on the healthy similar to those of the disease; just as a diseased organ is more sensitive to its ordinary stimulus than a healthy one; witness the excessive sensitiveness of the inflamed eye to light of the inflamed ear to sound, of the inflamed skin to touch. No theory, then, was required to justify small doses of the homoeopathic medicine; they were the outcome of experience and observation.

We may say, then, that as long as Hahnemann remained in Leipzig attached to the Medical Faculty of the University as an extra-mural yet academical lecturer and teacher of medicine, he presented his medical system in a truly logical manner, quite devoid of theory of hypothesis; indeed, in all his writings up to this time, he inveighs against theory and speculation in medicine.

So utterly opposed was he to hypothesis, that he ridiculed the idea of our ever obtaining a knowledge of the proximate causes of disease. Thus in §§ 5 and 6 of the first edition of the *Organon* we read: "It is allowable to think that every disease must depend on an alteration in the interior of the organism, but this can only be surmised by the reason from what the external phenomena reveal concerning it; but it is not in itself cognizable in any way whatever. The invisible morbid alteration of the health in the exterior (symptom-complex) together constitute what is called disease; both make up the disease itself." This teaching is curiously emphasised and expanded in the corresponding paragraphs of the second edition thus: "It is allowable to think that every disease presupposes an alteration in the interior of the human organism. But this can only be dimly and delusively surmised by the reason from what the morbid symptoms reveal concerning it; but it is not in itself cognizable, still less infallibly cognizable in any way whatever. The invisible morbid alteration in the interior and the alteration of the health of the exterior observable to our senses (symptom-complex) together constitute to the eye of Creative Omnipotence what is called disease; but the totality of the symptoms only is the side of the disease turned towards the physician; this alone is observable by him, and is the sole thing he can know, or needs to know, in order to enable him to cure." We fondly think we know something more about the essence of disease now, and talk learnedly about increase and diminution of the inhibitory power of vaso-motor nerves, reflex action, cell-proliferation, bacilli, bacteria, and microbes, of which Hahnemann and his contemporaries knew nothing; but it is doubtful if we can improve on Hahnemann's dictum, that we can only know diseases by their morbid symptoms. As our instrumental aids to diagnosis improve, we are able to make additions to our knowledge of symptoms; but the revelations of the stethoscope, the pleximeter, the thermometer, the sphygmograph, the microscope, and chemical reagents, are merely additions to the sum of observable symptoms in disease; and the same methods must be applied to the investigation of the morbid states produced by medicines on the healthy, if we would keep pathogenesy abreast of pathology, and ascertain the most exact *simile* of the disease in the agents we employ for its cure. The more complete our knowledge of the artificial symptom-complex in medicinal diseases and of the natural symptom-complex in real diseases, the better shall we be able to employ medicines for the cure of diseases. Even should our improved methods enable us to determine with certainty the actual pathological changes in disease – which they are far from having yet done – Hahnemann will still be right in saying that diseases are only cognizable by their observable morbid symptoms, for it is only through the symptoms that we can infer the pathological state, or as he words it: "the invisible morbid alteration in the interior." As far, then, as we are concerned the observable symptoms constitute the disease, and when we have ascertained everything about a disease by means of our senses, aided by all the instruments we can employ, we have ascertained the disease itself. This is no theory; it is a bare statement of fact.

Thus, as long as Hahnemann lived in Leipzig, his teachings were free from hypothesis and speculation; he kept to the firm ground of observation and experience, and made no excursions into the treacherous quicksands of conjecture. In fact, he constantly denounced speculation and hypothesis as will-o'-the-wisps leading only into the quagmires of uncertainty and self-deception. But Hahnemann was forced to leave Leipzig in 1821. He accepted from the Duke of

Anhalt-Köthen, an asylum in the petty capital of the petty duchy. He exchanged the pleasant and varied life in the literary and commercial capital of the kingdom of Saxony for the dull monotony of a fifth-rate provincial town, whose inhabitants gave him no welcome, in fact, insulted him to such a degree that for years he never crossed his own threshold unless to visit his one patient, the Duke, but took the air in the narrow strip of garden attached to his house. In Leipzig he enjoyed a large and lucrative practice, where he had constant opportunities of testing his method in all sorts of acute and chronic diseases. In Köthen he had actually no practice among the townsfolk, and never visited a patient, except his patron. The only practice he had was occasional consultations by letter, and a few rich patients, the subjects of chronic diseases who, attracted by the fame of his name, paid short visits to Köthen in order to consult him. He was no longer surrounded by the crowd of admiring disciples, whom he taught and with whom he used to work almost every day, and who amused him every evening with cheerful conversation over pipes and small beer. He was relegated to the society of his wife and daughters, excellent persons, no doubt, in their way, but not of much use to him in a scientific point of view. He was thus driven in upon himself, as it were, with plenty of time to cogitate on the meanness and injustice of the colleagues who had conspired to effect his ruin in Leipzig, and who would have rendered it impossible for him to earn his bread, had not the charity of an amiable prince offered him a paltry post with the mild dignity of *Hofrath*. *Otium cum dignitate* he might now be said to possess, but the *otium* was torture to a man of his active mind and habits, and the *dignitas* was rather given than received by him. Deprived of his practice, torn from the society of his friends, no longer able to superintend an admiring circle of devoted and enthusiastic fellow labourers in the construction of his indispensable *Materia Medica*, the sense of having been unjustly treated by colleagues, by whom he felt that he ought to have been honoured and respected, gnawing like a canker-worm at his heart; conscious as he was of having done more for scientific therapeutics than any physician of the past or present, of having found the way to truth in medicine and of having trodden it all alone;[iii] in his enforced solitude and isolation, as he grew old he took to the dangerous courses of spinning hypotheses, which being uncorrected by discussion with other minds and incapable of being tested by experience at the sick-bed, he came to consider as truths of equal value with the great fundamental truth he had slowly and painfully elaborated by experiment and observation. We see this fatal tendency to speculation and dogmatism in the works and revised editions he published during his exile in this Patmos of Köthen. From a close and diligent observer of nature in the prime of his life, he became a seer of apocalyptic visions in his old age.

---

iii "In these investigations I discovered the road to the truth, which I had to tread all alone, far away from the beaten highways of traditional medicine." – Preface to the first edition of the *Organon*.

Unmindful of what he had formerly said, that it was impossible to ascertain the pathological process that took place in the hidden interior of the organism, he now tells us that disease consists in an alteration of the vital force, which he seems to regard as a distinct entity. This notion of a vital force presiding over the functions of organic life is as purely a hypothesis as the *archœus* of Van Helmont, with which, in fact, it is identical. I am far from denying the value of speculation, imagination or hypothesis in scientific matters when used to explain observed facts, but there is always a danger of regarding a hypothesis as a proved truth; and if the hypothesis should be false, it will surely vitiate all the reasoning founded upon it. The hypothesis of a vital force is now generally regarded as false, consequently a theory of disease founded on it can find no acceptance in the present day. When Hahnemann wrote, the vital-force hypothesis was a universal belief; so it may be said that Hahnemann was not to blame in adopting the belief. But, as a scientific man, he was to blame in adopting any belief at all. *knows*, he does not *believe*. He could not know that there was a vital force; he was not justified in believing in the existence of what he could not know. He should have stuck to this original declaration, that what takes place in the hidden interior of the organism is unknowable, and remained faithful to his own maxim, that the physician has only to do with observable and ascertainable phenomena, which indeed is identical with the first aphorism of Bacon's *Novum Organum*.

The idea of an immaterial vital force being the cause of diseases by its derangement, naturally led to the theory that medicines, by the processes of trituration and succussion, became divested of their material substance, and their powers thereby liberated; they became spiritual immaterial forces without a substratum of matter. And this idea he now promulgated, though he had formerly declared that, however much diluted, there must still remain some material stuff in the dilution. And the two opposite and conflicting statements stand side by side in the last edition of the *Organon*.[iv]

The hypothesis of the liberation of the spirit of the medicine by the pharmaceutical processes he employed, in the end suggested to Hahnemann this other hypothesis: that the power of the medicine was increased by dilution. To express this idea, "dilution" became "dynamisation," and it is curious to observe that, again side by side with this new idea of the increase of potency by dilution, the last edition of the *Organon* retains the statement originally made in the first edition, that the power of a medicine decreases by dilution in a regular mathematical progression.

In the solitude of his Köthen exile Hahnemann elaborated his wonderful theory of chronic diseases. He tells us that the subject had occupied him since the year 1816; but he never breathed a syllable of it, even to his most intimate friends, until

---

iv See §cclxxx, note, and §cclxxxvii, note.

the year 1827, when he summoned to his side two of his most faithful disciples – Stapf and Gross – and to them he communicated his theory that all chronic diseases, excepting those produced by unhealthy surroundings, evil habits and improper medicinal treatment, were owing to three chronic miasms, syphilis, sycosis and psora, the two former causing one-eighth, the latter seven-eighths of all chronic diseases. Similar views as regards the origin of many chronic diseases from psora had already been enunciated by Hoffman, before Hahnemann's birth, by Autenrieth in 1808, and by Wenzel in 1825; so the idea was not absolutely novel, and Hahnemann took it up and developed it to an extent undreamt of by his predecessors in this line. I will not attempt to show the plausibility of the theory, that has already been fully done by Henderson, in his reply to Simpson, by Dr Hughes in this place, and by myself on a former occasion. I would only remind you that it is a mere theory, and as such inconsistent with Hahnemann's oft-repeated denunciations of pathological theories and speculations. In 1828 Hahnemann published the first three volumes of his first edition of the Chronic Diseases. In the first volume this theory is set forth with great elaboration, and in the editions of the *Organon* published after this date, he introduced this theory of chronic diseases among his aphorisms. In the other two volumes he gave a number of pathogeneses of new medicines, which he termed "anti-psorics," this term involving another theory, viz.: that these medicines had a specific antagonism to the theoretical *psora*, which was again a departure from this former doctrine, that treatment should not be directed against the hypothetical cause of the disease, but against the actual disease as revealed to use by its symptoms.

Another innovation was introduced in the method he employed for ascertaining the pathogenetic effects of these new medicines. They were not proved, like the former medicines in the *Materia Medica Pura*, by testing them on himself and his band of zealous co-operators. The symptoms recorded were all obtained by his own observations – no names of fellow-provers are mentioned. He could not and did not attempt to prove the new medicines on the healthy. The symptoms he gives were those observed during the administration of these medicines to patients. What an uncertain, what an impure source, this is, needs no argument to prove. It cannot be said that this mode of ascertaining the effects of drugs was exactly a novelty to Hahnemann, for he indicates it already in the first edition of the *Organon*, §cxix: "But how are we able to discover the symptoms of the medicine even in diseases, especially chronic ones, among the symptoms of the original disease, is a subject of higher art, and should be left to masters in observation only." That he did not trust to this doubtful source for ascertaining the effects of his earlier medicines is sufficient obvious; but we now find him employing it to the exclusion of what in the previous paragraph he declares to be the most important method. viz.: trials of medicines on himself by the accurately observing and unprejudiced physician.

In Köthen he also fixed on the 30th dilution as the standard dose of every homoeopathic medicine, for every disease, in every constitution, at every age. He says he was led to select this dose by innumerable experiments. But as his experiments would require to be made with every dilution, in every disease and at all ages, it is obvious that no man's life would be long enough to test even one medicine in this way; especially when it is remembered how various are the characters of every case of a disease called by a particular name, how diverse are the idiosyncrasies of patients, what a difference of sensitiveness is to be met with among them. We must therefore regard Hahnemann's dictum, that the 30th dilution is the best in every case, as an arbitrary maxim, not founded on experience, and therefore purely hypothetical. In the first edition of the *Organon* he laid it down as a rule for the dose that it should be so small as just to be able to cause a slight apparent aggravation of the disease. But his was evidently an impossible problem, as no one could have gone on trying all kinds of doses in a disease until he found the one that caused a very slight apparent aggravation, more especially as, with all possible attention and even expectation, there are few who have ever observed this so-called "homoeopathic aggravation" in disease from any dose, great or small. Nor is there any reason for diluting medicines at all, if we are to accept as true what Hahnemann tells us in the last edition of the *Organon*, §cclxx, note, viz.: that precisely the same medicinal power can be communicated to an undiluted medicinal solution by continuous shaking for half an hour, as by diluting it up to his standard limit. "I dissolved," says he, "one grain of soda in one ounce of water mixed with alcohol in a phial which was thereby filled two-thirds full, and shook this solution continuously for half an hour, and this was in dynamisation and energy equal to the 30th potency." Were this so, the homoeopathic pharmacy would be very much simplified. There would be no sense in expending time and labour in making dilutions through thirty phials with accurately measured quantities of alcohol. One grain of the crude drug dissolved in an ounce of fluid and shaken continuously for half an hour would furnish us with a preparation precisely similar in potency to the standard 30th dilution.

Unfortunately, as we cannot help perceiving, Hahnemann, during his residence in Köthen, was too apt to accept as truths many speculations of his own, and even some crude suggestions of others, the accuracy of which he did not sufficiently test. Thus we find him in 1833, when preparing for the press the last edition of the *Organon*, eagerly accepting Ægidi's proposal to give medicines no longer singly and alone, as he had hitherto taught, but in combination; and it was only owing to the remonstrances of some of his oldest disciples that he refrained from adding a paragraph recommending these double-remedies (*Doppelmittel*), the admission of which would have been a serious misfortune to homoeopathy, and a complete departure from his former teachings

A careful consideration of Hahnemann's writings during his period of banishment at Köthen forces us to the conclusion that his expulsion from Leipzig was an unmitigated misfortune for homoeopathy. It was during this period that he introduced all those surprising doctrines that have rendered his system so repugnant to the intelligence of educated physicians. He then abandoned the safe and fruitful path of observation and experiment for the hazardous and unprofitable way of speculation and hypothesis, the folly of which he had previously demonstrated. He adopted the hypothesis of disease being a derangement of the vital force; of the spirit of a medicine being liberated from the matter; of the increase of power of a medicine by trituration and succussion; of the origin of chronic diseases from three fixed miasms; of the antipsoric power of certain substances, and of a certain dilution being the appropriate dose for all medicines in all diseases. Had Hahnemann remained in Leipzig, attached as an office-bearer, a lecturer, a sort of extra-mural professor in the Medical School of that city, engaged in extensive practice among patients of all sorts, surrounded by an attached circle of intelligent students and practitioners, his mind not embittered against his medical brethren by their injustice and persecution, we may safely say that he would never have abandoned his original method of investigation and observation and his Newtonian boast: *"hypotheses non fingo."* The hypotheses he spun out of his imagination in his solitary old age at Köthen would probably never have occurred to him in his busy Leipzig life, or, at least, they would have been subjected to the wholesome criticism of a number of intelligent and independent minds, and their hollowness exposed in the fierce fire of discussion. The grand truths of his immortal discovery would have been cultivated with assiduity. The evidence in favour of the excellence of his therapeutic rule would have been multiplied and assured. The acquisitions of pathology and physiology would have been utilised in the reformed therapeutics, the improved methods of research would have been applied by him to both natural and medicinal diseases. Rational therapeutics would have been engrafted on medical science. Hypothesis and speculation would have found no place in the new therapeutics, or, at least, they would have been kept within due bounds and not elevated to a creed. The dogmatism and intolerance that are so conspicuous in the writings of the septuagenarian hermit would never have been developed in the society of sharp-witted and independent companions. Homoeopathy would have remained what Hahnemann originally declared it to be, "rational medicine" *par excellence*, and its practitioners would not, as now, be handicapped in medical controversy by having to defend, explain away or repudiate a number of crude speculations which are not of the essence of homoeopathy, but which are clustered like parasites around that great therapeutic discovery, and which serve only to hide its fair proportions by their unwelcome obtrusiveness.

It is no doubt true that Hahnemann insisted on his hypothetical doctrines being accepted as of equal certainty and value with his doctrines that are founded on experience and reason; but we are not bound to accept them, or to accept anything that has not been proved and is incapable of experimental proof, and is not satisfying to our reason. Now the soundness of the therapeutic rule *similia similibus curentur* is capable of proof, and has been experimentally proved thousands of times, and it commends itself to our reason. The proving of medicines on the healthy, the single remedy and the small dose are necessary corollaries to the therapeutic rule; but the homoeopathic aggravation, the dynamisation of medicines by pharmaceutic processes, the original of seven-eighths of all chronic diseases from one miasm, the antagonism of certain drugs to the fanciful *psora*, the possibility of ascertaining the pure effects of medicines by giving them in small doses to the sick, the identical dose of all medicines in all diseases – all these teachings may bear the stamp of genius and show great originality of mind, but that is not the question. We have to determine if they are true by an appeal to experience and reason, as we appealed to experience and reason in the matter of the therapeutic rule, *similia similibus*; and if they do not stand the ordeal, we must reject them, even though they be Hahnemann's teachings – *magis amica veritas!* Hahnemann did not submit these, his later teachings, to the ordeal of discussion and experiment. His disciples have done this, and have more or less rejected the hypothesis of the Köthen period. But the rejection of what is hypothetical in Hahnemann's teachings does not affect that which is practical and experimental.

His discovery of the general therapeutic rule, *similia similibus curentur*, his immense and self-denying labours to render the application of this rule possible by proving medicines on himself and others, so far excel all that had previously been done for therapeutics, that the heroes of medicine of ancient and modern times sink into insignificance beside him; indeed, disappear altogether from the field of therapeutics; and it is a case of Hahnemann first, the rest nowhere.

What, let me enquire, have the greatest physicians of the past done for practical medicine?

Hippocrates, the so-called "Father of Medicine" – on the *lucas a non lucendo* principle, as he did almost nothing for medicine proper, and might rather be called the father of therapeutic nihilism – is hardly remembered for anything except his saying: "Art is long, life is short," which is but the weary wail of disappointment and failure.

Herophilus, whose name is indelibly inscribed on our *dura mater*,[v] though he discovered that human beings had a pulse, could not find the cause thereof, though he is said to have dissected 600 living human beings; but his therapeutical teaching was most disastrous, for it is believed that he was the author of the maxim, that diseases being compound, they required compound medicines –

---

v *Torcular Herophili*, the name of a confluence of venous sinuses in that membrane.

which was *similia similibus* of the wrong sort – and he was thus the parent of complex prescriptions, which have been the bane of the medical art ever since.

Erasistratus is now only remembered as the physician who got the largest fee on record for one prescription, nearly £25,000, which must make him an object of envy to all self-respecting physicians.

Galen is credited with the enunciation of the therapeutic rule *contraria contrariis curentur,* which being exactly and entirely wrong, was, of course, held to be the *ne plus ultra* of medical wisdom down to Hahnemann's time.

Dioscorides is said to be the father of *Materia Medica*. He arranged medicines in an arbitrary classification, according to their hypothetical qualities, as hot, cold, moist, dry, which has no foundation in nature, and therefore his book remained the classic text book, and his classification of drugs was retained down to quite recent times, as I have shown in my quotations from the *Doron Medicum.*

Paracelsus came very near to discovering the truth, but as he wrapped his doctrines in mystic language, and neglected altogether the true way to discover the fitting *similia* by testing medicines on the healthy, preferring to trust to his imagination, the school he founded had no substantial back-bone, and was lost in a cloud of mazy hypotheses. Much of Paracelsus' treatment was conscious homoeopathy, much of that of his predecessors and successors ahs been unconscious homoeopathy; many a physician has been homoeopath, *malgré lui,* or practised homoeopathy, as M. Jourdain spoke prose, *sans qu'il en sût rien;* but none has taught that the homoeopathic was the general rule of therapeutics.

Van Helmont may be looked upon as the inventor of the vital force, which he called *archæus,* and he thus set men's minds on a wrong track, which they persistently followed for many years. Hahnemann himself could not avoid it when he took to theorising on the nature of disease. Van Helmont was not without merit in exposing the futility of the therapeutics of his day, but he was only great in destruction, and did little or nothing in the way of construction.

Harvey was a great physiologist, and his grand discovery of the circulation of the blood formed a noteworthy epoch in medical history, but his contributions to therapeutics were *nil*. Nor was his merit in his discovery so great as Hahnemann's in his, for in Harvey's day some happy guesses at the truth respecting the circulation of the blood had already been made, and men's minds were prepared to receive it, whereas there was nothing of the sort in Hahnemann's case.

Sydenham is often called the English Hippocrates. While he sighed for specifics, and wrote uncommon good sense about the desiderata of therapeutics, he bled like Sangrado, and wrote prescriptions containing nearly four-score ingredients. He will be remembered as having declared: "*sine opio nolo esse medicus.*"

Stahl recast the doctrine of Van Helmont, altering the name of "archæus" to "animal spirits," but his therapeutics consisted mainly of bleeding and evacuants, and he denounced cinchona bark as a mischievous drug.[vi]

Hoffman defended cinchona from Stahl's depreciation of it, and accounted for its success in ague by its tonic properties. The rest of his therapeutics was equally conjectural, and, indeed, he seems to have thought that diseases were best let alone, for he wrote: *"fuge medicos et medicamenta si vis esse salvus;"* but perhaps he only intended this as a warning against other doctors, not himself; for he carried on a traffic in secret nostrums like many of his great contemporaries and predecessors.

Boerhaave professed the doctrine of *contraria contrariis*, but explained it as we have seen the rule *similia similibus* explained in our own time. Thus he says: "Contraries are removed by contraries – not by such means as are directly opposite or contrary to the disease present, but by such remedies as will afterwards manifest their effects contrary to the cause of the disease. If a hot drink produce perspiration in fever, then give a hot drink, for that will cool the body, which is what we want to do. If the primary action of opium is constipating and of rhubarb laxative, and the secondary the reverse according to the principle of reaction, then opium may be the remedy in constipation and rhubarb in diarrhœa." Hahnemann himself might almost have accepted this explanation.

Haller is chiefly known to us by his recommendation to test medicines on the healthy human body, before proceeding to experiment with them in diseases – but there is no record of his having carried his recommendation into practice.

Cullen was great in nosology, or the classification of diseases. He was a stout defender of theory in therapeutics, and it was the unsatisfactory character of his theory to account for the curative action of bark in ague that led Hahnemann to reject theory and consult experiment in order to ascertain the true rule of practice.

John Hunter made no notable contributions to therapeutics, but, as Fredault has pointed out, he first suggested the idea that one disease attacking the organism at a point where another disease is, cures the latter. This notion was

---

vi Among the works attributed to Stahl's principal disciple, Michael Alberti, I find one with the significant title, *De curatione per similia*, which is said by a writer in the *British and Foreign Medico-Chirurgical Review* for July, 1871, to be the key-note of homoeopathy. But I strongly suspect this writer never saw the work in question, and only made a guess at the subject. I believe, too, that Alberti never wrote such a work, for though I have not been able to find it in the British Museum, I have looked through scores of works attributed to him by Haller and the catalogue of the British Museum, and found that they were all merely inaugural theses of candidates for the degree of MD. in the school of Halle, of which Alberti was president. It is thus that Haller has been enabled to father upon Alberti no less than 372 separate works, whereas I believe his extant writings do not amount to more than a dozen. Most of the essays falsely ascribed to him are the usual crude lucubrations of inexperienced students, and I have no doubt this one is of the same character.

further developed by Hahnemann, and forms the basis of his attempted explanation of the method of cure by homoeopathic remedies. From this germ, too, sprang Hahnemann's hypothesis of an apparent aggravation in all cases preceding the curative action. In Trousseau's *"médicine substitutive"* the same idea is apparent.

John Brown constructed a complete system of therapeutics, founded on a double theory of disease and medicinal action. In spite of these merits it failed to obtain general acceptance, though its partisans in Göttingen heroically endeavoured to get it into the heads of its opponents by cracking their skulls with cudgels.

Rasori and Broussais, the contemporaries of Hahnemann, both tried their hands at constructing systems of therapeutics, the simplicity of which was admirable, but the results of their practical application were disastrous, though they are not yet altogether abandoned in their native lands.

The retrospective glance I have cast, with much aid from our Russell's admirable *History*, at the most prominent representative men of the past history of medicine, shows us not a single name among the heroes of medicine connected with any real advance in therapeutics - which is, after all, the sole object of medical science - until we come to Hahnemann. What strikes us most is, that the homoeopathic therapeutic rule was not discovered, or at least suspected to be a general rule for treatment, by any of the illustrious and thoughtful men who adorned the medical schools of the past. Now that we know it, it appears so simple and obvious. But so did the way to make an egg stand on its end appear after Columbus had shewn how to do it. Hahnemann's is the one name in the whole history of medicine connected with a rational, simple and efficacious system of therapeutics, based on the solid foundation of impregnable facts.

Hahnemann has not yet obtained a universal recognition of his true place in medicine; but even among those who most persistently ignore claims and who affect to treat him as a dreamer or a charlatan, the influence of his genius is conspicuous by the change he has wrought in their practice. The sanguinary and cruel treatment of disease has almost been abolished. Bleeding, whether local or general, is now rarely, very rarely, resorted to, though ominous signs of a desire to rehabilitate the long disused practice have lately appeared in the medical periodicals. Possibly, doctors have fondly imagined there has been again a "change of type" back to the old state of things when diseases were "tolerant of blood-letting," but since homoeopathy has taught them better, they will hardly find that patients have resumed their tolerance of phlebotomy. Blistering and cauterisation are scarcely ever heard of. Mercurial salivation is only practised in holes and corners. Complex prescriptions are generally allowed to be unscientific, though still too often written; but the pedantic jargon of *base, adjuvant, corrigent* and *excipient* has passed away, and the true reason of the multiplication of the ingredients in the prescription is frankly acknowledged; and that reason is the same as impels the sportsman to put a number of shots in his cartridge, to wit, that if some miss others may hit. Many of the most scientific physicians practise a more than Hippocratic nihilism, under the euphemistic name of "expectancy." Remedies derived from the homoeopathic *materia medica* are furtively introduced into practice and given on homoeopathic principles in fractional doses. No opposition is offered to their introduction, provided the proposer makes no mention of the source of his inspiration, and can make it appear from some futile experiments on frogs or rabbits – which seem to furnish different results to every different experimenter – that they promote or destroy the inhibitory influence of some nerves, or that they retard or accelerate the movements of a heart removed from the body, or do something equally instructive. Anything of this sort suffices to give a kind of physiological imprimatur to a remedy, and so render it a welcome and valued addition to the old-school *thesaurus medicaminum*, but its true source is well known to all who choose to enquire. The most popular modern works on therapeutics, such as those of Ringer and Phillips, are in the main mere *réchauffés* of homoeopathic practice. New pharmaceutical preparations are constantly being introduced under the names of "granules," "parvules" and "dosimetric medicines," which homoeopathy may accept as sincerest flattery, they being a close imitation of her pharmaceutical preparations. Almost the only relics of pre-Hahnemannic therapeutics that still survive are purgatives and sedatives, and the use of these, I am bound to admit, is as frequent as ever. Indeed, to invent or introduce a new purgative salt, powder, pill, water or lozenge, or a novel narcotic, is a sure way to fame and often to fortune. The great Virchow, whose fame overtops that of every living medical scientiate, as Mont Blanc does the Alps, does not scruple to certify publicly to the "invariable and prompt success" of the purgative water called "Hunyadi Janos," which is merely a strong solution of Epsom and Glauber's salts; and at the last International Congress he had the temerity to assert that no medicine discovered by the Hahnemannian method of physiological proving on the healthy human body could be even distantly compared for therapeutic utility to *chloral hydrate*, which was discovered in his laboratory by experiments on the lower animals, and which promises to be as destructive to health and life as opium itself.

The vaunted success of this mode of discovering the powers of drugs by torturing stupid frogs and rabbits with them will hardly have the effect of convincing us of its superiority over the Hahnemannian method of testing them on intelligent human beings, more especially when we observe the exceeding diversity of opinion with regard to the mode of action of almost every drug arrived at by our most intelligent vivisectors. Take, for example *aconite*. From a series of experiments on frogs, one observer is convinced that it acts primarily by paralysing the peripheries of the motor nerves; another, that it produces its effects by its action on the medulla oblongata; another, that it paralyses the central nervous system;

another, that it paralyses both central nervous and muscular systems; another, that it first augments excito-motor functions and sensations, and only paralyses them secondarily; another, that it paralyses the sympathetic nerve; another, that it paralyses the terminations of the pneumogastric; another that it stimulates the inhibitory centre of the pneumogastric; another, that it paralyses all nitrogenous tissues; another, that it first paralyses the sensory, then the motor part of the spinal chord; another, that it acts directly on the protoplasm. You may accept which of these conclusions you like, but will not find any of them of the slightest use in practice. On the other hand, Hahnemann's experiments with *aconite* on human beings have furnished us with a series of objective and subjective symptoms which have proved of the greatest value in enabling the practitioner to cure many of the most dangerous and fatal diseases to which humanity is subject, and which will prove equally valuable to all future generations. When we compare the relative value to the sick and suffering of Hahnemann's mode of investigating the powers of medicines by testing them on the healthy human being, with that adopted by our modern physiologists by experimenting with them on tortured and mutilated reptiles, we shall surely arrive at the conviction, that in order to obtain useful information with regard to medicinal agents, "the proper study of mankind is man" – not frogs.

Every now and then the patient world is excited, and the medical world is fluttered, by the announcement of some wonderful discovery in anatomy, physiology or natural history that, we are told, will revolutionise the art of medicine and make possible the cure of diseases hitherto deemed incurable. The latest fad of this sort is the ingenious speculation of Pasteur, who, though no medical man, has propounded a new pathology which has fascinated a credulous profession and a large portion of the semi-scientific public. According to him, all diseases are divisible into two classes, those in which a microzoon has been found, and those in which one will be found. And it was authoritatively announced that the universal microzoocide was discovered in carbolic acid, which we were informed kills bacteria, vibriones, bacilli, micrococci, microbes, and all other morbific vermin, and yet, like a celebrated insect powder, is "perfectly harmless to animal life." So the logical inference was that carbolic acid was the universal remedy. But it gradually transpired that some of these minute organisms, so far from being destroyed by carbolic acid, increased and multiplied themselves amazingly under carbolic acid dressings, and that almost all their varieties could exist in the organism without causing disease; and more astonishing still, it was shewn by Rossbach[vii] that an inorganic chemical ferment of vegetable origin, free from foreign organisms, when introduced into the blood of a healthy living animal, caused this blood to swarm with bacteria in countless profusion in an incredibly short time; and

---

vii *Medical Record*, Aug. 1882, p. 311.

further, it was found that carbolic acid was not so "harmless to animal life" as had been represented, for some surgeons have had to give it up, because it poisoned not only their patients – which might be borne with equanimity, for patients are used to be poisoned, as eels are to be skinned – but even their illustrious selves, which was intolerable. A recent attempt in the Paris hospitals to apply the carbolic acid treatment to the cure of typhoid fever was followed by disastrous consequences, the mortality having been something shocking even to the allopathic mind and conscience[viii].

These continual announcements, that at length something has been found that is certain to do wonders in the way of curing disease, never seem to get beyond the stage of hope or prophecy – like man, medicine "never is, but always to be, blest." They remind me of Mr. Snodgrass attitude on a certain memorable occasion, when he made a feint of pulling off his coat and announced that he was just going to begin, but never did actually begin. Medicine in the Snodgrassian attitude is not a very imposing spectacle, more particularly when some candid friend like James Johnstone whispers in its ear that it would have been better for the sick if the whole race of physicians and apothecaries had never existed; or like Sir Astley Cooper, who said that the art of medicine was "founded on conjecture

---

[viii] The "carbolic craze" must be near its end when one of the most intelligent surgeons and successful operators can thus write of it: "I have shown in my published writings that carbolic acid has done much more harm than good; perhaps it would have been better if we had never heard of it." – Lawson Tait, on the *Uselessness of Vivisection. Proceedings of Birmingham Phil. Soc.*, vol ii, p. 127. Another surgeon, Dr Keith, of Edinburgh, if possible still more distinguished for successful operations, spoke thus at the International Medical Congress of 1881; "For some time I have not found the carbolic spray necessary, and have not used it in my last 27 cases, all of whom have recovered easily. With every possible care, the spray has not in my hands, prevented the mildest septicaemia, and its effects on the kidney were sometimes disastrous. I have frequently seen kidney haemorrhage follow long operations, and two deaths in hospital patients were occasioned, I believe, by carbolic poisoning . . . I have given it up, believing that, on the whole, it did more harm than good." – *Trans. of the Intern. Med. Congress of 1881* vol. ii, p. 235.

But the fertile genius of M. Pasteur has not rested contented with the mere cure of diseases by destroying their *microbes*. He conceived the grand idea of cultivating these *microbes* to harmlessness, taming or civilising them, so to speak, and then inoculating them into the bodies of animals liable to catch the virulent disease from uncultivated *microbes*. In this way a mild form of the disease would be produced and the animal protected from the graver form, as vaccinated children are protected from small-pox. This idea has been developed by an enthusiastic disciple to the length shown in the following quotation:- "Considering the results already obtained, we are justified in hoping that some day science will gain possession of the viruses of all diseases in the world, and will transform them into their own peculiar vaccines [*i.e.*, cultivate and tame their *microbes*.] And then, instead of waiting for the onslaught of contagious diseases, the human and animal populations may be protected against them by anticipatory inoculations of their viruses modified by cultivation into prophylactics." (Dr Bouley, *Le progrès en médécine par l'experimentation*, p. 438.) When that time comes it will be all up with doctors both human and veterinary, so they will do well to make the most of their present opportunities before all disease-producing *microbes* have been cultivated into innocuousness.

and improved by murder;" or like Virchow, who flatly denies that we have any rational therapeutics, and that in spite of his eulogium of chloral and Hunyadi Janos; or like Osterlen, the author of a standard work on *Materia Medica*, who says that when physicians reflect that medicines are powerful substances which may easily become poisons, they will confine themselves to the treatment of diseases by hygiene and dietetics. Thirty-six years ago Sir John Forbes wrote thus of the condition of old physic: "Things have arrived at such a pitch that they cannot be worse. They must mend or end." They have not mended – why have they not ended? Because old physic, like some other condemned female offenders, always asserts, as a plea for a respite, that she is pregnant with some wonderful new idea. And she can always get a jury of respectable matrons impanneled, led on by Professor Tyndall or some other *amicus curiæ*, who are ready to swear that they believe her to be really in the family-way this time, and about to be delivered of a precious offspring that will be of inestimable value to the patient world. But nothing ever comes of it. The poor old creature is hopelessly barren, never indeed was other than an epicene monstrosity.

When time, the great healer, shall have allayed the anger and prejudice of the profession against the importunate reformer who rudely routed them out of their fool's paradise of contented self-sufficiency, and dared to lay an impious hand on the cherished maxims of traditional routine, and to throw doubts on the value of their methods and medicines; when the generation who hate Hahnemann because they are conscious of having acted unjustly towards him shall have passed away; when the bulk of the profession shall have acquired that "lucidity," which Matthew Arnold has too flatteringly credited them with; when the enthusiasts who have burlesqued some of the most purely theoretical speculations of his old age and foisted on our rational therapeutics their fluxion potencies[ix] and their grotesque

---

ix Those who call themselves "Hahnemannists" do so apparently on the *lucus-a-non-lucendo* principle. Their teachings and practice are in almost every particular at complete variance with, if not the exact opposite of what Hahnemann taught in his *Organon* and elsewhere. Thus, Hahnemann directs that dilutions of medicines shall be made with alcohol in as many separate phials as there are dilutions, each phial receiving one drop of the previous dilution in 99 drops of pure spirit, and being shaken vigorously to ensure thorough admixture. The Hahnemannists have rejected all this, and make all their dilutions with ordinary service water with all its impurities, in one single bottle, no shaking being administered, but the bottle being merely inverted at each so-called dilution. Whereas Hahnemann fixed the 30th dilution as the limit of his preparations, the Hahnemannists carry on their un-Hahnemannic processes to the 10,000th, 100,000th, 1,000,000th and even higher figures. Whilst Hahnemann by precept and example taught us to investigate the properties of substances that either have or may reasonably be expected to have a powerful action on the human frame, the Hahnemannists devote their energies to proving common articles of food, such as white sugar and skim milk, or allied nutritious substances such as milk-sugar and bitch's milk, or mystic imponderables, such as sun's or moon's rays, and diluted magnetic force. Lastly, though Hahnemann taught that the remedy was to be selected by reason of the perfect correspondence of its ascertained effects with the totality of the symptoms of the disease, the Hahnemannists teach the novel doctrine of choosing the remedy from some one arbitrarily selected peculiar symptom, which

and often loathsome preparations, such as *Lac caninum, Lac defloratum, Saccharum album, Syphilinum, Sycotinum, Gonorrhin, Leucorrhin, Sol, Luna, Nix,* &c., by which they show themselves to be the lineal descendents of those who introduced into ancestral medicine the *Aqua aurea, Oleum philosophorum, Album Græcum* and *Nigrum,* bezoars, murderer's bones, sympathetic ointments and amulets – when these enthusiasts shall have discredited themselves by their absurdities; when a new generation of earnest and unprejudiced enquirers shall have arisen, who will be capable of winnowing the golden grains of truth from the chaff of fanciful speculation, what position will Hahnemann occupy in the domain of medicine?

He will be known to all future ages as the physician who first taught that diseases must be treated by medicines which have an elective affinity for those parts of the organism that are the seat of the morbid process,[x] that it is only by testing medicines on the healthy that their affinities can be learned, and that they must be administered for curative purposes in disease in quantities too small to produce collateral disturbances. In one word, Hahnemann will be acknowledged to be the one, the sole founder of rational therapeutics, the *facile princeps* of true physicians, whose mission it is, as he says, "to restore the sick to health." The

---

they euphemistically term a "key-note." Now, all these innovations and novelties in doctrine and practice may be improvements or otherwise, but they are not what Hahnemann taught, they are in fact entirely different, I may say utterly opposed to what he taught, and it is difficult to comprehend how their authors can arrogate to themselves the title of "Hahnemannists," which to the common understanding implies that they are *par excellence* and the only true followers of Hahnemann; while they denounce as "mongrels" and unworthy to be considered as true homoeopathists those who still obey Hahnemann's directions in preparing their medicines, in not exceeding the 30th dilution, in prescribing real medicines, and in being guided as much as possible by the totality of symptoms in the selection of remedies; in short, who comply with the teaching of Hahnemann as long as these were deduced from experiment and observation, though they may refuse assent to the hypothetical doctrines of his old age.

x "There can surely be no ground for doubting that, sooner or later, the pharmacologist will supply the physician with the means of affecting, in any desired sense, the functions of any physiological element of the body. It will, in short, become possible to introduce into the economy a molecular mechanism, which, like a very cunningly contrived torpedo, shall find its way to some particular group of living elements, and cause an explosion among them, leaving the rest untouched." These words of Professor Huxley in his address to the International Medical Congress, 1881, convey the idea of an eminent scientific authority as to the *desiderata* of scientific medicine. They exactly express what homoeopathy is doing, and has to a great extent fairly accomplished. It has supplied the physician with medicines whose mode of action on the organs and functions of the body he has experimentally ascertained, and enabled him to send a "molecular mechanism" to any spot in the organism where disease may be lurking, leaving all other parts and organs untouched. And yet neither old physic nor her scientific dry nurse perceive that homoeopathy has done for medicine what science requires. While they talk of the right way to be pursued by the medicine of the future they fail to take notice that this right way has been followed with success for more than two generations by the despised disciples of Hahnemann, whose methods they must pursue if they would place their art on the basis of scientific truth.

history of medicine may be ransacked in vain to find any figure at all comparable to him. He stands out in bold relief as the first, the only one who brought order into the chaos of therapeutics, who transformed medicine from a wild wilderness of hypothesis and caprice into a blooming, fruitful garden of regularity and beauty. It was not so much by intellectual greatness, it was not by superhuman intuition that he accomplished his great reform, it was by his innate love of truth and abhorrence of specious falsehood, by his firm resolve to accept nothing as true that did not stand the test of experiment, even though it were hallowed by the tradition of millenniums. And having once discovered the clue, he pursued it with a singleness of mind, with a self-sacrificing diligence that grudged no toil and shirked no pains, and was not to be diverted from its object by an promise of ease or honour, nor yet by the sneers of the heads or the persecution of the tail of the profession. The greatness of his aim, to relieve the sufferings of the fellow-man, was at once his stimulus and his reward. When he found that his efforts to perfect the medical art procured him only insult, calumny and persecution at the hands of his colleagues, he never condescended to reply to the hostile and unfair criticism that were passed upon his work, and he offered no resistance to the machinations of his foes, even when they sought to ruin him and deprive him of his means of earning his bread. Rather than sacrifice one jot or tittle of what he held to be necessary for the practice of his system in all its purity and integrity, he sacrificed himself. In his behaviour under persecution he displayed an antique heroism. He had his weaknesses and his faults, he would have been more than human if he had not. As Balzac well says: "Quelque grands que puissant être les grands homes connus ou inconnus, ils ont des petiteses par lesquelles ils tiennent à l'humanité." But his weaknesses only showed themselves in his old age, and during his exile and enforced solitude. He then became too prone to accept without sufficient examination any idea that occurred to himself or others that he fancied would contribute towards the development and perfection of his method. He grew intolerant of the criticism and opposition of his own disciples with regard to matters of minor importance. No such faults manifested themselves during his prime and when he lived in the world. They were the natural consequences of the harsh treatment of his colleagues, of his old age and enforced solitude, when he had ample time to brood over the vast importance of his discovery and the criminal folly of those who rejected it without enquiry, and sought to discredit its author by detraction, calumny and persecution. The wonder is, not that he manifested some irritation under these circumstances, but that he showed so little.

When the experience and observations of intelligent and impartial enquirers shall have purged his system of the adventitious and repulsive excrescences that have gathered about it, the great truths he taught will come out more conspicuously and clearly, and the united voice of the profession will acknowledge that the merit of having indicated a general rule for the curative employment of medicine in disease, and of having rendered the application of this rule possible by ascertaining the true powers and qualities of medicines, is Hahnemann's and Hahnemann's only. Hahnemann told us that the true rule of therapeutics is *similia similibus curentur* – let likes be treated by likes – when Hahnemann shall have obtained his true place in medicine, the actual practice of the medical world will be expressed by the words *similia similibus curantur* – likes are treated by likes.

References

1 Hahnemann, S. *Organon of Medicine* (trans Dudgeon, RE)., London, W.Headland 1849, (revised); Birkenhead. Hahnemann Publishing Society, 1893.
2 Hahnemann, S. *The Lesser Writings* (trans Dudgeon, RE), London, W.Headland 1852.
3 Hahnemann, S. *Materia Medica Pura*, Liverpool, Homoeopathic Publishing Society, 1880.
4 Hahnemann, S. *The Chronic Diseases, their Specific Nature and Homoeopathic Treatment*, 5 volumes (trans. Hempel, C.), New York, Radde, 1845.
5 Hahnemann, S. *The Chronic Diseases, their Specific Nature and Homoeopathic Treatment*, 4 volumes (trans. Hempel, C.), New York, Radde, 1846.
6 Hahnemann, S. (trans Tafel, LH), *The Chronic Diseases, their Specific Nature and Homoeopathic Treatment 2nd edition*, 4 volumes, Philadelphia, Boericke & Tafel, 1896.
7 Clarke JH, 1904, Obituary, Robert Ellis Dudgeon MD, *The British Journal of Homoeopathy*, October 1904.
8 Clarke, JH. *Odium Medicum – The Times Correspondence*. London; The Homoeopathic Publishing Company. 1888.
9 Dudgeon, RE. *Hahnemann, the Founder of Scientific Therapeutics Being the Third Hahnemannian Lecture*, London, E Gould & Son 1882.

11

HAHNEMANN'S WORK AND RESULTS

Introduction

A less controversial and less well-known scholar was Alfred Pope, a man of principle. His essay is thorough and careful, and one based on the logic of science. He shows that Hahnemann's work is based on observation, which is given as a reason for its endurance. The essay speaks for itself with clarity and there is no need for further commentary. Biographical material about Pope in the form of an obituary is there to reinforce the authority of the essay.

> **About Alfred Pope**[1]
> Alfred Crosby Pope was the eldest son of the Rev Alfred Pope, minister of Spencer Street Chapel, Leamington, and was born in that town on 11 September 1830. Educated at a private school in Leicester and at Mill Hill Grammar School, he commenced the study of medicine at the University of St Andrews in the winter session 1847–48, but in the summer of 1848 he proceeded to the University of Edinburgh, where he went through the usual curriculum, passing his intermediate in 1850 and going up for his final in 1851. At the latter there can be no doubt that Pope's answers were considered perfectly satisfactory by all his examiners until it became whispered about that he was interested in homoeopathy and meant to study it seriously! Then, although his examination was virtually over, he was heckled by Dr (afterwards Sir Robert) Christison, especially in the matter of dosage and his attitude towards homoeopathy; this was repeated with variations by Professor Syme, and the result was a foregone conclusion. Pope was asked to attend next day at 4 p.m., when there was to be an *extraordinary* meeting of the Medical Faculty; after the meeting terminated, instead of receiving his diploma of MD, Pope "was informed by Dr Balfour, the Dean of Faculty, that he was desired by the Medical Faculty to announce to me that they were not satisfied with my examination, and in the second place, that they were not satisfied with the line of practice I meant to adopt."[i]

---

i *British Journal of Homoeopathy*, 1850, 9. pp. 612 & 615.

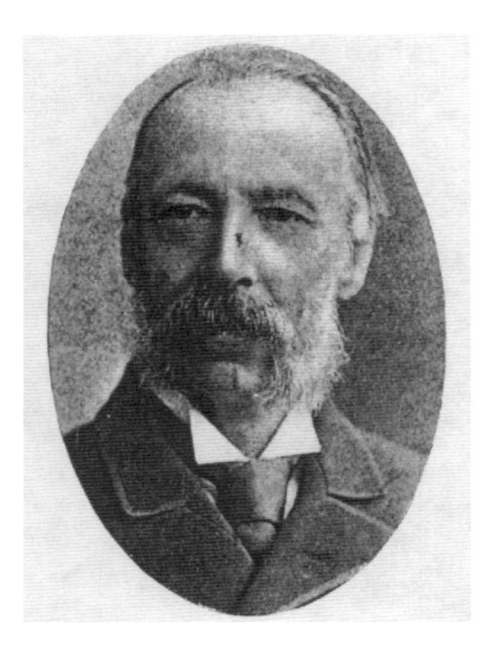

Figure 11.1 Alfred Pope (1830-1908)
Reproduced with permission of Homéopathe International & Dr Robert Séror.

In a word, the degree, which would have been granted without question to any other candidate, was refused, to the lasting shame of the University of Edinburgh. Bitterly as Pope was called upon to suffer in his own person for conscience' sake, he had the satisfaction before many years were over of seeing the celebrated amendment to the Medical Bill, with its special "clause for the protection of homoeopathists," brought forward and carried by Lord Ebury at the third reading of the Bill in the Upper House,[ii] and after having once more "run the gauntlet" in the Lower House, being finally placed upon the statute-book, where it remains to this day as the charter of our liberties. In 1852 the degree of M.D. was conferred upon Pope by the Hahnemann Medical College of Philadelphia, and in 1856 he became M.R.C.S. of Eng. Having married and settled in practice in York in 1859, Pope became a frequent contributor to the pages of the *Monthly Homoeopathic Review*, mostly in the shape of unsigned articles, and in April, 1865 he joined the editorial staff of the *Review*, his colleagues of that day being Dr John Ryan and Dr William Bayes. It is in his capacity as joint editor of the *Review* that Dr Pope will be best remembered by the present generation of homoeopathists, and a list of his unsigned articles contributed to the pages of the *Review* during an editorship extending over more than forty years would be a compendium of the history of homoeopathy in Britain during that period.

---

ii Vide leading article on The Medical Act, *British Journal of Homoeopathy*, 1857, 16. p. 29.

Pope joined the British Homoeopathic Society in 1862, was elected Vice-President in 1873 and 1874, and President in 1881. In 1880 he was appointed Lecturer on Materia Medica to the London School of Homoeopathy.

Many of the lectures there delivered were from time to time published in the pages of the *Monthly Homoeopathic Review*, and afford to this day some of the best reading in materia medica of which our school can boast. The pity is that they have never been republished in book-form.

Pope was Vice-President of the International Homoeopathic Convention held in London in 1881, and at the Leeds Congress of 1895 he was chosen by an overwhelming majority as President of the International Homoeopathic Congress to be held in London in 1896

Although Pope's health had been failing for years, the end came unexpectedly, for he was out for his usual drive within an hour of his death. The end was speedy and painless.

Hahnemann: his work and its results[2]
By Alfred Pope 1830-1908

We assemble here to-day to recall, once more, the memory of "a man of genius and a scholar" - of a physician who, during the final decade of the last and the earlier years of the present century, originated, conducted, and ultimately accomplished a work, the influence of which is felt, the results of which may be seen wherever the science of medicine is studied or the art thereof is practised.

The teaching of Hahnemann was both negative and positive. While, on the one hand, it was iconoclastic, on the other it was reconstructive. At a time when the necessity for what were termed heroic measures, venesection, mercurialism and purgation, more especially, was almost undisputed throughout the profession, and was accepted as inevitable with the most implicit faith by the public, Hahnemann asserted, and, what is much more to the purpose, demonstrated their worthlessness as curative agencies, and the positive danger to human life involved in the use of them. That the conclusions he arrived at and urged upon the attention of his professional brethren were sound, the rusty state of the surgeon's lancet at the present time, and the complete abandonment of the art of cupping as a source of livelihood, the rarity with which the induction of salivation is advised in acute disease, and the comparative infrequency with which an active purgative is prescribed under similar circumstances, afford abundant evidence. In short, well nigh everything which he denounced, in the therapeutics of his day, as being worse than useless for the purpose of cure, is repudiated on the same ground by the physicians of our own time.

The teaching Hahnemann, however, was, as I have said, not simply negative, it was also positive. While seeking to destroy such therapeutic methods as were injurious he was no less industrious in endeavouring to design and build up such as gave proof of being salutary. His efforts as a great teacher of medicine were not restricted to the eradication of error; they were, with even greater ingenuity, earnestness, and persistency, devoted to the planting of truth.

It is to this the positive side of Hahnemann's work, and to the results which have flowed, and are still flowing from it, that I propose, as I trace the leading events of his life, to draw your attention this afternoon.

Christian Friedrich Samuel Hahnemann was the son of a poor man, earning a small and precarious living by painting on porcelain for the proprietors of the celebrated Meissen Works, in the Kingdom of Saxony. In the town of Meissen he was born, either on the 10th or 11th or April, 1755 – tradition says it was the former – the parish register, I understand, testifies to its being the latter date. From his earliest years his education was the object of his parents' most zealous care. For the acquisition of knowledge of every kind, especially for such as is linguistic, his capacity might fairly be deemed precocious; no language, indeed, whether ancient or modern, seemed to come amiss to him. So great had been his diligence, that, when at the age of twenty he passed from the Grammar School of his native town to enter upon the study of medicine at the University of Leipzig, he was not only a well matured classical scholar, familiar with Greek and Roman literature, but also with the still more recondite Arabic and Hebrew; and likewise with the modern tongues of England, France and Spain. A sum of twenty thalers was all the money his father was able to bestow upon him when he left his roof, and it was by teaching ancient and modern languages, and by translating, into his native German, books written in them, that he was enabled to provide himself with the necessaries of life while at the University.

After two years of hard work at Leipzig, Hahnemann entered at the University of Vienna. At the conclusion of an *annus medicus* at this renowned seat of medical learning, he accepted the post of physician and librarian to the Governor of Transylvania at Hermanstadt. It was during his stay here, that he gained that deep insight into the phenomena of intermittent fever, which stood him in such good stead in after years. In 1779 he graduated at the University of Erlangen, whither he was attracted by the low scale of frees demanded of a student on proceeding to a degree. He now received the appointment of medical officer of health at Gommern; and, having occupied it for a couple of years, he removed to Dresden. Here he formed an intimate friendship with Dr Wagner, then one of the leading hospital surgeons of the day. It is not a little significant of the impression his professional attainments at this time had made upon the minds of Dr Wagner and his colleagues, that Hahnemann was selected to perform the hospital duties of his friend during the time when a long illness precluded him from undertaking them.

Research and literary work ever continued to occupy a large share of his attention. The most important of his contributions to medical literature at this period being his celebrated essay *On Arsenical Poisoning* – a work which remained for many years the chief authority on the subject of which it treated, one which Sir Robert Christison, in his *Treatise on Poisons* published nearly fifty years afterwards, styled "elaborate," and one from which he quoted repeatedly. Ample evidence this of the thoroughness of his investigations, the soundness of his conclusions, and the importance attached to his work by those best qualified to judge of its merits.

Thus when the year 1790 opened, Hahnemann had been a constant student of ancient and modern medical literature for fully fifteen years; he had enjoyed the advantage of listening to the teaching and observing the practice of some of the most eminent physicians and surgeons of his generation in Leipzig, Vienna and Dresden. During twelve of these years he had diligently made use of extensive opportunities for applying the touchstone of experiment to the results of all this study and observation. This all decisive test, the test of clinical experiment, the only test of any moment in estimating the value of therapeutic methods, forced upon him the conclusion that the principles of drug prescribing which then dominated the practice of medicine were, in their results, generally useless, in many others injurious, and in all uncertain. At this time he had arrived at precisely the same point as that reached by the late Sir John Forbes, in 1846, when in his celebrated article *Allopathy, Homoeopathy, and Young Physic*,[iii] he uttered his conviction that in "the condition of physic," "things have arrived at such a pitch that they cannot be worse. They must mend or end," and, he added, "we believe they will mend." Hahnemann, indeed, saw no prospect of any mending, and resolved at once that, so far as he was concerned, they should "end." He declined the responsibility of any longer prescribing mixtures of drugs of doubtful vale and uncertain effects to persons suffering from severe disease. To practise medicine without prescribing drugs, at a time when no one so much as dreamed of the art of nursing ever superseding that of medicine-giving, was impossible; to order *Placebos* did not comport with his ideas of honesty; to look upon drugs as "mere aids to faith in the weary time," after the manner of Dr Moxon, was, from his point of view, not only untrue, but treating a most serious matter as a burlesque. Hahnemann believed in the power of drugs. He felt that when given they could not fail of doing evil, if no advantage was derived from their being taken. In his letter to Hufeland, *On the Great Necessity for a Regeneration in Medicine* (Lesser Writings, p. 581), published in 1808 – a letter which forms a kind of *apologia pro*

[iii] Forbes, J, ed., *British and Foreign Medical Review*, or *Quarterly Journal of Practical medicine and Surgery*, Vol xli. 1846,

suâ vitâ during the previous eighteen years – he gives his expression to this conviction in the following terms:-

> "To become," he writes "in this way" – that is, as he puts it in a previous passage, to treat his "suffering fellow-creatures with unknown medicines," – unknown because they are "the subject of numbers of contradictory opinions that have been repeatedly refuted by experience;" "with unknown medicines which being powerful substances, may, if not exactly suitable, easily change life into death, or produce new effects and chronic ailments, which are often much more difficult to remove than the original disease. To become, in this way, a murderer or aggravator of the sufferings of mankind was, to me, a fearful thought – so fearful and distressing was it, that, shortly after my marriage, I completely abandoned practice, and scarcely treated anyone for fear of doing him harm, and, as you know, occupied myself solely with chemistry and literary labours."

With such materials as, alone, were within his reach, Hahnemann then refused any longer to attempt to relieve suffering or to cure disease. He betook himself to the study of chemistry, a science in the investigation of which his numerous and valuable contributions to Crell's *Annalen* prove him to have been one of the most proficient workers of his time, and furthermore he laboured hard at the translation of medical works for the Leipzig booksellers.

In a frame of mind eminently calculated to appreciate and sympathise with the opening chapter of Cullen's celebrated *Treatise of the Materia Medica* – the chapter entitled *The History of the Materia Medica, with some account of the Chief Writers upon it* – this classical work was placed in his hands to be rendered into German.

In the brilliant address delivered here four years ago on an occasion similar to the present, Dr Burnett referred to the influence which the study of Cullen had had upon the mind of Hahnemann, at this stage of his history, as being greater than is generally supposed. Here I am sure that Dr Burnett is right. There was much in common between the Scotch Professor and his German translator. Both were intimately acquainted with the past, and the then recent medical literature of all countries. Both were fully convinced of the unsound basis upon which the supposed knowledge of the actions and uses of drugs rested. Both were dissatisfied with the methods employed to acquire a more accurate knowledge of the actions of drugs. And yet, again, both were vitalists, both regarded a vital principle as that through which drugs operated upon the body.[iv] On the practical method necessary to render the employment of drugs safe and useful, however, their views differed, and that widely.

Cullen regarded the mode of studying Materia Medica as capable of being mended. Hahnemann, on the other hand, felt that it must undergo an entire

---

iv Cullen WA, *A Treatise of the Materia Medica*. Edinburgh, C Elliott, 1789, vol.1, p. 59.

change. Cullen looked upon the general indications of disease as being all-sufficient for directing the prescription of drugs. Hahnemann saw, in such a trust, the origin of many of the most disastrous results of the practice of medicine as he found it. Hence it arose that Cullen, though far more precise and critical than his predecessors in the study of that department of medicine of which he was, during nearly half a century, the leading authority in Great Britain, kept to the old lines, classifying drugs according to their crude qualities as astringents, tonics, emollients, corrosives, stimulants, sedatives and the like; and leaving the physician to select his remedy or remedies from one or other of these classes, according as the prevailing pathological theory might suggest. Herein Hahnemann saw merely a perpetuation of the old sources of error, the old causes of therapeutic failure. From these he had, by his retirement from practice, cut himself adrift for all time. That he had done so he makes abundantly clear in a foot note which he appends, in his translation of Cullen's *Materia Medica*, to an expression, on the part of the author, of a fear that public opinion might be offended by his disparagement of ancient writers. In this note Hahnemann, after declaring his complete sympathy with Cullen on this point, says, "We must tear ourselves away by very force from these worshipped authorities, if we, in this important part of practical medicine, are ever to be able to cast off the yoke of ignorance and superstition. It is," he adds, "high time that we did."

An attempt on the part of Cullen to explain the curative power of *cinchona bark* in intermittent fever by its tonic action on the stomach, suggested a fallacy to the mind of Hahnemann. This supposed explanation remind me not a little of a similar effort made a few years ago to interpret the *modus operandi* of *Ipecacuanha* in the cure of some cases of vomiting, by imagining it to exert a tonic influence upon the sympathetic system generally. Cullen set forth his view in the following sentence:–

> "We proceed therefore upon the supposition that the bark possesses a tonic power, and that the action of this power in the stomach sufficiently explains its operation in preventing the recurrence of the paroxysms of intermittent fever: for I see no foundation" he adds, "for referring it to any mysterious and unexplained specific power; which, however, some writers seem still disposed to maintain."

In reply to this Hahnemann wrote:–

> "By uniting the strongest bitters with the strongest astringents, you may get a compound that, in a small dose, shall possess much more of both qualities than the *bark*; yet you will never, in all eternity, obtain a fever specific from such a compound."

The error in Cullen's hypothesis confirmed Hahnemann in his opinion that the action of bark in intermittent fever was specific, that there existed, between the *bark* and the fever, some relation which did not exist between it and other so-called vegetable tonics. To solve the nature of this relation was now the question before him. How could he, how could anyone, know what the natural action of a drug was, save by taking it when in health? He could see no other method. Haller and Stoerck had endeavoured to study the action of drugs in a similar manner, but their researches had proved fruitless. Nothing daunted by their failure, Hahnemann, whose experience in intermittent fever in the Hungarian marshes had rendered him thoroughly familiar with its various phases, proceeded to dose himself with the *bark*. As he did so he found some of the more marked subjective phenomena of the disease, he knew so well, arise in his own person. Then occurred to him the enquiry, did the doctrine that some diseases are best cured by similars – set forth by Hippocrates two thousand years before, noted now and again by more than one medical author during the ages that followed, deliberately expressed by Stahl early in the then rapidly expiring century and still more recently suggested once again by Stoerck – did this doctrine supply the means of solving the nature of the relations subsisting between specific remedies and the cases of disease they cured? Did it suffice to explain the recoveries, here and there, recorded in medical literature, and distinctly traceable to the use of one or other drug? Was this the bond that in the future was to unite the study of drug action and the investigation of disease? Was this the missing link which was to make the then separate chains of pathology and therapeutics one and undivided in the time to come? This was the kind of question which Hahnemann, in 1790, set himself to answer.

Ere any distinct conclusion, worthy of publication to the profession, could be arrived at, a large amount of research had to be gone though; and not a few, but *au contraire*, a very considerable number of experiments had to be performed – and that on himself. Hence it was not until six years later that in the essay entitled, *On a New Principle for Ascertaining the Curative Power of Drugs*[v3] Hahnemann gave to the profession – through Hufeland's *Journal* – his mature conviction that the principle which lay at the root of successful drug selection was that expressed by the formula *similia similibus curentur*. During these six years, as the light dawned upon him, as experiment and research gradually convinced him that he was on the right track, he resumed the practice of his profession, and, as his references to cases in his subsequent papers show, he did so with encouraging success. After an exhaustive and utterly destructive criticism of the measures previously made use of to ascertain the remedial properties of drugs, Hahnemann arrived at the following conclusion:–

> "If I mistake not," he says, "practical medicine has devised three ways of applying remedies for the relief of the disorders of the human body.
>
> "The *first way to remove or destroy the fundamental cause of the disease*, was the most elevated it could follow. All the imaginings and aspirations of the best physicians in all ages were directed to this object – the most worthy of the dignity of our art."

---

v Hahnemann S, *Lesser Writings* (trans Dudgeon RE). London: W Headland, 1851; p. 295.

And, again, he describes the removal or destruction of the fundamental cause of disease as an "object above all criticism, though the means employed were not always the fittest for attaining it." The prevention or destruction of the fundamental causes of disease has, in our day risen into a distinct department, and that one of the greatest importance and public utility. It has advanced just in proportion as the sciences of chemistry, physiology, and pathology on the one hand, and of geology, mechanics, and engineering have progressed on the other. The imperfections of these branches of knowledge, when Hahnemann lived, rendered what we now understand as preventive medicine impossible. At the same time, it is interesting to note how fully alive he was to its importance.

He next describes the method which seeks to remove the symptoms present, by medicines which produce an opposite condition, e.g., constipation by purgatives, &c.

He refers to the *third way* in which remedies have from time to time been sought for chronic diseases, and acute diseases tending to chronic, which should not cloak the symptoms, but which should remove the disease radically, in one word, for specific remedies - the most desirable, most praiseworthy undertaking that can be imagined. Thus, for instance, they tried *arnica* for dysentery and in some instances found it a useful specific.

"But what guided them?" he adds. "What principle induced them to try such remedies? Alas! only a precedent from the empirical game of hazard, from domestic practice, chance cases in which these substances were accidentally found useful in this or that disease, often only in peculiar unmentioned combinations, which might perhaps never again occur, sometimes in pure simple diseases.

"It were deplorable, indeed," he continues, 'if only chance and empirical *apropos* could be considered as our guides in the discovery and application of the proper - the true - remedies for chronic diseases, which certainly constitute the major portion of human ills."

Such being the position in which Hahnemann found the so-called specific remedies of his time, his next business was, if possible, to ascertain how their true action might be discovered. He proceeds as follows:-

"In order to ascertain the actions of remedial agents for the purpose of applying them to the relief of human suffering, we should trust as little as possible to chance, but go to work as rationally and as methodically as possible. We have seen that for this object the aid of chemistry is still imperfect, and must only be resorted to with caution; that the similarity of *genera* of plants in the natural system; as also the similarity of species of one *genus* give but obscure hints; that the sensible properties teach us mere generalities, and these invalidate by many exceptions; that the changes that take place in the blood from the admixture of medicines teach nothing; and that the injection of the latter into the blood-vessels of animals, as also the effects on animals to which medicines have been administered, is much too rude a mode of proceeding to enable us therefrom to judge of the finer actions of remedies. Nothing then remains but to test the medicines we wish to investigate on the human body itself."

He then proceeds to show that the testing of medicines on the human body had, in all ages, been recognised as essential to the understanding of their action, but that this testing had hitherto been pursued in a false way – viz., on the sick.

He next argues that, in order that any real progress may occur in therapeutics, two questions must be answered: "*First*, what is the pure action of each (drug) by itself on the human body? *Secondly*, what do observations of its action in this or that simple disease teach us?"

The answer given by Hahnemann to the second of these enquiries is that which chiefly concerns us at the moment. He tells us that the requisite material is "partly obtained in the practical writings of the best observers, of all ages, but more especially of later times. Throughout these, the as yet only source of knowledge of the powers of drugs in disease is scattered; there we find it faithfully related how the simplest drugs were employed in accurately described diseases, how far they proved serviceable, and how far they were hurtful or less beneficial."[vi]

A standard which will enable us to judge of the truth and value of such observations "can," he presently observes, "only be derived from the effects that a given medicinal substance has by itself in this and that dose developed in the healthy human body."[vii] (*Ibid*, 311.)

He then asserts that the principle which such observations foreshadow and lead up to, is contained in the following axioms:-

> "Every powerful medicinal substance produces in the human body a kind of peculiar disease; the more powerful the medicine, the more peculiar marked and violent the disease.

> "We should imitate nature, which sometimes cures a chronic disease by superadding another, and employ in the (especially chronic) disease we wish to cure that medicine which is able to produce another very similar artificial disease, and the former will be cured – *similia similibus*."

I would in passing note here, that on this, the first occasion on which Hahnemann distinctly formulated the principle of *similars*, he at the same time offered a hypothetical explanation of it – one to which in his later years he declared that he attached no value – and one, I may add, that has never met with much, if any, acceptance, from any one.

This essay discloses very fully the mode of study, and the line of thought arising out of it, which led Hahnemann to those therapeutic conclusions with which his name will be for ever associated.

---

vi Hahnemann S, 1851, *op. cit*, p. 310.
vii *Ibid*, p. 311.

Observe, in the first place, that the principle of drug selection, which was to form the basis of prescribing, was derived from an investigation of recorded instances of drug action on healthy human beings, as seen inter alia in poisonings, and these were compared with histories of cases and diseases which the same drugs had been observed to cure.

Secondly, – While by this method of enquiry Hahnemann aimed at the discovery of *specifics*, it was not specifics for generic forms of disease, but specifics for individual cases of generic forms of disease, that he hoped to obtain.

On this very important point he thus expresses himself:

> "Now when I entirely deny that there are any absolute specifics for individual diseases in their full extent, as they are described in ordinary works on pathology, I am, on the other hand, convinced that there are as many specifics as there are different states of individual diseases, i.e., that there are peculiar specifics for the pure disease, and others for its varieties, and for other abnormal states of the system."[viii]

Then, *lastly*, throughout this essay, the appropriate dose of a medicine selected on this principle is described as moderate or small – as one in which the drug "could not perceptibly develop the same phenomena;" but, save in illustrative cases, its size is nowhere expressly defined, neither is there any idea of a uniform dose for all drugs suggested.

In the course of the following year, in an essay published in the same journal, he urged the employment of only one medicine at a time, and earnestly protested against prescriptions directing the concoction of mixtures containing a variety of ingredients. "The more complex our receipts," he says, "the more obscure will it be in medicine."[ix] – Again, in 1800, in a preface to a translation by him of a *Thesaurus Medicaminum*, the author of which was a member of the London College of Physicians, he enforced the same principle.

During these ten years, while collecting the materials for and publishing the essays I have quoted from, Hahnemann resided for a time in the neighbourhood of Leipzig, and for a period had charge of a lunatic asylum at Georgenthal, in the Thuringian Forest, when the recovery, while under his care, of Klockenbring, a celebrated Prussian statesman, excited considerable attention throughout Germany. He afterwards lived for a short while in one or two small German towns, ultimately settling in Königsglutter about the year 1797. By this time his therapeutic views had, as I have shown, taken a definite shape. He now felt himself on ground sure and safe when prescribing, and once again entered heartily into the practice of his profession. His success excited the jealousy of his medical neighbours, and as each prescription contained but one medicine, and that in a very small dose, a perfect uproar was created among the apothecaries of the place, who

---

viii *Ibid*, p. 306.
ix *Ibid*, 371.

felt, and not unreasonably, that their craft was in danger. Ultimately, he found it impossible to entrust the members of the Apothecaries Guild with the dispensing of his prescriptions, and in self-defence was compelled to prepare them himself. This was illegal; and he sought, by giving his medicines gratuitously, to bring himself within the letter of the absurd German law which, by prohibiting the physician from dispensing, placed him and his patients at the mercy of the druggist. At the instance of his professional brethren, the Guild of Apothecaries prosecuted him for doing so, and succeeded in their action. Had Hahnemann been content to bow the knee at the shrine of the pestle and mortar, he might have resumed practice and doubtless have fared well. He, however, was not made of the right material for a compromise of that or of any other kind which called upon him to sacrifice one jot or tittle of what he believed to be true; what he was convinced was essential for the recovery and safety of the sick. Deeply regretted by a large proportion of the inhabitants of the town, he left it, only to find himself exposed to precisely similar treatment at the hands of the druggists in the several towns in which he attempted to reside between 1799 and 1810, when he returned to Leipzig, whence, after a brilliant career of twelve or thirteen years, he was again obliged to sacrifice himself rather than submit to the demands of the same trade element.

During the years of weary wanderings that passed, between his expulsion from Königsglutter and his return to Leipzig, Hahnemann was chiefly engaged in making researches into the recorded effects of drugs, and performing experiments with them, not upon cats and dogs, not vicariously, but upon himself. The object of these experiments was to discover the indications given by medicines of the disturbing influences they exerted upon the functions of the body – the human body. During this period he published, together with several others, two very remarkable essays; one entitled *Æsculapius in the Balance*, and the other *The Medicine of Experience*. Both appeared in Hufeland's *Journal*.

In the latter portion of the former he delivered himself of a powerful argument against the dispensing of medicines being restricted by law to the members of the Apothecaries' Guild – the chemists and druggists of Germany. He pointed out, and that in a very striking manner, that the results of such legislation had proved it to be detrimental to science, degrading to the physician, and injurious to the sick; and that so far from being to the advantage of the public, it had but one purpose, one end – the enrichment of the apothecary.

In his *Medicine of Experience* he still further elaborated his therapeutic method. This essay formed the groundwork of his well known – albeit little understood, and consequently much misrepresented – *Organon der Heilkunst*, published in 1810.

Hahnemann had been repeatedly charged with and blamed for having in these two essays, and in all his subsequent writings, alluded to his professional brethren who differed from him in terms of bitterness and intolerance; in language which, it is said, nothing could justify. Is this true? Remember, it is impossible to allege anything of the kind against Hahnemann prior to the appearance of these essays. That in them and in later papers he did asperse the motives and denounce the methods of practice of the medical men and medical writers around him in words and tones that nothing could justify us in adopting nowadays, is true enough; but recollect that from 1799, and onwards to the end of his life, he was, through the influence of his professional brethren, made the victim of a relentless persecution, both material and moral; through their influence, during twenty years and more, he was repeatedly prevented from practising his profession; was driven from town to town in search of a livelihood; by them he was, during the last forty years of his life, studiously and grossly misrepresented, not only in doctrine, but in motive, and held up to public scorn and infamy in all the medical periodicals of his country, and in scores of pamphlets besides. Think of this, and while doing so, reflect upon its cause – the demonstration, after long years of patient investigation and experiment, of a mode of enquiry into the action of drugs and a method of using them in disease, which not one of those who harassed him professionally and opposed him in the press ever attempted to examine, much less practically test – and then tell me who there was who ever lived, who is there living now, who, having undergone such outrageous treatment as this, would have written and spoken regarding the authors of it otherwise than Hahnemann wrote and spoke of them?

It is very easy – a very simple process indeed – for us to sit at home in comparative ease, no one daring to interfere with our teaching and mode of practice, and describe Hahnemann's counter attacks upon the members of his own profession as highly improper, very indecorous, and so on; but, at the same time, it is nothing less than unjust so to do.

Before anyone presumes to cast a stone at Hahnemann on this score let him first of all ask himself how he would have felt; how he would have expressed himself; how he would have acted, had he been called upon to endure what Hahnemann endured!

Hahnemann may have erred – I hope that he did err, and at this distance of time can believe that he was mistaken in the estimate he formed of the motives of his medical brethren – but had he, treated by them as he was, regarded these motives as other than he did would have been something more than human.

The year 1810 saw Hahnemann once more in Leipzig. Hither he came not merely to practise the art of medicine but to teach the science and art of therapeutics. His chief desire, the coping stone of his ambition, was to attain a position from which he might communicate to his professional brethren the lessons he had learned during the preceding twenty years. It was no sudden fancy, no crude theory, no untested method that he had to lay before them, but the outcome of twenty years of reading and experiment – twenty years of reflection and clinical experience with which he was anxious to indoctrinate them.

The study of the action of drugs by the light of experiments on the healthy. The clinical application of drugs directed by the principle of similars. The prescribing of medicines so administered in small doses – in doses which would not perceptibly develop the same phenomena. The exhibition of medicines singly, uncombined with any others. These were the views which, after twenty years of diligent enquiry, Hahnemann felt convinced lay at the root of all successful therapeutics. These were the views he so earnestly desired to teach.

Further, these views represent the whole of what we now describe by the word homoeopathy. In after years, as his experience expanded, as his observations multiplied, they were expressed in more minute detail; his directions for conducting experiments with drugs were more carefully precisionised; his instructions for the examination of patients and the selection of the most completely similar remedy were rendered more fully and more exactly; the measurement of the dose, which he esteemed the safest and most efficient, was in later years stated more categorically than it was at any time prior to his return to Leipzig. While these alterations in detail, or rather I should say developments, were in progress, his first principles, those which formed the foundation of Hahnemann's method, never changed. Homoeopathy remained the basis of his teaching until the day of his death, forty-three years later. Aye, and the therapeutic principles enunciated by Hahnemann at the close of the last century are the therapeutic principles of those who to-day are prepared to acknowledge that to the best of their powers they openly and undisguisedly treat disease homoeopathically. The experience of the last ninety years has taught us much, very much, in matters of detail; it has added immensely to our knowledge concerning the action of drugs; it has done a great deal to facilitate our selection of them in disease; it has shown us that in posology Hahnemann was needlessly minute, and that his dogmatism thereon was a mistake. But, in his definition of the fundamental principle of therapeutics, this same experience has abundantly proved that Hahnemann was right; that one better calculated to help the physician in controlling disease has been so much as proposed.

For a medical doctrine – and above all a therapeutic doctrine – to endure without any change, save in minor matters of detail, and not only so but to be ever taking deeper root, ever spreading wider and yet more widely during early a century is, in these times, when fashion is a power in medicine, when hypothesis succeeds hypothesis with marvelous rapidity, when the medicine which is confidently prescribed in a large number of cases during one year, is all but forgotten during that which follows, – such endurance I contend is strong evidence of its truth.

What, we may well ask, is the cause of this endurance – whence comes so much vitality? Its cause is to be found in the fact that Hahnemann's teaching was based upon experiment. He appealed to nature for his information, not to his imagination. He recognised experience, as Herschell says, as "the fountain of all our knowledge of nature," as the "only ground of all physical enquiry." He appealed to facts in the first instance, and then, not to hypothesis, not to theory, but to a strictly logical deduction from them. His work was not performed hastily: Hahnemann knew how "to labour and to wait." Six years elapsed ere he published a part of his conclusions, and ten had nearly sped their course before he felt himself justified in communicating the principles of his entire method to his professional brethren.

In 1810, as I have said, Hahnemann settled in Leipzig, not only to practise medicine but to teach it. That he might do so in a legal manner it was necessary that he should obtain the rank of *Privat Docent* at the University. To do so, it was required that he should defend a thesis before the Medical Faculty. Doubtless, those who in Leipzig were opposed to his views, thought that he would fall before a trial of intellectual strength with the learned members of the Medical Faculty of their University. If so, bitter and great indeed was the stock of disappointment that lay in store for them!

The thesis that Hahnemann prepared and defended was entitled *De Helleborismo Veterum*.[x] In it he described the ancient mode of using *hellebore* in the treatment of chronic disease, discussing a variety of questions arising out of this therapeutic method in a manner which renders the entire essay one of the most remarkable exhibitions of genuine scholarship in the whole range of modern medical literature. One of the most thorough scholars of his time, a friend of the late Professor Henderson, of Edinburgh, described it as "remarkable for the display of extensive reading in the ancient authors, and not only those immediately connected with his own professional pursuits, but also in the classical writers of antiquity," and familiar as this gentlemen was with the most learned physicians of Europe, he added: "I know very few medical men possessed of the same amount of learning".[xi]

"This Thesis" Dr Dudgeon informs us,[xii] he defended on the 12th June, 1812. "It drew," he adds, "from his adversaries an unwilling acknowledgement of his learning and his genius, and from the impartial and worthy Dean of the Faculty a strong expression of his admiration."

When I read this remarkable production, admire the marvelous acuteness of its criticism, the logical precision of its argument, and reflect upon the vast extent of research, the close study of the almost countless folios its preparation must have involved, together with the intimate acquaintance with Roman, Greek, and

---

   x Hahnemann S, 1851, op. cit.

   xi Henderson, W, *Homoeopathy fairly represented. A reply to Professor Simpson's Homoeopathy misrepresented*, Philadelphia; Lindsay & Blakiston, 1854. p. 138.

   xii Dudgeon RE, *Lectures on the Theory and Practice of Homoeopathy*, London: Henry Turner, 1853, p. 32.

Arabian writers its author displays throughout its pages, and then turn to the estimate formed of him by the puny and superficial critics, the shallow-pated pamphleteers and other blind guides of professional opinion during the last thirty or forty years, and see him held up by them as a laughing-stock to the profession and the public, described as a quack, and represented as being well-nigh everything that is infamous – language fails me wherewith I might adequately express my feeling of contempt for his detractors.

Having become a *Privat-Docent*, Hahnemann commenced to lecture on the science and art of medicine. Here at last he was in his right position; here he was, emphatically, the right man in the right place.

Many physicians and students of medicine from different parts of Germany attended his lectures. From among those of them who appeared to him to be most competent and trustworthy he selected his associates in the series of pharmacological experiments in which he was engaged. During his residence here he published the results of these experiments in his *Materia Medica Pura* – a *Materia Medica* which was pure in the sense that it was simple relation of observations of fact; pure in the sense that it was all free from hypothesis.

Once again, however, this "man of genius and scholar," as Sir John Forbes so aptly called him, was compelled to break up his home, to sever his connection with the University with which he was associated, and to depart out of the city he loved so well – and all this at the bidding, and in order to preserve intact the commercial interest of its drug-dealers. His large and constantly increasing practice, together with the numerous disciples he was making, excited the envy and jealousy of his professional neighbours, and by them the Apothecaries' Guild was again induced to prosecute him – as they had elsewhere done aforetime – for giving medicine to his patients. Their cause succeeded; and being prevented from practising in the only way in which he felt that he could practise with any justice to himself or advantage to those who sought his advice, he left Leipzig never to re-enter it. The Duke of Anhalt-Köthen, a warmly attached friend of Hahnemann, invited him to reside in the capital of his limited dominions, gave him the rank of Hofrath (Councillor), and appointed him his physician. To Köthen, then, he removed, and there for fourteen years he lived, studied, wrote and practised; and there he was, during this time, visited professionally by large numbers of invalids from all parts of Europe. In 1835, he married a second time, and responding to the entreaties of his wife removed to Paris, where he speedily found himself the centre of a large consultation practice. Here he died in 1843, at the age of 87.

In looking back over a career so long, so laborious, so active, and so eventful as Hahnemann's, who can hesitate to regard it as a grand one? Grand in its object – the perfecting of the art of healing. Grand in the learning and self sacrifice brought to bear upon the attainment of this object. Grand in its utter contempt for the obstacles placed in the way of its pursuit. Grand in the unwearying energy which characterised it throughout. And, above all grand in the stainless honesty which rendered him proof against any and every temptation to deviate, by so much as a hair's breadth, from a course traced out by painful experiment and deep and constant thought; a course, the truth and value of which was deeply engraven upon his conscience by clinical observation – one entered upon and adhered to from as pure a sense of duty as ever animated a martyr.

Yes, Hahnemann's was a grand career. The more the events which marked it progress are known, the more the doctrine he taught is studied and clinically tested, the more conspicuous will his true greatness appear. "His name" wrote Sir John Forbes, "will descend to posterity as the exclusive excogitator and founder of an original system of medicine as ingenious as many that preceded it, and destine probably to be the remote, if not the immediate cause of more important fundamental changes in the practice of the healing art than have resulted from any promulgated since the days of Galen." (*Brit. And For. Med. Rev.*, xli.)

These prophetic words have already been partially fulfilled; and if therapeutics is ever to become a true science, if the art which is to grow out of it is ever to become safe and useful, they will be far more than fulfilled in the future.

The work which Hahnemann took in hand – that to which his whole life was dedicated, that from the prosecution of which neither the sure prospect of professional advancement (would he but consent even to appear *stare super antiquas vias*) nor the most relentless persecution could make him swerve – was the laying the foundations of the science of pharmacology – "the science of the action of remedies;" that which the *Lancet* the other day defines as one "which deals with the modifications produced in healthy conditions by the operation of substances capable of producing modifications" (*Lancet*, Aug. 16, 1884.) Aye, and he went further than this. He built upon these foundations. He bridged over "that wide and deep gulf which" (we have been lately told) "has always been fixed" "between the pharmacologist labouring to elucidate the mysteries of the subtle actions of drugs upon the complicated and intricate human organism, and the therapeutist struggling to apply these results to the successful treatment of disease." The writer of the article in the *British Medical Journal* (Aug. 9th, 1884) from which this sentence is quoted, proceeds to say: "We believe, however, that signs are not altogether wanting which lead us to see that this gulf is beginning to fill in, and that, in the not very remote future, it will be successfully bridged over." Gentlemen, this gulf has been spanned: the bridge which crosses it has stood for well nigh a century! When nearly ninety years ago Hahnemann proved that it was the similarity between the action of a drug and the nature of the morbid process constituting individual disease, as revealed by the symptoms arising from the administration of the one and marking the occurrence of the other, as being the relationship between the two that could alone direct the therapeutist how to avail himself of the labours of the pharmacologist, *he constructed this bridge!* From that day to this, direct evidence has been constantly accumulating in all parts of the world that its foundations were well and truly laid, and that the erection they supported was substantially and firmly built.

In more recent times this direct evidence has been largely supplemented by such as is indirect. Physicians there are who would fain persuade us that there is no general principle which can guide us in the treatment of disease, who (as did a distinguished pathologist and popular clinical teacher a couple of years back at the College of Physicians) assure us, with much apparent confidence, that the notion that there is any medical doctrine in reference to therapeutics is "a device of the enemy" – and yet their daily practice, a goodly proportion of their every day prescriptions, bears testimony to the fact tat the bridge – the medical doctrine by which Hahnemann united the labours of the pharmacologist and those of the therapeutist – is no mere phantom, but a stern reality, a reality of the deepest interest to the physician, of the greatest importance to the patient.

"I believe," said Dr Burney Yeo, at King's College, a few weeks ago (*Med. Times*, May 17th, 1884), "I believe that the homoeopathists have, in many instances, called attention to the value of drugs which had been too much neglected." This sentence is a distinct testimony to the truth of the principles taught by Hahnemann. It affords striking, albeit most unintentional, evidence that there is doctrine in reference to therapeutics. Were it otherwise, how could the homoeopathists have been attention to the value of these drugs? Beyond the method of Hahnemann they had no means of ascertaining the therapeutic value of drugs, which was not within the range of the knowledge possessed by the bulk of the profession.

Yes; homoeopathists have called attention to the value of drugs which had been too much neglected; and they have been able to do so simply because they studied the physiological effects of these drugs – *more Hahnemanni* – and applied them in practice in the treatment of disease as the law of similars dictated.

Then again, who, but through the hint supplied by this principle would, on studying the physiological effects of *arsenic*, have inferred its power over cholera? Who, knowing the kind of influence excited in the bowels by *corrosive sublimate* would, but for this principle, have though of giving such a drug in dysentery? Who for any reason, save this, would have suggested that *Ipecacuanha* would prove a remedy in vomiting, or *Camomile tea* in infantile diarrhœa? What but a thorough consciousness – silent and unexpressed though it be – of the reality, as a medical doctrine of the principle of similars, would ever have prompted Dr Sidney Ringer to test the value of *pilocarpine* in the night sweats of phthisis? Who but one long and practically familiar with the physiological effects of drugs, as set forth in Hahnemann's *Materia Medica Pura* and similar works, and their prescription in disease as the principle of similars suggests – could ever have written that well-known work entitled *Materia Medica and Therapeutics – Vegetable Kingdom*?

a production regarding which the *British and Foreign Medico-Chirurgical Review* said, that its "teachings were accepted with something like admiration by the profession," and that "the newer matter it contained was wholly taken from two sources, the later German researches and homoeopathic literature." The writer then describes the author as a "man preaching pure homoeopathy, and yet his teachings are accepted with something like admiration by the profession." This the writer traces to a want of knowledge of their subject on the part of the critics. But there can be no doubt that these teachings were regarded with admiration because they stood the clinical test. They stood the clinical test because they had been derived from a medical doctrine that is true – and that medical doctrine is the one wherewith Hahnemann enabled the therapeutist to avail himself of the labours of the pharmacologist.

It would be easy, did time permit, to multiply very many fold illustrations of the therapeutic products of the application of the principle of similars to the selection of remedies daily utilised by those physicians who denounce Hahnemann as a visionary and a fanatic, and represent his teaching as having been "injurious to medical science." No amount of declamation, however passionate, nor of theoretical objections, however ingenious, can obliterate the fact that the drugs I have named, and many more beside the, owe their position as remedies in the forms of disease in which they are hourly prescribed solely to the method of investigating the properties of drugs set forth and carried out by Hahnemann, coupled with the doctrine of drug-selection propounded by him. This being so, it is simply puerile to deny the existence of a therapeutic doctrine; it is misleading to tell us that there is no general principle which can guide us in the treatment of disease; while to state that the principle of similars has proved "injurious to medical science" is contradicted by the experience of every physician who avails himself of the most direct of the practical improvements which have taken place in therapeutics during the last twenty years. The fact that there is such a principle – such a doctrine in therapeutics – is being demonstrated every day.

Neither is there anything calculated to excite our surprise that there should be such a doctrine or principle. It has been looked for, longed for, hoped for by many thoughtful physicians during the last two or three centuries. It was such a principle, such a doctrine, that Sydenham anticipated when he said: "The method whereby, in my opinion, the art of medicine may be advanced turns chiefly upon what follows, viz.: that there must be some fixed, definite, and consummate *methodus medendi*, of which the common weal may have the advantage."[xiii] It was of such a principle, such a doctrine as this, that Professor Alison, of Edinburgh – in complete ignorance of Hahnemann's work – felt the necessity, when he declared that: "the increasing efficacy of our art must depend on the progress which may

---

xiii *The Works of Sydenham*, London; Sydenham Society. 3rd Edition 1848, vol 1, p. 17.

yet be expected in the discovery of specifics." Still more clearly, much more pointedly was it, that Sir Thomas Watson, in his address at the Clinical Society in January, 1868, referred to such a doctrine, such a principle as this, when appealing for "authentic reports of trials with medicinal substances upon the healthy human body" he urged that, taken together with careful clinical observations, "such trials must lead at length – tardily, perhaps, but surely – to a better ascertainment of the rules, peradventure to the discovering even of the laws by which our practice should be guided, and so bring up the therapeutic and crowning department of medicine to a nearer level with those other parts which are strictly ministerial and subservient to this."

These words depict with remarkable accuracy the spirit which animated Hahnemann, when between 1790 and 1796 he devoted himself to the task which he afterwards so thoroughly accomplished, and equally exactly do they describe the result he achieved. It is in a spirit similar to this that those who are satisfied neither with the teaching of Hahnemann nor with the present state of therapeutics must work, if they would improve the art of medicine "in that department" of which the President of the Section of Medicine, at the Belfast meeting of the British Medical Association the other day, told his hearers "we know least."

The inauguration this year of a Pharmacological Section by this Association is calculated at first sight to inspire with hope those physicians who are, above all things, anxious to see "the therapeutic crowning department of medicine" placed on "a nearer level with those other parts which are strictly ministerial and subservient to this."

But, alas, a brief glance at the statement of the means of therapeutic research relied on by the President to render the contributions of the section valuable is more than sufficient to dissipate any hope of improvement from this quarter. He directed the members of the section to three "means of therapeutic research."

First, to experiments on animals. – This is a method of enquiry regarding which Cullen observed – and his remarks are as true to-day as when they were first penned a century ago: "this is a very proper measure," he says, "in investigating the powers of all untried substances, and may give a proper caution with regard to the trial of the same upon the human body, but it can go no further." This, I would here note, was the object with which Dr Murrell dosed his cats with the nitrite of sodium, respecting which so much sensational writing appeared early in the present year. Cullen continues: "For it is well known that the effects may be very different in the two subjects, as some substances act much more powerfully, and others more weakly upon the human body than upon those of brutes; and therefore we can draw no certain conclusion from the effects of substances upon brute animals till they are actually tried upon human beings."[xiv] It is perfectly true

---

xiv Cullen WA, op cit, vol. 1, p. 153.

that experiments with drugs upon the lower animals have a value, but this is not seen, as Cullen says, until they have been "actually tried upon human beings." Their value consists in their displaying the material alterations produced by a given drug in the body of an animal poisoned by it, and the comparison of these with the symptoms to which it gives rise both in human beings and in the brute creation during life.

When a healthy person takes *tartar emetic* experimentally for some time, the oppression over the chest which arises, the bruised and sore feeling which pervades it, and the profuse expectoration of white frothy mucus which is painfully coughed up, all suggest the existence of a congested lung, similar to that which sometimes follows an exposure to cold; but it is eminently satisfactory to know from the experiments of Majendie, Richardson and Molin, that such a condition is revealed *post mortem* in animals poisoned with it.

Thus while such experiments taken alone are insufficient for clinical purposes, when undertaken as supplementary to a more precise method of enquiry, they are in some instances at least, both interesting and instructive.

In the *second* place, Dr Maclagan referred the section to "statistical observation of the results of treatment." As, however, he concludes that for this purpose statistics "are not only valueless but have been in the past positively misleading," it would be unnecessary for me to remark upon it, were it not that in a sentence or two later in his address, he says of statistics that "they have no place in therapeutic research." This is not correct.

For the purpose of ascertaining the relative importance of different remedies in the same form of disease, they are, indeed, of no value, and may well be set down as misleading, for as Dr Maclagan truly points out the same form of disease varies greatly in different persons. Take so simple and well defined a disease as pneumonia, for example. It would be useless to attempt to gauge the relative value of *Phosphorus, Bryonia,* and *Antimonium tartaricum* in its treatment by statistics. Some cases will derive advantage from the first of these medicines, others from the second, and others again from the third. But to conclude that, because out of a hundred cases of pneumonia, sixty were benefited by *Phosphorus,* thirty by *Bryonia,* and ten by *Antimonium tartaricum,* therefore *Phosphorus* is the best remedy in pneumonia would be in the highest degree fallacious.

On the other hand, when we use statistics to test the relative value of methods, plans, and principles of treatment, they do furnish useful information, provided that they are compiled by observers competent for the task and honest in its performance; that the cases are numerous; that they occur at the same time, in the same locality, and among persons occupying a similar social position. By comparing, by the aid of statistics of this kind, the results of treating a given disease, or series of diseases, by medicines prescribed empirically, antipathically, and homoeopathically it is quite possible to arrive at a very definite conclusion as to which method or principle of drug selection proves most generally successful. Such is the place of statistics in therapeutic research.

The *third* mode of research – individual observation – is, says Dr Maclagan, "that on which we have to rely." Individual observation of what Dr Maclagan does not state. Pharmacology, we have been told, deals with "the modifications produced in healthy conditions by the operation of substances capable of producing modifications." If this is so – and most certainly it is so – the individual observations should consist in experiments with drugs upon healthy persons. There is not, however, a single sentence in this address leading any one to suppose that this is what its author meant. Diseases are, it is concluded, due to the presence of germs, and the individual observation alluded to is, I must presume, to be devoted to the discovery of germicides. But how these articles are to be gone in search of Dr Maclagan gives no hint.

After all, the "individual observation" on which it is supposed that "we have to rely" in therapeutic research amounts to nothing more than the plan "of acquiring the knowledge of the virtues of medicines by experience" discussed by Cullen. In commenting upon it, Cullen says: "An experience of the effects of substances upon the living human body" – and here he referred, as is abundantly proved by what follows, to the sick and not to the healthy body – "an experience of the effects of substances upon the living human body is certainly the only sure means of ascertaining their medical virtues; but the employing of this experience is extremely fallacious and uncertain, and the writers on Materia Medica abound with numberless false conclusions which are, however, supposed or pretended to be drawn from experience." True as this was in Cullen's time, it is no less so to-day.

While, then, the establishment of a Pharmacological Section by the British Medical Association is evidence of a desire, on the part of the members "to find a clue" as Dr James Smith expressed it at Belfast, to "the labyrinth" of the "modes of action of remedies," the means so far proposed to discover it are unhappily as inadequate to the purpose as they are wanting in originality.

To find "this clue," the British Medical and all other Associations are shut up to taking the course suggested by Stahl and emphasised and carried out by Hahnemann. None ever proposed or attempted has proved so certain, so abundantly fruitful a source of knowledge of "the modifications produced in healthy conditions by the operation of substances capable of producing modifications" as this has done. So far as we know at present there is no other means than this by which we can detect the organs and tissues for which different substances have an affinity, none by which we can hope to learn the kind of action they exert upon them.

When this kind of knowledge is obtained, and it is sought to utilise pharmacological facts for therapeutical purposes, how will this, the practical end, be accomplished? "We must admit," said Dr Bristowe, three years ago – "we must admit the truth of the homoeopathic view of the relations between medicines and diseases before we can admit the special value of investigations conducted only on the healthy body." (*Brit. Med. Journ.*, 13th Aug, 1881.) Precisely so. And as the "special value of investigations conducted on the healthy body" is admitted by all the more eminent students of pharmacology in Europe and America, it needs little of the gift of prophecy accurately to forecast the therapeutic issue of pharmacological enquiry.

Of one thing I am certain, and it is this, that if any physician or body of physicians will pursue his or their investigations into the actions of drugs upon the healthy human organism in the manner carried out by Hahnemann eighty and more years ago, and urged upon the profession in our own land some fifteen years since by one whose authority in medicine was, aye and still is, justly held in the highest esteem – urged upon the profession by the venerable Sir Thomas Watson – and then, having done so, if he or they will compare the results of his or their observations with the phenomena of those diseases the drugs experimented with have been known to cure, he or they will have abundant reason to feel assured that the law of similars is no *ignis fatuus* – is no fitting subject for a trifling joke – but that there is good, solid ground for believing in its reality.

I am here reminded of the words of Professor Burden-Sanderson, that, "in judging of a therapeutical method the one and only criterion is success." This being so, the clinical test must follow the pharmacological enquiry. The application of this test will – so runs the testimony of many thousands of physicians who have practised homoeopathically during the last eighty years – so runs the testimony of some nine or ten thousand who are actively engaged in doing so to-day – the application of this test will transform any pre-existing hesitation of the value of pharmacology, *plus* the principle of similars, into an abiding confidence in their united value; will convert any doubt that may have been felt respecting the truth of homoeopathy into a firm conviction of its paramount importance as a therapeutic method; will assure the investigating physician that through it he can obtain a power of control over disease that previously he had never dreamed of possessing.

That we know aught of this method, that we are in actual possession of this increased control over disease, is the direct result of the life work of Hahnemann.

When we think of the constancy and consistency with which he sought and wrought it out, all undeterred by the gravest and most serious obstacles that could beset a scientific and clinical investigator – when we reflect upon the genius and scholarship he brought to bear upon his enquires, the courage and self-sacrifice with which he pursued them, Hahnemann presents himself to us as, what in very deed he was, one of the most genuine heroes who ever devoted a life to the ascertainment of truth in medicine, or ever laboured to diminish the physical suffering disease entails upon mankind!

Tunbridge Wells, October 1st, 1884.

References

1 Obituary, Alfred Crosby Pope MD MRCS, *The Homoeopathic World*, 1908, 1 May.
2 Pope, A, Hahnemann: his work and its results. The fifth Hahnemannian lecture, London, *Monthly Homoeopathic Review*, 1884, 29:1, 1-27.
3 Hahnemann S, *Lesser Writings* (trans Dudgeon RE), London: W Headland, 1851; p. 295.

12

CLARKE ON REVOLUTION

Introduction

This is another stirring paper, onwards and upwards and over the medical barricades, Dr John Henry Clarke on his horse right behind Hahnemann leading the fight!

For a further insight into how Clarke developed his ideas after studying under Hughes the reader is referred to an exchange of letters about Clarke's *Dictionary*.[1]

> **About John Henry Clarke[2] (see also Chapter 15)**
>
> John Henry Clarke was a scholar and an industrious writer who collected material from around the world. His best friends included James Compton Burnett, Thomas Skinner, and Robert Cooper. They regularly dined together and after Cooper's death they became known as the Cooper Club. Each of the members could themselves be the subject of a lecture. Clarke wrote the *Dictionary* because of his own laziness so that he would not have to search so hard in his books if he had it all in one place. So he wrote down everything they said at dinner and the *Dictionary of Practical Materia Medica* is full of symptoms with (B) and (RTC) as sources.[3] In fact you cannot discover much about how Burnett prescribed from his own prolific writings, you have to read him with one eye on Clarke to see the real reasons for his prescriptions. Also some of Burnett's one-liners finished up in Clarke's *Clinical Repertory*.[4] His *Dictionary* was presented to American colleagues at a conference in Atlantic City with the sentiment 'Hands Across the Sea'.[5]
>
> You may not have realised that Skinner was a high potency man and the hospital staff in the 1870's were mainly 3x'ers. When Clarke became a true Hahnemannian under the influence of Skinner all offices became closed to him, hence the club and its brilliant publications. His obituaries make it clear that he used all the potencies as needed, and that when he was later offered honours within the Society he refused them[6]. Clarke wrote some philosophy and his *Constitutional Medicine*[7] is the only clear and original

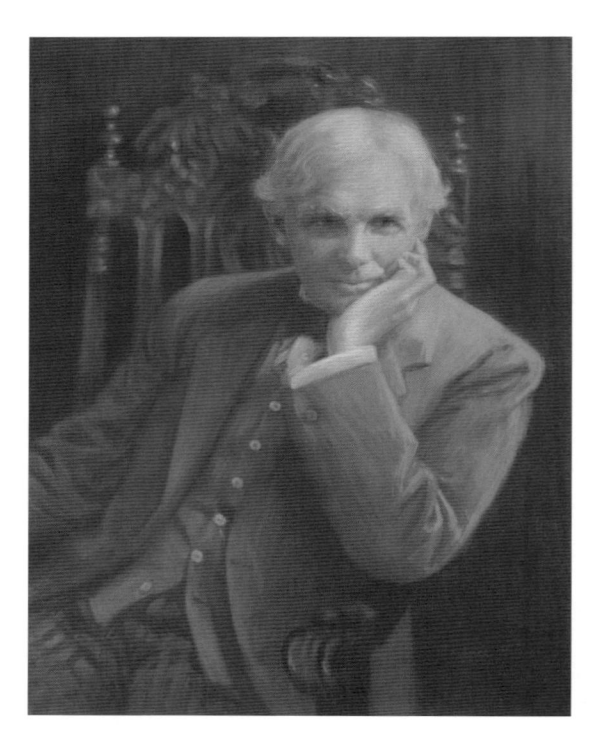

Figure 12.1 John Henry Clarke (1851–1931)

Reproduced with the permission of CAMLIS, Royal London Homoeopathic Hospital.

summary of the obtuse ideas of the celebrated von Grauvogl and his infamous *Hydrogenoid Constitution*.[8] He was Editor of the famous journal, *The Homeopathic World*, from 1885 to 1898, and again from 1923 until his death in 1931. He wrote many books, some of which are still in print.

Clarke did not confine himself to homeopathy. He wrote about diet and lifestyle,[9] and became interested in William Blake.[10] He was an anti-vivisectionist, taking the scientific imperative of homeopathic medicine further into the moral sphere. This was by all accounts an area where apparent moral clarity was obfuscated by political alliances, which may appear improbable today.[11]

There was a view among certain antivivisectionists at that time that there were too many Jews involved in medical research. Clarke went so far as to work for an organisation devoted solely to the purposes of anti-Semitism and similar propaganda. He took the chair at its foundation meeting.[12,13] There were very close ties between this organisation, the Britons, who later became the British Union of Fascists, and the London Anti-vivisection Society. Clarke served as treasurer and vice president for the Britons. Until his death Clarke was at the heart of all this and wrote many booklets with titles such as *The Call of the Sword*,[14] *England under the heel of the Jew*,[15] *White Labour versus Red with a Synopisis of the Protocols*[16] and *Democracy and Shylocracy*.[17] Lebzelter shows how Clarke was left to manage the organisation when the president went to court to defend a libel action by Sir Alfred Mond, which was lost. Clarke wrote of the 'need to expel man of alien blood and alien instincts'. He also argued that Prussia and Germany were Judaic nations and that the First World War was one of Jewish finance aimed at an overthrow of the Christian civilisation of England.

Clarke was a significant figure in the development of homeopathy and I cannot see how this revelation changes that. I have now known about this information for some 30 years, having stumbled upon it by chance and have not understood how to deal with it. I still refer to his books and study them avidly. Knowing the context does not seem to change my need to study but sometimes I wonder who he really was.

One medical historian, Frank Honigsbaum noted that many figures from the world of unorthodox practice joined right wing political groups.[18] There was much overlap with the Eugenics Society, with hindsight this can be seen as a hint of what was to follow after Clarke's death. Proctor suggests that 'the early racial hygiene movement was not a monolithic structure but a diverse blend of both Left and Right, liberals and reactionaries'.[19]

The revolution in medicine[20]
by John H Clarke

Ladies & Gentlemen
One hundred years ago the art of medicine still lay wrapped in Cimmerian night. The power of the dark ages, which the protestant revolution had rolled away two hundred years before from other pursuits and avocations of men, unfettering the intellect in science and the conscience in the moral world, still lingered like a trailing, inky cloud after a storm over all that concerned the treatment of sick humanity. No ray of reason pierced the impenetrable fog of theory on conjecture in which the ministers of healing moved, blindly led by blind tradition, and blindly worshipping the fetich, authority. Now and again the bolder spirits had ventured, like Paracelsus, to rise in revolt against the ruling powers of darkness; but in their attempts to break the rusted and corroding chains of authority - chains, which to the generality were a glory instead of a shame - they had succeeded in breaking only themselves. Systems of treatment based on fanciful theories of disease had risen, had had their day, and had sunk into their native night. Discoveries in anatomy and physiology had been made - and had left the practice of medicine

no better than before. A century and a half had passed since Harvey wrote the treatise which contained his grand induction of the circulation of the blood – and induction, be it here remarked, honestly made from anatomical observations, and not, as is commonly alleged, from the observation of vivisected animals, – thus completing the work of Servetus, Realdus and Cesalpinus, who had been before him in the field and had paved his way. But Harvey did not dream of saying a word against the prevalent custom of bleeding for almost every disease – or, indeed, of suggesting any improvement in the healing art. So absolutely without effect on practice had Harvey's great discovery proved to be, that in the succeeding generation the physician in ordinary to the son of Harvey's master, the second Charles, published a work[i] on "mummiall quintessences," among which a quintescence to be distilled "in the month of June or July" out of a "great quantity of overgrown old toads" was one the least objectionable.

1786

In the year of our Lord, 1786, when the Old Régime in France was rapidly approaching its tragic end, and when the man who was destined to master the wild forces of the impending revolution, and to lead them through the length and breadth of Europe, overturning thrones and dynasties and shaking to their foundation the social and political institutions of the western world, was a young lieutenant of artillery in his nineteenth year, – in this year a man who was born to inaugurate a very different revolution – to put an end to the reign of Darkness in the world of medicine, – already twelve years the great soldier's senior, was a general medical practitioner in the town of Dresden, dreaming as little as the other of the great part in the world's history he was to be called upon to play. At this date Hahnemann was innocent of homoeopathy.

Hahnemann

I must not trench too much on the ground so ably occupied by my predecessors in this place, who have spoken of Hahnemann, *The Man and the Physician, Hahnemann as a Medical Philosopher,* as the *Founder of Scientific Therapeutics,* and of *Hahnemann and his Works*; but it will not be possible for me to avoid it altogether. And though some of the ground may be old, the recent publication in English of the great work by the lamented Dr Ameke, of Berlin, *Homoeopathy: its Origin and its Conflicts,* translated by Dr Drysdale, of Cannes, and edited by Dr Dudgeon, opens up much that is both valuable and new.[ii]

---

i Bolnest, Edward. (Physician in Ordinary to King Charles II) *Aurora chymica, or, A rational way of preparing animals, vegetables, and minerals for a physical use,* London: Printed by Tho. Ratcliffe, and Nat. Thomas, for John Starkey: 1672.

ii Ameke W, Drysdale AE (trans), Dudgeon RE (ed), *History of Homoeopathy, its Origins; its Conflicts, with an appendix on the present state of university medicine,* London, E Gould for British Homoeopathic Society. 1885.

Who, it may be asked, was Hahnemann, that he should set himself to revolutionise the most conservative of arts, the profession in which the worship of ancestors was observed with a piety more than Chinese?

Samuel Hahnemann was the eldest of a family of ten born to a painter on porcelain, of Meissen, in Saxony. His father, whose means were none too ample, destined the boy to follow the same trade as himself. But when God has special work for a man in this world He does not leave his upbringing entirely in the hands of his parents. As a child Hahnemann shewed an intense passion and a wonderful aptitude for learning. When his father removed him from school (as he did for long periods together), with the aid of a clay lamp of his own construction the child continued his studies in this chamber at night after the less congenial labours of the day. But his teachers would not part with such a scholar without making great efforts to retain him. At last they prevailed on the father to allow the boy - whose health had given way under the combined effects of hard manual labour and chagrin - to follow his bent, they offering to forego all fees for his instruction. Such was the confidence he inspired that when only in his twelfth year Herr Müller, the principal of the Meissen School - of whom Hahnemann always speaks with the greatest veneration and affection, - commissioned him to teach to others the elements of Greek. At the age of twenty he removed to Leipzig to begin the study of medicine, his last school essay being entitled "The Wonderful Construction of the Human Hand." As showing his appreciation of his father's treatment of him, much as he had been thwarted and opposed, a note of Hahnemann's, written years afterwards, may be quoted here:

"In Easter, 1775, my father sent me to Leipzig, with the sum of twenty thalers - the last money that I ever received from him. He had to bring up several children on his limited income, and this sufficiently excuses the best of fathers."[iii]

Thus the struggle with adverse circumstances began in Hahnemann's childhood; and there can be no doubt that this early lesson in enduring hardness formed one of the most important elements in the training for his after life. At Leipzig the struggle continued. Hahnemann supported himself by teaching and by translating for publishers whilst he diligently attended the medical classes of the University. Here his fees were remitted by virtue of a kind of Government foundation instituted for the benefit of poor and deserving students. After two years spent at Leipzig he removed to Vienna in order to study medicine practically, since Leipzig possessed no hospital. At Vienna he attended the Hospital of the Brothers of Charity, in the Leopoldstadt, under Quarin, the Physician in Ordinary to the Emperor. Like most of his preceptors, Quarin conceived a great liking for the young Hahnemann, for whom he showed his partiality by taking him with him

---

iii Ameke W, Drysdale AE (trans), Dudgeon RE (ed), *History of Homoeopathy, its Origins; its Conflicts, with an appendix on the present state of university medicine*, London, E Gould for British Homoeopathic Society 1885. p. 151.

on his visits to private patients. "He singled me out," says Hahnemann, "loved and taught me as if I were his sole pupil in Vienna, and even more than that, and all without expecting any remuneration from me."[iv] To the genuine teacher a pupil of Hahnemann's kind is in himself a sufficient reward. It is to Quarin's lasting honour that he discovered Hahnemann's worth; and the love and the care he bestowed on his pupil were seeds sown in a fertile soil. A post of resident physician and library custodian to the Governor of Transylvania, obtained at Quarin's recommendation, enabled Hahnemann to replenish his scanty resources, and at the same time to pursue his practice and his studies. In 1779 he took his MD degree at Erlangen, where the graduation fee was lower than at Leipzig; thence he returned to his home, and after a short residence at Dessau removed to Gommern in 1781. Two years later he married Henrietta Küchler who shared with him for nearly fifty years the storms, the labours and the trials of his life. He now removed to Dresden, where we have already seen him, and where he remained for about six years practising his profession as best he might, and making good use of the electoral library.

A reformer not a destroyer

If a man would inaugurate a new and better era in any department of human affairs, it is first of all necessary that he should master what there is of good in the old. He comes not to destroy but to fulfil. So Hahnemann, long before he commenced the work by which he is now almost exclusively known, had made himself in all the branches of his art, and even in those which are now regarded as subsidiary branches, not merely proficient, but one of the first authorities of his time. Chemistry at this day owes to Hahnemann's genius, among other things, the discovery of the best test for metals in solution; and the apothecaries, who were destined to be the first to cast the legal stone at him, possessed in his *Pharmaceutical Dictionary* – a work of immense labour, learning and research, which took him years to complete, – their most valuable and most indispensable friend. His early writings prove him to have been far in advance of the men of his day. The practices of "fashionable physicians" he freely criticised; and in place of their violent measures he praised the virtues of cold water and fresh air in a way that would surprise modern sanitarians who imagine that hygiene is a discovery of the latter half of the nineteenth century. His learning in all that concerned his Art was unrivalled. No writer of eminence, living or dead, escaped his wide reading and scholarship, whilst his wonderful memory retained for his use almost everything that he read.

---

iv Ameke W, Drysdale AE (trans), Dudgeon RE (ed), *History of Homoeopathy, its Origins; its Conflicts, with an appendix on the present state of university medicine*, London, E Gould for British Homoeopathic Society. 1885. p. 152.

In the valley of the shadow
But before Hahnemann was ready to enter on the external conflict he must first feel the power of the darkness in his own soul and conquer it there. In spite of his great powers and high intelligence, - nay, rather by very reason of them - the seemingly never-ending night of medicine oppressed him to the dust. Where smaller and less sensitive natures could live and move without discomfort a Hahnemann could not breathe. At last he could bear it no longer; he had reached, he thought, the "Everlasting No" of medicine, and he gave up the practice in despair. Removing from Dresden in 1789, he came again to Leipzig, and there supported himself and his family by working as a literary hack, enduring the hardships of extreme poverty rather than continue to kill his fellow-creatures - as he felt he was doing - in accordance with the rules of his art. But illness in his own family recalled him to himself. He felt, as he believed in the goodness of God, that there must be a real healing art, if only it could be found.

Dawn
This was the darkest hour before the dawn. Just then Hahnemann was engaged in translating Cullen's work on *Materia Medica* from English into German; and when he came to that part of the work which deals with Peruvian Bark, he was dissatisfied with the attempt Cullen made to explain the curative action of the drug in ague. It occurred to Hahnemann that if he were to try the effect of the drug on himself in health, he might obtain some information as to its action in disease. He therefore took an ordinary dose of the powdered bark. Within a short time he was seized with an attack of the chills and fever indistinguishable from a fit of ague. Thinking this might possibly be a genuine attack of ague and not the result of the dose, after a little delay, he repeated the experiment, and again the same result followed. He had now no longer any doubt; and the exactness of his observation has since been confirmed by numberless similar experiences. Bark cured ague: and bark could also cause the very counterpart of ague in the healthy. This was the first ray of light which heralded the coming dawn. Further experiments on himself with bark and other drugs proved that this was no isolated experience, but an instance of a general rule: that there was a definite relation between the action of a drug on the healthy and its action on the sick, and that by knowing the one the other might with certainty be predicted.

With the breaking in of light upon his own mind Hahnemann was restored to hope and life.

But unlike certain modern discoverers who are eager to rush before the public with every idea that comes into their minds lest another should come before them and claim the priority (which is not really worth the claiming), Hahnemann took care to make sure his ground before he made any definite announcement. His translation of Cullen was published in 1790. For six long years he worked at the subject before he published his famous Essay *On a New Principle for ascertaining the Curative Properties of Drugs*, in which the homoeopathic principle was first clearly made known to the world. The essay was published in the leading medical periodical of the day, *Hufeland's Journal*, and it bears to the practice of medicine much the same relation that Harvey's essay on the *Motion of the Heart* bears to physiology. The essay excited much comment at the time of its appearance, as it was bound to do, but no one suspected it then of being heretical, whilst its great originality and power were acknowledged on all hands. It was not until he had laboured still three-and-twenty years in developing his system, had collected around him an enthusiastic band of disciples, and had won the confidence of a large circle of patients, that his medical brethren – and especially the apothecaries – became alive to the dangerous nature of his teachings and practice, and put in operation against him the favourite engine of the Dark Ages – persecution.

The new light which had dawned in this way upon Hahnemann's mind shed its rays before and after; illuminating and explaining much of the experience of the past, as well as indicating the path by which advance was to be made in the future. In numbers of the cases of cure recorded in ancient writings, as Hahnemann shewed, the drugs which had been given had removed conditions the like of which they were capable of causing when administered to those in health.

In this *Essay on a New Principle* Hahnemann formulates his conclusion thus:-

> "Every powerful medicinal substance produces in the human body a peculiar kind of disease, the more powerful the medicine, the more peculiar, marked and violent the disease."

> "We should imitate nature which sometimes cures a chronic disease by superadding another, and employ in the (especially chronic) *disease we wish to cure, that medicine which is able to produce another very similar artificial disease, and the former will be cured; similia similibus.*"

This proposition has never been shaken. Denied it has frequently been; misrepresented it still is; disproved it cannot be.

Hahnemann had now his foot upon the solid ground of fact. The weakness of all previous systems of treatment that had been proposed lay in their having been founded on the quicksands of theory. If Hahnemann had first sought to find some supposed explanation of the fact made plain to him, and if he had then sought to build up a system upon the explanation instead of upon the fact, his system would have fared no better than the others. Facts are durable things; explanations are always changing.

On his own body Hahnemann "proved" a large number of drugs; that is to say, he took them in substantial doses when in health and observed the effects that followed. These he noted as they occurred and made no attempt to explain them, simply labelling them what they were, "positive effects." Drugs, like human beings, are apt to be at times a little inconsistent in their actions. For instance, *Belladonna* will cause some persons to perspire profusely, and will make the skin of other persons dry. Like a sensible man, Hahnemann, instead of trying to reconcile these inconsistencies, or to find an ingenious explanation of them, preferring, as smaller men are wont to do, his own explanation to the facts, simply set down both as "positive effects." An observer of the old school seeing one of these effects would immediately dub the medicine a "sudorific," and another seeing the opposite effect would be equally certain to dub it "anti-sudorific;" and each would go away satisfied that he possessed a scientific understanding of the drug's action, and for ever after use it according to the name he had given it, ignoring as exceptional all contradictory experiences. So it has been; and so it is to this day among those who reject Hahnemann; and hence the confusion that prevails in the works of orthodox writers on materia medica, to the distraction of the unhappy student who is compelled to learn their contents – for examination. Hahnemann swept away all these delusive names, embodying at the best only partial experiences, and suffered the much abused drug to write out its own character in the symptoms and changes it produced in his healthy body; he performing the simple clerical duty of writing, so to speak, to the drug's dictation. By so doing, Hahnemann has made it possible for us to know the actual powers, the very characters in fact, of hundreds of substances now in daily use in homoeopathic – and allopathic! – practice.

At the time when his essay was published Hahnemann was a physician of the highest standing and repute (which no one then thought of questioning), and in the forty-second year of his age. A physician who knows nothing but drugs is, properly speaking, no physician at all; but a physician who does not know how to use drugs is a man without his right hand. Hahnemann was no one-sided enthusiast – he was an accomplished physician in all other matters apart from his knowledge of drugs and his skill in the use of them; and he was thus in every way qualified to lead the reform in the most important of all the divisions of the doctor's art – the treatment of the sick by drugs. For the question of drug-action barred the way of all progress; and so long as the practice of drug administration remained unreformed, so long as the absurd theories and the high-sounding, delusive terms in which they were embodied held dominion over the physicians' minds, the inauguration of a better era was impossible. But now that the light had come to him, Hahnemann was fully equipped and ready to enter on his life's great work, for which all before then had been a preparation. He was not alone in bewailing the state of the practice of his time, nor was he alone in his discernment of the curative powers of drugs; others, like Von Stoerk, had possessed an insight of a limited kind into the properties of drugs, and saw the necessity of giving them singly, before Hahnemann. But there was none who saw a way out of the darkness until he came; there was none who was able to gather up the good and shew how it might be recognised and distinguished from the mass of the bad. He alone possessed the genius, the talent, the learning, the faith and the fortitude that were needed to withstand all the powers arrayed against him, to lead all those who would follow him into a region of light, and to compel all those who refused to follow, to cease at least to do evil, if they would not learn to do well.

The threefold work

Cleansing the Augean stable

Hahnemann's work was of a three-fold kind. He had first to clear his ground of the rubbish of ages, taking care to preserve everything of value that lay concealed among the heaps; he had to build a new edifice on the ground he cleared; and all the time he had to defend his work and himself against the attacks of his numberless foes, the blind lovers of darkness, the pharisaic sticklers for the old order, right or wrong. For, as there were those in the days of Plato who would rather be in error with him than be right with any less authority; and, as, in Harvey's time, almost all his professional brethren declared that they would rather be wrong with Galen than be "circulators" with Harvey; so at the beginning of this boasted nineteenth century of ours – and I fear not at the beginning alone – the medical profession were almost unanimous in preferring to slay with Galen *secundum artem* – according to the most approved rules of their art – than to heal with the revolutionary Hahnemann. And verily they did slay *secundum artem*, as we shall presently see.

The only measure most relied on by the physicians of Hahnemann's time in their endeavours to combat disease was blood-letting. Next in importance to this came the administration of complex mixtures, the prescriptions for which were regarded as in themselves works of art to be compiled as carefully as a sonnet, almost as much for the admiration of awe-struck apothecaries as for any possible good the compounds might do to the patients. Hahnemann's keen eye soon perceived the folly and the wrong of both of these fashionable measures. In 1791,[v] just when the idea of homoeopathy had taken possession of his mind, we find him writing of blistering and bleeding in this philosophical strain:-

> "It is the common delusion that the sores produced by vesicating agents only remove the morbid fluids. When we consider that the mass of the blood during its circulation is of uniform composition throughout, that the exhalents of the blood vessels give off no great variety of matter under otherwise identical conditions; no rational physiologist will be able to conceive how a vesicating agent can select, collect and remove only the injurious part of the humours. In fact the blister under the plaster is only filled with

---

v Translation of *Monro's Materia Medica*, Vol. II., p. 275. Ameke, p. 76.

a part of the common blood when it is drawn from a vein. But according to the insane idea of these short-sighted doctors, venesection, too, draws off the bad blood only, and continued purging only evacuates the depraved humours. It is terrible to contemplate the mischief which these universally held foolish ideas have caused."

In the following year, 1792, Hahnemann's sentiments on this question brought him for the first time into open conflict with his professional brethren. He alone of all men had the courage to criticise publicly the medical treatment of the Emperor Leopold II of Austria, who died *secundum artem*, in this way:

> "The monarch was on the 28th of February attacked with Rheumatic Fever" – This is the report of Lagusius, the Physician in Ordinary to the Emperor, with a running commentary (in the brackets) by Hahnemann; – 'and a chest affection [which of the numerous chest affections, very few of which are able to stand bleeding? Let us note that he does not say pleurisy, which he would have done to excuse the copious venesections if he had been convinced that it was this affection.] and we immediately tried to mitigate the violence of the malady by bleeding and other needful remedies [Germany – Europe – has a right to ask: which?]. On the 29th the fever increased [after the bleeding! and yet] three more venesections were effected, whereupon some [other reports say distinctly – *no*] improvement followed, but the ensuing night was very restless and weakened the monarch [just think! it was the night and not the four bleedings which so weakened the monarch, and Herr Lagusius was able to assert this positively], who on the 1st March began to vomit with violent retching and threw up all he took [nevertheless the doctors left him, so that no one was present at this death, and indeed, after this, one of them pronounced him out of danger]. At 3.30 in the afternoon he expired, while vomiting, in the presence of the Empress."[vi]

Commenting on the case elsewhere Hahnemann said: "His physician, Lagusius, observed high fever and swelling of the abdomen early on February 28th; he combated the malady by venesection, and as this produced no amelioration, three more venesections were performed without relief. Science must ask why a second venesection was ordered when the first produced no amelioration. How could he order a third; and, good Heavens! how a fourth, when there had been amelioration after the preceding ones? How could he tap the vital fluid four times in twenty-four hours, always without relief, from a debilitated man who had been worn out by anxiety of mind and long continued diarrhœa? Science is aghast!"[vii]

But bleeding was not to be abolished at one blow. Hahnemann strove against the practice with all his might, and for years the neglect of bleeding continued to be the chief sin of homoeopathy in the eyes and mouths of its opponents. But except in the practice of Hahnemann and his followers bleeding continued to the

---

vi Ameke W, Drysdale AE (trans), Dudgeon RE (ed), *History of Homoeopathy, its Origins; its Conflicts, with an appendix on the present state of university medicine*, London, E Gould for British Homoeopathic Society. 1885. pp 88–89.

vii *ibid* p. 88.

be the favourite method of treatment; and it was only when the immeasurably and incontestably superior statistics of homoeopathic over the ordinary treatment emboldened some practitioners of the unreformed faith to leave their patients without any medical treatment at all that they began to perceive the truth of Hahnemann's teaching – that bleeding was slaying. When they left their patients to Nature their death-rate fell in an amazing way, though it still remained distinctly higher than that of homoeopathists. It is now the fashion to ascribe the discontinuance of bloodletting to certain experiments on animals performed by Marshall Hall. This is a very pretty story, and quite good enough for those who wish to believe anything rather than the truth of their indebtedness to Hahnemann; but the wise know well that great reforms are not brought about in that way. Another ingenious device for robbing Hahnemann of his credit due is the theory advanced by some that diseases have changed their type since his time, and that the Sangrado bleeders of the past were quite right in their bleedings, and that Hahnemann was quite wrong in denouncing them. This is another pretty story; but the race of blood-letters is not yet entirely extinct, and the results the modern Sangrados have to show bear a striking resemblance to those of their forerunners, notwithstanding the supposed "change of type" in disease. Witness the case of Count Cavour. On May 29th, Cavour was taken ill, in the midst of his parliamentary duties, with chills, followed, after some hours, by pains in the bowels and vomiting. He was bled the same night, and again the next day both morning and evening. On the 1st of June he was again twice bled. On the 2nd of June the wound in the arm re-opened during an effort, and further bleeding took place. On his doctors attempting to bleed him again (this time at the request of Cavour himself, who though that nothing else could relieve him of his sufferings, which were really the result of the bleedings he had already been subjected to) no blood would flow. Quinine was then given. Cavour asked that it might be given in pills, instead of in solution, because he knew from experience that the solution would make him vomit. The doctors would not consent to this, and violent sickness ensued. The next day he was cupped and blistered, but the blisters could not be made to rise. King Victor Emmanuel, who visited the minister, proposed to his doctors that they should open a vein in his neck. This proposal there were about to take into consideration, when they were saved further trouble by the death of the that patient. Cavour died suffering from unquenchable thirst[viii] It may fairly be said Cavour resisted the treatment he received better than the Emperor Leopold, although the illness of the latter occurred before the supposed "change of type" of disease had been discovered. The proposal of Victor Emmanuel to still further deplete the already bloodless man met with a singular nemesis when some years

---

viii   Ameke W, Drysdale AE (trans), Dudgeon RE (ed), *History of Homoeopathy, its Origins; its Conflicts, with an appendix on the present state of university medicine*, London, E Gould for British Homoeopathic Society. p. 261. 1885

later, within the memory of us all, he himself perished – *secundum artem* – of his sanguinary doctors.

These historic examples will serve to show how firmly rooted in the medical mind was the idea that blood-letting was a necessary thing, and how much courage it demanded on Hahnemann's part to depart from the received tradition. His attitude on this question caused him to be denounced as a murderer – for denying his patients the "benefits" of blood-letting! – throughout the medical world, and cost him the friendship of some of the ablest physicians of the day who had previously been on terms of closest intimacy with him.

Hahnemann early emancipated himself from the dominion of the complex prescription; but it cost even him a severe struggle. It was considered then the highest mark of proficiency to combine a large number of ingredients in the same prescription, arranging them artistically under the imposing names of basis or principal, *adjuvans, corrigens, dirigens* and the rest, – which were supposed to "assist," "correct" and "direct" the action of the ingredient in chief. When Hahnemann had the courage to prescribe only one thing at a time, he could not help feeling a little ashamed of the mean opinion the apothecaries were sure to form of him, the apothecaries who made up the prescriptions being paid in proportion to their length. The opinion of the apothecaries with regard to Hahnemann did not improve with time.

In 1797, the year following that in which his epoch-making *Essay on a New Principle* was published, Hahnemann contributed another notable paper to Hufeland's *Journal*, entitled, *Are the Obstacles to Certainty and Simplicity in Practical Medicine insurmountable?* In this article he delivers himself as follows:

> "Who knows whether the *adjuvans* or the *corrigens* may not act as *basis* in the complex prescription, or whether *excipiens* does not give an entirely different action to the whole? Does the chief ingredient, if it be the right one, require an *adjuvans*? does not the idea that it requires assistance reflect severely on its suitability, or should a *dirigens* also be necessary? I thought I would complete the motley list, and thereby satisfy the requirements of the schools.
>
> "The more complex our prescriptions are the darker is the condition of therapeutics ... How can we complain of the obscurity of our art when we ourselves render it obscure and intricate?"[ix]

In the same year in which he first publicly attacked bloodletting, 1792, Hahnemann shewed his courage in departing from the evil traditions of his profession in another matter of great importance. In his day, and long after his day, it was the custom to treat lunatics as if they had been wild beasts. Hahnemann protested

---

ix Ameke W, Drysdale AE (trans), Dudgeon RE (ed), *History of Homoeopathy, its Origins; its Conflicts, with an appendix on the present state of university medicine*, London, E Gould for British Homoeopathic Society. 1885 p. 78.

against the wickedness of this practice, and his cure of the Hanoverian Chancellor Klockenbring by gentle means is a matter of European history. "I never allow an insane person," say Hahnemann, "to be punished either by blows or any other kind of corporal chastisement, because there is no punishment where there is no responsibility, and because these sufferers deserve only pity and are always rendered worse by such rough treatment and never improved."[x] After his complete cure, Klockenbring, "often with tears in his eyes," shewed Hahnemann "the marks of the blows and stripes his former keepers had employed to keep him in order."[xi]

Thus Hahnemann anticipated another of the improvements in medical practice fondly imagined to be a discovery of recent years and credited to Englishmen. All honour to the English doctors for the work they did, and the reform they brought about; but the originality is not theirs – it belongs to Hahnemann.

Constructive and defensive

Hahnemann did not spend all his powers in fighting the abuses of his time. All the while, he was assiduously working out his idea, testing the action of medicines on his own healthy body, and building up his system on the solid ground of his observed results. In the year, 1810, he had so far perfected his system that he was able to publish his celebrated *Organon*, in which he set forth in detail what he had briefly sketched in his *Essay on a New Principle*, fourteen years before. In the following year he applied to the University of Leipzig for permission to teach medicine under its authority. The Senate of the University were not very well disposed to entertain his request, but they said that if he would write a thesis, and defend it before them, his request should be granted. Hahnemann readily complied, sending in his *Helleborism of the Ancients*, a work of such extreme merit that his censors could not find in it a single fault, and granted him the licence to teach forthwith. For eight years he continued thus to teach and to practise, aided now by an enthusiastic band of disciples, and supported by a large section of the public. But there was growing feeling of jealousy among his professional brethren, and the apothecaries came to like him less and less. For Hahnemann had discovered that besides the great advantage there was in giving only one drug at a time – a very grave sin of itself in an apothecary's eye – there was no need to give a poisonous dose of even that one drug in order to obtain its curative effects. This was altogether too much for the equanimity of the apothecaries. Their craft was in danger. One medicine at a time, and not much of that! – how was a poor apothecary to live? On the principle of securing the greatest good to the greatest number – apothecaries being many and Hahnemann only one –

---

x *ibid* p. 67

xi Ameke W, Drysdale AE (trans), Dudgeon RE (ed), *History of Homoeopathy, its Origins; its Conflicts, with an appendix on the present state of university medicine*, London, E Gould for British Homoeopathic Society. 1885. p. 67.

they determined to extinguish Hahnemann. There was a law in Germany forbidding a physician to make up his own prescriptions. This proved an admirable opportunity for the boycotting proclivities of the trade. They refused in a body to dispense any prescription of Hahnemann's, and when he dispensed his own medicines, even though he made no charge for them, they put the law in force against him, and so procured his banishment from Leipzig in the year, 1819. He was then in the sixty-fifth year of his age. After long and painful wanderings from state to state, he at last found an asylum in the little town of Köthen, under the egis of the friendly Duke of Anhalt.

Unexpected allies

When Hahnemann went into exile he left behind him enthusiastic disciples to carry on his work and develop his system. Hahnemann might be exiled, but homoeopathy was not extinguished. And homoeopathy had allies little reckoned on by its foes. Epidemics in their courses fought for homoeopathy. Contagious fevers which swept off the patients of the old school doctors spared those of Hahnemann and his followers. Perhaps the most potent ally homoeopathy has ever possessed has been the dreaded cholera. It is often said that homoeopathy is all very well for children, and for mild diseases in adults; but no stretch of allopathic ingenuity can make of cholera a mild disease, or a disease peculiar to children. Yet it remains on the testimony of their own witnesses - allopathic doctors appointed under Government authority and prejudiced against the system of Hahnemann - that wherever homoeopathy and allopathy have been tried in epidemics of cholera side by side, the results of the homoeopathic treatment have proved immeasurably superior to those of the allopathic. This is a fact which it remains for our opponents to explain; they cannot explain it away.

Hahnemann, ere he left Leipzig, had already made his work's foundation sure, and had rendered impregnable the house of his fame. Thirty-three years had passed over his head since we first found him at Dresden. The storm of the French revolution had burst and had passed. Napoleon had had his day and had fallen from his high estate. Amidst all the political turmoil of his time, and the storms of his own life, Hahnemann had accomplished a work which was destined to bring about a revolution fraught with the happiest consequences not to Europe only, but to the whole civilised world.

The revolution and the man

1786 & 1886

Let us now come to our own day and compare the darkness of 1786 with the comparative light of 1886. In the sixteen years and upwards during which I have been connected with the medical profession as student or practitioner I have never once seen a patient bled. In all truly civilised countries bleeding now occupies the very last instead of the first place among the means of cure. The habit of prescribing a number of drugs in the same mixture is not yet by any means extinct, especially in country districts; but the practice of giving one drug at a time is rapidly gaining in favour even among allopathists, and no one now dreams of skillfully building up a prescription of *basis, excipient* and the rest, as in itself a work of art. The leaders of the allopathic section are approaching the "Everlasting No" of prescribing, – the point Hahnemann reached in 1789 – for they openly declare that they have little or no faith in drugs; and when one of them succeeds a homoeopathist in the care of a case of acute disease he thinks the best thing he can do is to give the patient no medicine at all. The effect of the revolution in medicine, of the deliverance from the tyranny of this Dark Ages, has been felt in every home in Christendom. The lancet, the leech, and the fearful concoction are no longer the haunting terror they once were from the cradle to the grave. Douglas Jerrold's death-bed appeal to the doctor who insisted in cupping him – "Why torture a dying creature, doctor?" has been answered by Hahnemann – Why indeed?

An abler pen than mine has sketched the debt of the children to "The great Deliverer."–

> "Children," says Miss Cobbe, "noticing the busts of Hahnemann in the shop windows, may be properly taught to bless that great Deliverer who banished from the nursery those huge and hateful mugs of misery – black founts of so many infantile tears – mugs of sobs and sighs and gasps and struggles unutterable, from one of which Madame Roland drew the first inspiration of that martyr spirit which led her onward to the guillotine, when she suffered herself to be whipped six times running, sooner than swallow the abominable contents."[xii]

The influence of Hahnemann is everywhere. It presses like an enveloping atmosphere, and, like an atmosphere, so insensibly that it may be unperceived. We find it in the home; in the hospital; we find it in allopathic books. It may be denied; and even by those who have consciously helped themselves to his works it may be ignored; but it is there, and history will not fail to declare it.

Medical dogberry's

I know it is the fashion to say that the improvement must have come with the growing enlightenment of the age; but the answer to the simple-minded persons who make this statement – and who remind me of worthy Dogberry, when he said, "to read and write comes by nature," – the answer to them is, that with all the growing enlightenment of the previous centuries, the improvement did not come, and until Hahnemann pointed out the way no one had any notion how medicine was to escape from the darkness of erroneous theories, and the chains of dead

---

[xii] *Sacrificial Medicine*, in *The Peak in Darien*, by Frances Power Cobbe, p. 196.

Authority. It was only by the immeasurably superior results of Hahnemann's treatment over their own that the opposing section were, "at long and last," as the Scotch folk say, induced to give up their barbarous practices, and to leave the sick man at least a chance of getting well. Those who like may believe in the wonderful effects of Marshall Hall's vivisections: the deliverance of medicine from bondage was wrought by the heroic struggles of Hahnemann for light, begun in his childhood, and carried on during long years of privation, of labour and of persecutions, and maintained with a fortitude rarely seen among the sons of men, and never seen except when founded, as Hahnemann's was, on a mighty faith in the goodness of God, and in his own commission. This is the kind of thing, and this only, which can bring about such a beneficent revolution as this century has witnessed in medicine; and sine the world is not altogether under the dominion of evil, a career like that of Hahnemann can never be wasted or lost.

The man

Such was Hahnemann, and such was his work. The discovery that he was an ignorant charlatan is one of the many remarkable allopathic discoveries – not to say inventions – of the last half century. In his own day his works were too well known to admit of such slanders gaining credence. Base motives and his criminal neglect of blood-letting were the chief stones thrown at him then. But Hahnemann was not to be destroyed by persecution, and he was too great a man to make any querulous complaint of that which he endured. "I care nothing," he says, in 1828, "for the ingratitude and persecutions that have pursued me on my wearisome pilgrimage; the great objects I have pursued have prevented my life from being joyless."[xiii] And on his death-bed, when it was remarked that Providence owed exemption from suffering to him who had already suffered so much in his efforts to relieve others, he replied with all his old fire, "Why should I expect exemption from suffering? Every one in this world works according to the gifts and powers which he has received from Providence, and *more* or *less* are words used only before the judgment-seat of man, not before that of Providence. Providence owes me nothing. I owe it much. Yea, everything."[xiv]

That Hahnemann had faults and failings I do not deny, any more than I deny that there are spots on the face of the sun. But we do not refuse to own that the sun warms us and gives us light because we have discovered the spots; and to see them at all we require to look through darkened glass. There may be some persons dim-signed enough to see the spots – and even to see spots where there is none –

---

xiii Hahnemann S, *Chronic Diseases* (trans Tafel, LH), Philadelphia, Boericke & Tafel, 1996. & Ameke, p. 163.

xiv Ameke W, Drysdale AE (trans), Dudgeon RE (ed), 1885 *History of Homoeopathy, its Origins; its Conflicts, with an appendix on the present state of university medicine*, London, E Gould for British Homoeopathic Society. 1885, p. 167.

without such help, and foolish enough to deny that the sun shines. Such, it seems to me, are those mentally pur-blind persons who see so plainly the defects (real or imagined) in Hahnemann's character that they cannot bring their magnanimity to allow him any credit at all.

Some there are who cannot see a hero, even when placed fairly before their eyes. Their insect range of vision is so narrow and so low that they see nothing clearly that is much greater than themselves; and their minds are so much in subjection they will not believe in anything they cannot see. But these are not the men to measure Hahnemann. His fame lives not in their breath. His fame has firm foundations; it is sure as the everlasting hills. It may be hidden from little minds by the little reputations of to-day, as the snowy peak of some sky-piercing giant may be hidden from view by hillocks close at hand; but as, when distance levels meaner heights, the monarch of the range towers over all the scene, so as years roll on will the name and fame of Hahnemann tower over the plains of history, when the little reputations of to-day shall have mingled indistinguishably with the common dust.

Our inheritance

The revolution not complete
But great as the work of Hahnemann is, and great as is the revolution he has brought about, the revolution is not yet complete. It is true, there are in the United States of North America upwards of 10,000 practitioners of medicine following in the footsteps of Hahnemann, and all the world over the positive – as well as the negative – benefits of the new method are known. It is true, also, that allopathic professors, after filling their books with the records of their labours in torturing dumb brutes, and endeavouring in vain to extract from these some therapeutic pabulum wherewith to allay the cravings of their famishing pupils, are fain to present them with a dish of crumbs furtively swept from Hahnemann's floor. But this by no means contents us. As Hahnemann's heirs, much remains for us to accomplish. He has shown us the better way; it is for us to go forward. We must develop our inheritance, and defend it against the attacks, overt and covert, of those in power in the profession. We must make our case plain to the people, who are the ultimate judges and masters of either medical school.

Medical ethics
There is much talk in these days about Medical Ethics. In the minds of our opponents medical ethics is an invention of recent date, expressly or mainly designed for the purpose of putting down homoeopathy. Ladies and gentlemen, the only principle of medical ethics I know, is the good of the people; and for each individual doctor the people are represented, first and foremost, by his individual

patients; and after that, according to his powers, by the world at large. The profession exists for the people. But this is scarcely the view of the allopathic section. In this country strong men – yes; even strong Scotchmen! – dare not do the thing they own to be right, because, forsooth! their college says they must not: and this is what they understand by medical ethics. Over the Atlantic, in the Land of Freedom, the same "code of medical ethics" holds sway; and because some have ventured to rebel against the old commandment of the dark ages of medicine, "Thou shalt extinguish the light," – which is, being interpreted into the language of to-day, "Thou shalt boycott homoeopathy." – fierce civil war has broken out in the allopathic ranks.

En avant!
So long as this state of things continues – so long as the allopathic materia medica remains the most hated and hateful of the studies of the medical curriculum; so long as its professors present their students with the torturings of dumb creatures as the only source of progress in the art of prescribing, and slander Hahnemann whilst they steal homoeopathy, and for the most part mar what they steal; so long as the student is hindered from following the dictates of his own conscience by the pressure of authority and professional opprobrium; – so long must we be at work and in arms. There is a comfortable maxim of which we are all very fond, "Truth is great and will prevail." Yes; but also – lies are great, and at present *they* prevail; and unless we walk in Hahnemann's steps, and endeavour with all our might to set forth the truth as it should be set forth, lies will prevail to the end. Truth is worth working for and fighting for; and truth demands it. We may sit at home cosily repeating our beautiful maxim, like the American editor in the time of the war, who could not fight – much as he liked fighting – because he had to remain at home to announce from day to day the inspiring news that "the Government were about to take vigorous measures to put down the rebellion;" but if we all do this, the liberation of medicine will never be complete – the lies will prevail to the end. The same strenuous efforts, the same faith and fortitude which enabled Hahnemann to accomplish all he did, are demanded of us, according to our measure, to maintain what he began. We lament that our powers are so small, and our numbers so few; we wish with all our hearts that the great men opposed to us (and their greatness we do not call in question) would bring their great powers to work the rich field which is altogether too vast for us to overtake, instead of using the weight of their names to resist our efforts and to dissuade those who would from following in the better way. Still we are not discouraged; we are doing what we can. Our little hospital here stands out as a witness for the truth, and though we could wish that it were larger, and our own skill more worthy, we have no reason to be ashamed of the position it holds among the institutions of the metropolis. Its wards are open for the inspection of those who wish to learn; and

for those who have time to attend regular classes provision is made for systematic teaching in the school of medicine with which the hospital is combined.

We are doing what we can; and we hope to do yet more in the time to come. The revolution is progressing. But the progress is slow; and those who hate knowledge are many. Our work is for truth and justice and light. To all who love Justice and are not afraid of truth we look for help in our endeavour to break down what still remains of the tyranny of darkness in medicine, and to hasten the coming of the perfect day of liberty and light.

References

1. Hughes R, Clarke, JH. *A Dictionary of Practical Materia Medica: some criticisms and a reply.* (Letters) *The Homoeopathic World* 1902; April.
2. Treuherz, F, Homoeopathy around the world: travels and tribulations. *The Homoeopath*, 1991; 11:3.
3. Clarke, JH. *A Dictionary of Homoeopathic Materia Medica*, 2 vols, London, Homoeopathic Publishing Company, 1900-1902.
4. Clarke, JH. *Clinical Repertory*, London; Homoeopathic Publishing Company, 1904.
5. Burford, G. The Clarke Memorial Meeting, *BrHomJ*, 1932, 22.1: 115-143.
6. *Homoeopathy* 1932, 33 & 73-74 which reprints the notice from *The Times*, and *Homoeopathic World* 66:1, January 1932.
7. Clarke JH. *Constitutional Medicine*, London, Homoeopathic Publishing Company, nd.
8. von Grauvogl, E., Shipman, G. trans. *Textbook of Homoeopathy 1865*, London, S Compston, 1870.
9. Clarke, JH. *Vital Economy or How to preserve Your Strength*, London; T. Fisher Unwin, 1908.
10. Clarke, JH. *God of Shelley & Blake*, London; Watkins, 1930.
11. Roth. JA. *Health Purifiers and their Enemies*, New York, Prodist, 1967, p. 32.
12. Benewick, R. *Political Violence and Public Order*, London, Allen Lane, 1969, pp 42-44.
13. Lebzelter, G. *Political Anti-semitism in England 1918-1939*, London, Macmillan/St Antony's, 1987, pp 42-44.
14. Clarke JH. *The Call of the Sword*, London; The Financial News, 1917.
15. Clarke JH. *England under the heel of the Jew*. London; Judaic Publishing Company, 1918.
16. Clarke, JH. *White Labour versus Red, with a Synopisis of the Protocols*, London; The Britons and The Judaic Publishing Company, 1922.
17. Clarke, JH. *Democracy and Shylocracy*, London, Judaic Publishing Company.
18. Honigsbaum, F. *Division in British Medicine*, London; Kogan Page, 1979, p. 169.
19. Proctor RN. *Racial Hygiene: Medicine Under the Nazis*, Cambridge MA; Harvard University Press, 1988.
20. Clarke, JH. *Revolution in Medicine being the 7th Hahnemann Oration delivered at the London Homoeopathic Hospital*, London; Keene & Ashwell, 1886.

13

MORE COMMENTARY FROM DUDGEON

Introduction

Robert Ellis Dudgeon (see Chapter 10) waxes lyrical with optimism in the following commentary, he writes about Hahnemann's letters but rather than seeing the enemy round every corner he insists that homeopathy and the ideas of Hahnemann will survive:

> What remains to us of the schools founded by Galen, Paracelsus, Sydenham, Boerhaave, Van Helmont, Stahl, Cullen, Brown, Broussais? They are nothing but mere nominum umbre, but Hahnemann lives and flourishes in scores of colleges and universities, in hundreds of hospitals and dispensaries, in thousands of qualified and busy practitioners, and in millions of lay adherents in every civilised country in the world.

He shows how each sceptic whom he cites has misrepresented Hahnemann's ideas. We have much to learn from Dudgeon about how to converse constructively with our enemies. Would that we had his education, scholarship and literary style.

The Hahnemann Oration[1]
By Robert Ellis Dudgeon 1820-1904
Delivered at the opening of the London Homoeopathic Medical School, 3rd October, 1887

A series of letters from Hahnemann to a patient, ranging from 1793 to 1805, has lately been disinterred from some secret hold of the patient, a respectable tailor of Gotha, who died in 1851, at the advanced age of 92, which would lead us to surmise that his life was not shortened to any considerable degree by the ministrations pre- and post-homoeopathic of his illustrious physician (see Chapter 2).

These letters, which have appeared in the *Monthly Homoeopathic Review*, extend over a most interesting period of Hahnemann's career. They first show him residing in Gotha, where, being on term of intimacy with the editor of a quasi-scientific popular periodical, he communicated to the editor his views on the treatment of insanity by non-restraint and kindness, which was in consequence warmly advocated by the editor in his paper.

This proposed plan of treating insane patients without the strait-waistcoats, chains, blows, and tortures to which these unfortunate beings were subjected in every existing asylum, excited the scorn and contempt of all the clique of alienists, or mad-doctors; but it recommended itself to the judgment of Madame Klockenbring, the wife of the Hanoverian Chancellor, whose reason had been unsettled by a lampoon from the pen of the celebrated *litterateur* and play-writer Kotzebue, who himself fell a victim to the political fury of the student Sand.

Klockenbring, who had been treated by the most renowned alienists of Germany in the barbarous manner then prevalent, had gone from bad to worse, and his devoted wife, being struck by the novel plan she read of in the aforesaid periodical, opened communications with the editor, who referred her to Hahnemann as the author of the new treatment. Hahnemann at once offered to undertake the treatment of her husband; but as he had no locality suitable for the reception of such patients, the Duke of Saxe-Coburg-Gotha, who seems to have taken a warm interest in Hahnemann, and to have been favourably impressed with the humane and rational character of his views, gave up to him a wing of his Georgenthal castle, in the Thuringian forest, which was fitted up for the reception of the distinguished patient. After a treatment extending from June, 1792, to March, 1793, that is nine months, Klockenbring returned to Hanover perfectly cured of his insanity. Hahnemann had not yet begun his therapeutic reform, and was only known to the profession as the author of orthodox works on medicine and chemistry, so that there was no prejudice against him as an innovator in therapeutic matters, and therefore it might be supposed that this cure, which created a great sensation throughout Germany, would have led to the acceptance or dispassionate consideration of his views on the treatment of insanity. But those who think so are little aware of the conservative spirit of the medical faculty. The traditional cruel treatment went on in the asylums as before. The alienist clique denied, of course, that the cure was owing to the system pursued, which was opposed to that advocated by all the best authorities. Hahnemann was duly abused for opposing his insignificance as a comparatively unknown and obscure practitioner to the effulgent authority of the great alienists of past and present times, who had laid it down as an incontrovertible maxim that fetters, scourges, strait-waistcoats, and general bullying and cruelty were the only correct methods of treating the insane. He was accused of charging an exorbitant fee for his services, viz., 1,000 thalers, equal to £150. Such a fee would, of course, have been considered as very moderate had it been demanded by one of the leading alienists for a nine months' treatment, even had the patient been uncured, rendered more insane, or done to death; but that it should be claimed by a man who had no reputation as an alienist, and probably few patients of any description, was shocking to all medical gigmanity, as it threatened to destroy the prestige of the illustrious incapables who had hitherto, unquestioned, laid down the law on the subject of insanity and its treatment.

Calumny and detraction effectually prevented any further trial of Hahnemann's bold and original method of treating the insane. No more insane patients came to Hahnemann, and so he was forced to give up his extemporised asylum, and to seek some other sphere for the exercise of his medical talents. It was not until many years had elapsed that the rational method of treating the insane, practically proved to be the true method by Hahnemann in 1793, was generally adopted in Germany. On my first visit to Vienna in 1841, the cruel treatment of insanity was prevalent, and insane patients were still received into the Eisenthurm, a dismal dungeon, as will be remembered by those who pursued their medical studies in the Kaiserstadt at that period. Pinel, in France, and Conolly, in England, enjoy the reputation of being the introducers of the non-restraint system into their respective countries; but to Hahnemann undoubtedly belongs the honour of having been the first to propose it and successfully carry it out in practice, though his name is never mentioned by any of the historians of this great reform. *Sic vos non vobis!*

It is very commonly supposed, or at least stated, by his ill-informed detractors, that Hahnemann, from his one experiment with *bark* in 1790, invented the whole system of medicine, which goes by the name of homoeopathy. Even Hahnemann's latest critic, Dr Lauder Brunton, alleges that his *bark* experiment is "the foundation-stone of his doctrine of homoeopathy," and he cites a passage from the Presidential Address of Dr Nankivell in proof of this preposterous statement. Of course this passage from Dr Nankivell's address proves nothing of the kind – indeed, it alleges just the contrary. Dr Nankivell says what we all know to be true, viz., that the result of Hahnemann's experiment with *cinchona bark* was what led him to investigate the effects of other drugs upon the human organism, in order to see if in them also the same, or some other relation between their effects on the healthy and the symptoms of the diseases they cured, could be discovered. It was not until after six years of patient investigation, observation, and research in the writings of medical authors of the past and of his own time that he cautiously and modestly expressed his opinion on an essay published in a medical periodical, that in many instances medicines caused effects on the healthy similar to those of diseases they were known to cure, and he stated his belief that many chronic diseases might be cured by giving medicines whose positive effects on the healthy corresponded with the symptoms of these diseases.

So far was Hahnemann from having invented his system of treatment all at once, that, as we learn from these old letters, he treated his patients with very material doses of medicine, prescribed in the usual manner from the druggist's shop up to 1799. His practice differed from that ordinarily pursued in that he usually gave but one medicine at a time, though he ordered several different medicines to be taken on the same day.

In 1805 Hahnemann published in Latin his *Fragmenta de viribus medicamentorum positivis*,[2] containing the knowledge of the positive effects of some drugs on the healthy human organism he had acquired by his own experiments and from the observations of others; and accordingly, we find in the last letter of the series written in that year unmistakable evidence that he then had adopted the plan of giving his single medicines in doses much smaller than those in general use, that he dispensed his own medicines – which the licensed apothecaries could not be trusted to prepare; and we know from other sources that he was then often guided by the similarity of their positive effects, which he had laboriously collected, to the symptoms of the disease he was treating. But it is also evident that, as we might expect from the imperfect records of the *Fragmenta*, he had not yet acquired the precision in prescribing which he only got many years later when his *Materia Medica* had become, by the aid of a zealous band of disciples, much more complete. For in this letter we find him sending several different medicines, numbered 1, 2, and 3, and directing if No. 1 failed, No. 2 was to be tried, and if still no effect was produced, the patient was to take No. 3.

These letters show how slowly and cautiously he proceeded, and how gradually his system was built up and perfected. They afford a complete refutation of the often-repeated allegation that homoeopathy is a system which Hahnemann thought out in his study and sprung at once on the profession and the world such as we now know it. Had it been a mere medical theory, such as all the systems hitherto promulgated, it would certainly like them have been introduced fully equipped and complete in all its parts. But it is no medical theory, it is what Hahnemann described it in the title of his great essay, the precursor of the *Organon*, which he published in 1806 – *The Medicine of Experience*. Every part of it was the outcome of many years of patient study and experiment, and therefore it was built up slowly and gradually, bit by bit, each bit being a true induction from carefully observed facts.

We also see from these letters how careful Hahnemann was to insist on an excellent system of bathing and exercise in the treatment of his patients, and this at a period when hygiene was utterly neglected or not yet thought of in Germany. We know that even before these letters were written Hahnemann had already published several works on hygiene. In fact, he may be said to be the founder of hygiene as well as of the non-restraint treatment of insanity.

It is curious to observe with what unteachable persistency the majority of the critics of homoeopathy misrepresent its essential characteristic, which Hahnemann expressed by the formula *similia similibus curentur* – let likes be treated by likes. The question arises in our minds: Do they do this wilfully or ignorantly? If wilfully, then we can have but a poor opinion of their honesty. If ignorantly then we must feel astounded at the rashness of authors who write on subjects with which they have made no effort to become acquainted. In charity let us believe that these critics imagined they were giving a perfectly truthful account of Hahnemann's doctrine, though probably they were only repeating what they had heard others say respecting it, or they had really evolved the idea of homoeopathy from their inner consciousness, as the German professor did his camel, and they had not a suspicion that their notion of homoeopathy was not quite correct. It is a widely prevalent fashion among old school practitioners to imagine that they know perfectly what homoeopathy is. Nothing is more commonly heard from the lips of an old-school practitioner than this: "We know all about it." But as a rule, these gentlemen, when subjected to cross-examination, betray their utter ignorance of the very fundamental principle of homoeopathy, and are unable to state it in intelligible, or at all events correct, terms.

Some of the greatest men in the dominant school have essayed to "dish" the homoeopaths by exposing the absurdities of the system, and it is pleasant to see how many of them have written, with *ex cathedra* dogmatism, the most ludicrous absurdities about a system they have either not studied or not comprehended. A few examples may not be without interest.

Andral, the greatest of Parisian clinicians and therapeutists, undertook a practical trial of homoeopathy in his hospital. He commenced by letting everyone know that he had no belief in the system, but he omitted to mention that he had no acquaintance with it, and had the vaguest idea of what might be the exact meaning Hahnemann attached to the formula, *similia similibus curentur*. He though it was to single out the most prominent and important symptom of the disease and to give for its cure a medicine that had shown its power to cause this single symptom. Andral's notion of homoeopathy might be considered very pretty, but it was as unlike the real thing as it could well be. Neither Hahnemann nor his disciples are responsible for the practice Andral was pleased to term homoeopathy. Andral might have used in extenuation of his ignorance that at the time he performed his experiments – 1833 – there was no French work on the subject of homoeopathy, even the *Materia Medica Pura* of Hahnemann being untranslated. But then we might expect that he would not announce that he had made a fair trial of homoeopathy when he could not be sure that he had a correct notion of what constitutes homoeopathy. It does not speak much for the honesty of the illustrious man that though the practice he had made trial of in the hospital of La Pitié was immediately repudiated by the followers of Hahnemann, he still went on appealing to it as a refutation of the pretensions of Hahnemann, and it is as little creditable to succeeding hostile controversialists that Andral's bogus experiments are invariably referred to as a complete refutation of homoeopathy.

Sir Benjamin Brodie was one of the most celebrated surgeons of this country. Someone thinking, no doubt, that because he was a renowned surgeon he must also be a great authority on everything connected with physic, asked him to give his opinion on homoeopathy, Sir Benjamin, highly flattered by this mark of confidence in his therapeutic knowledge – the more so probably because no one had hitherto supposed he had any – wrote and published a letter, which appeared in *Fraser's Magazine*. Naturally, he stumbles over the definition of *similia similibus*, which seem to be the *pons asinorum* of medical critics and lecturers. He says, "the plain English of it is that one disease is to be driven out of the body by artificially creating another disease similar to it;" and he then proceeds to pick to pieces this man of straw which is of his own manufacture. And yet Sir Benjamin tells us that he has read the works of Hahnemann and of several of his disciples, so that we are lost in amazement to see what a mess Benjamin has made of his studies of homoeopathy. John Hunter said something similar, viz.: that one disease – not necessarily artificial – will drive out another; and Trousseau describes a method he calls *Médecine substitutive*, which is precisely John Hunter's idea, or rather, I should say, precisely Sir Benjamin Brodie's idea of what homoeopathy is. But *similia similibus curentur* does not mean this at all. It is true that Hahnemann tried at one time to account for the cures made by homoeopathy in some such way as this of Hunter's and Trousseau's substitution of one disease for another. But the truth or falsity of this speculation no way affects the correctness of the therapeutic rule – *similia similibus curentur* – which is not a theory, and which can very well afford to do without any theory yet a while.

Another great authority in medicine, Dr C. J. B. Williams, formerly professor of Medicine and Physician Extraordinary to the Queen, Lumleian Lecturer, &c., &c., on retiring from practice, and having considerable leisure time on his hands, bethought himself that he could not better employ this leisure time than in writing his autobiography. The potentate who finds occupation for idle hands suggested to him that he should write something about homoeopathy in this autobiography, which he was well qualified to do in an unprejudiced and satisfactory manner, because having retired from practice he could have no hostile feeling against it, as its success could not do him any injury. Another qualification he had for the impartial treatment of his self-imposed task, was that he knew absolutely nothing about the subject. It is curious that a physician and lecturer on medicine should not have made himself at all events superficially acquainted with a system which occupies such a large and important place in medicine; but, perhaps, medicine is not singular in possessing writers whose dogmatism is in the inverse ratio of their knowledge. Here s what Dr Williams says: "The fundamental dogmas of homoeopathy are – (1) "*Similia similibus medentur*,' or 'like cures like.' Hahnemann, who ought to know something about the matter, says his therapeutic rule, which is not a dogma, fundamental or otherwise, is '*similia similibus curentur*,' – 'Let likes be treated by likes.' The second 'fundamental dogma' of homoeopathy, according to Dr Williams, is 'infinitesimal medication, involving the paradoxical and gratuitous assumption that an infinitesimally small (or any small) quantity shall have the reverse of the effect of a large quantity.' So far as I know, both of these, as absolute propositions, are utterly untrue." 'Infinitesimal medication' is neither a dogma nor a practice of homoeopathy. Hahnemann himself says, while disapproving of the excessive dilution of medicines proposed by a disciple, "there must be some end to the thing, it cannot go on to infinity." If some of Hahnemann's disciples, neglectful of his warning and advice, have carried the dilution of medicines to an extravagant length they yet are unable to assert that their practice in this matter is a dogma of homoeopathy, or even an essential principle of the homoeopathic system, and it has been distinctly repudiated and denounced by Hahnemann himself. Small doses can only, by an extravagant and strained use of words, be called "infinitesimal." But the dosage of homoeopathy, be it small or infinitesimal, does not involve the assumption that a small quantity shall have the reverse of the effect of a large quantity. Such an assumption has nothing to do with homoeopathy at all. I have seen it broached several times in allopathic periodicals, notably the *Lancet,* and it is certainly a pet dogma of our friend Dr Sharp, on which he has founded his brand new system of "antipraxy;" but that, as he tells us, is not homoeopathy – very much the contrary indeed. It is, he says, directly antagonistic to Hahnemann's homoeopathy, which it is destined to upset and extinguish altogether – somewhere about the Greek Kalends let us hope. So Dr Williams is as wrong as he can possibly be on both points, and we only wonder how he could have lived so long with homoeopathy growing up all around him, and have so utterly failed to learn what it is.

Another man of light and leading in the medical world, Dr W. T. Gairdner, Professor of Medicine in the University of Glasgow, in his address on medicine at the meeting of the British Medical Association in August last, made the following assertion: "The Brunonian system represented the treatment, not of one disease, but of almost all diseases as bound up with, and at the same time confined by, one formula or method, of which the practical outcome was the copious administration of alcoholic stimulants and of *opium*. Substitute infinitesimals for the very palpable and potent remedies of John Brown, and exactly the same remark may be made of the homoeopathic doctrine, also a revolutionary child of the 18th century." Now Dr Gairdner has had a good deal of experience in medical polemics, and has written several pamphlets and articles on the theme of homoeopathy which, indeed, displayed a plentiful lack of knowledge of the subject, but, as he was fully answered by competent writers, and set right where he was manifestly wrong, he ought by this time to know what homoeopathy is. But anything more hopelessly at variance with the facts than the passage just quoted it would be difficult to match. He is completely wrong as to the Brunonian system, which is not bound up with and confined by one formula or method, but is a system, like all previous and later systems – except homoeopathy – which starts a theory or speculation as to the nature of the disease, and adapts the treatment to this speculative nature of the disease. Thus all diseases are either sthenic or asthenic; if the former, they are to be treated with bleeding and antiphlogistics, if the latter, with stimulants, such as *alcohol* and *opium* – opium being, according to Brown, the most powerful of stimulants. The doctrine is simplicity itself; it only needs two provisos to make it as true as it is simple: first, that diseases should all be either sthenic or asthenic, and recognisable as such; second, that antiphlogistics are the remedies for the former, stimulants for the latter. No two things could be more unlike one another than the Brunonian system and homoeopathy.

Homoeopathy has nothing to do with speculation as to the nature of the disease, nor does it divide its remedies into antiphlogistics and stimulants, or make any other classification of them at all akin to this. Of course, Dr Gairdner knows this as well as we do, and it says little for his scientific spirit or his love of truth that, for the sake of obtaining a cheer from the ignorant bigots among his audience, he would peril his reputation as a teacher of medicine, and ruin his character for veracity – if he ever had one, for truthfulness, if we remember right, was not a conspicuous quality in his former controversial writings – by making such a curiously unveracious statement respecting homoeopathy. In another part of his address he praises Sir John Forbes for not refusing "to accept truth even at the hands of homoeopathists," and his audience would have merited equal praise had they refused to accept – well, the opposite of truth – even at the hands of Professor Gairdner.

But the most extraordinary misstatement in reference to homoeopathy was perpetrated by Dr Lauder Brunton in the preface to the third edition of his *Pharmacology*. Goaded by the repeated attacks made on him for conveying the remedies of the homoeopathic school into his work without any acknowledgment of the source whence he derived them, he promised a full reply to his critics and a statement of his opinion of homoeopathy in the preface to the forthcoming third edition of his work. In this preface he says, "The mere fact that a drug in small doses will cure a disease exhibiting symptoms similar to those produced by a large dose of the drug does not constitute it a homoeopathic medicine, for this rule was known to Hippocrates, and the rule, *similia similibus curentur*, was recognised by him as true in some instances." Was ever such an incorrect and illogical statement palmed off upon an expectant public? Of course, every one knows that the mere fact that a drug will cure a disease exhibiting symptoms similar to those produced by itself on the healthy constitutes it a homoeopathic medicine, and an illustration of the principle or rule *similia similibus curentur*. The dose has nothing to do with the principle, though, as a fact, in homoeopathic treatment a smaller dose than that which caused the symptoms in the healthy is usually required for the curative purpose. But the reason given for denying the homoeopathicity of the medicine administered on strictly homoeopathic principles is the most astounding part of the statement: "For this rule was known to Hippocrates and the rule *similia similibus curentur* was recognised by him as true in some instances!" How homoeopathy should not be homoeopathy because it was known to Hippocrates is a puzzler, and why because *similia similibus curentur* was recognised by Hippocrates as true in some instances its validity as the homoeopathic formula should be impugned, is as exquisitely absurd a *non sequiter* as has ever been committed by a medical author, and that is saying a great deal. Evidently Dr Brunton did not know what to say against homoeopathy, so he penned the paradoxical nonsense I have quoted in order to seem to be saying something against it; but if attentively examined the passage proves nothing against homoeopathy, but a great deal against Dr Brunton's power of dealing fairly with a great question of medical science. No wonder Dr Brunton says "I dislike controversy extremely," when it is evident he does not understand the elementary principles of fair discussion. How can we expect the rising generation of doctors to leave their medical schools with an accurate knowledge of the great medical reformation of this century when their teachers present them with such perverted views of the subject? And Dr Brunton is not only a teacher of Materia Medica at Bartholomew's Hospital School of Medicine, but likewise is, or was, and may be again, Examiner in Materia Medica to the Royal College of Physicians and other institutions for the manufacture of doctors, and editor of a monthly medical periodical called *The Practitioner*, in which every work brought out by the editor is praised up to the skies – a new form of "log-rolling" not contemplated by the American inventors of that operation.

It is tedious to repeat the inanities and misrepresentations respecting homoeopathy that have been uttered and written by men occupying prominent positions in established medicine, so I will not quote or comment on any more of them. Very few attempts at a fair estimate of homoeopathy have proceeded from the opposite camp, and these belong to a different period from the present. Sir John Forbes, Dr Andrew Combe and Dr Kopp have given the fairest accounts of the homoeopathic doctrine and method. The two latter were, by their studies, almost convinced of the truth of homoeopathy, and the first named, Sir John Forbes, would probably have accepted the homoeopathic rule as the best therapeutic guide had he not previously committed himself to the assertion that there was no truth in therapeutics, and that patients would do better to go without physic at all.

The sceptical spirit Sir John Forbes displayed has frequently possessed distinguished physicians in all ages. But never was this spirit so rife as in the present day. Sir William Gull, only a few weeks ago, deliberately confessed his almost entire want of belief in the curative power of drugs. Dr Moxon – lately dead – held out no hopes of therapeutics ever being better than empirical guess work, and he denounced the "rational method" in physic as the greatest curse to patients, leading us to infer that he was in favour of some *ir*-rational method which he did not describe. On the other hand, the *Lancet*, of September 17th last, asserts that rational medicine is the only scientific article, but it is a *lesé-majesté* against rational medicine to attribute to it any particular law. Any law that it may possess it must share in common with all other sciences, and it must conform to the laws of every other science, and all sciences must have the same laws. This may be very profound, but it is not very intelligible; indeed, it seems very like – not to put too fine a point on it – arrant nonsense. Imagine medicine being subject to the laws of gravitation, optics, mechanics, chemistry, mathematics, and the rest of the sciences, and having no particular law or laws of its own! *Empiricism* – which may other authorities of the old school say is just what medical treatment is – this learned editor declared to be the antagonism of science, and *experience* he sneers at, and maintains that science is in no way advanced by it. As his rational medicine is an impossibility, and he entirely discards the experience which has hitherto been the sole guide of old-school therapeutics, medicine must be in a parlous state indeed.

No speaker on the subject of medicine at the various schools which are now commencing their winter session will fail to deplore the backward condition of therapeutics and to prophesy its great advance in the immediate future. This lamentation and this prophecy have been repeated in the introductories with unfailing regularity ever since our medical schools were founded, and still the wail as to the backward state of therapeutics is heard as an obligato *miserere* to the *te Deum laudamus* for the anticipated astounding progress of therapeutics.

But as regards the prophecy of the great advance in the art of healing which is to occur in the near future, authorities differ as to the efficient agent in this vaccinated advance. Some see in the discovery of microbes the dawn of a glorious day for therapeutics. It has not as yet enabled medical men to cure diseases better than before; indeed, the microbes seem often more tenacious of vitality than their host, for occasionally the latter succumbs to the remedies intended to destroy the former, who continue as lively as ever. And there goes the renowned physician, Professor Semola, all the way from Italy to Washington, and tells the 2,700 doctors assembled there at the International Medical Congress, that "Bacteriology has produced no practical results in the cure of internal diseases. To consider bacteriology as the key to all pathology – to assume that these microbes are really at the bottom of all the mischief – is the chief error of to-day," on which the commentator in the *Daily News* plaintively exclaims. "Alas! it was the very acme of wisdom not so very many days ago." Others look to what they call "pharmacology" as the *deus ex machina*, which shall make of therapeutics an exact science, and we of course agree with them in this, for we, and Hahnemann before us, have always asserted that therapeutics is to be advanced through pharmacology, of which Hahnemann indeed was the founder. But we differ considerably as to how pharmacology is to be pursued. Hahnemann and his followers say it must be through their action on the healthy human being that the effects of medicines are to be ascertained, whereas the pharmacologists of the dominant school attempt to cultivate this science by experiments with drugs on other animals than man. Monkeys and dogs, rabbits and frogs, are the chief subjects of their experiments. But it may be safely said that thousands of experiments with drugs on wildernesses of monkeys, packs of hounds, warrens of rabbits, and morasses of frogs would throw little light on the effects of these drugs on man, and none at all on their curative powers on sick humanity. The inferior animals not being able to communicate with us by speech or signs, we can only observe the rude and rough chemical, mechanical and irritant effects of drugs on them, and it is not apparent how an observation of these effects could be of use in the treatment of disease to anyone, and more especially to one who refused to be guided by the homoeopathic rule. The pharmacologists of old physic have not fared very well at the hands of some great authorities on their own side; notably, Dr Wilks, Lawson Tait, and others, who deny utterly the advantage to therapeutics of the tortures inflicted on the poor brutes. Even Dr Whitlaw, who opened the section of pharmacology and therapeutics at the annual assembly of the British Medical Association this year, said, after damning pharmacology with faint praise, "the real work only begins where the pharmacologist leaves off." In that case it might be as well that the pharmacologist - of the established school - should leave off at once, for it is about time that real work was commenced. Dr Lauder Brunton is one of the greatest experimenters in this way. His favourite subject of experiment is the frog, of which he has vivisected and poisoned immense numbers; but, in his large work on *Pharmacology*, lately published, I cannot find a single instance where he was led to the remedial use of a drug by its effects on his more or less mutilated frogs. But, still, in spite of his repeated failures to elicit anything useful for the treatment of human diseases from his futile experiments on frogs, he goes on with them without stopping - a veritable medical Micawber - always hoping that something will turn up. But nothing ever does or ever will, and I venture to say that no remedy for the diseases of mankind has ever been or will ever be discovered by any number of experiments on lower animals. I will go farther, and maintain that no remedies for human maladies will ever be discovered by the opponents of homoeopathy by the most carefully conducted experiments on healthy men. Several distinguished men of the old school have proposed and even carried out experiments with drugs on healthy human beings, in the vague hope that something useful for remedial purposes would result from them, but when they have collected this pathogenetic material they are quite at a loss what to do with it, for they must not use it to treat diseases which present similar symptoms to those their drugs have produced, for that would be flat homoeopathy - Dr Lauder Brunton to the contrary notwithstanding - and they deny that there is any other principle showing the relation of drug action to disease. Only last week the editor of the *Medical Press* worked himself up into a towering passion at the very idea of being thought to care a straw about medical principles. "We ask the public to believe us," he exclaims, "when we assert that in our estimation the question whether the methods we employ are allopathic or homoeopathic is as far beneath us as not to be deserving of a thought." How very high up that editor must be – perhaps up a tree! So the material the Jörg's, the Frerich's, the Segin's, the Harley's and other old-school experimenters have painfully collected would be utterly wasted were it not greedily snapped up by our school and transferred to the pages of the *Materia Medica*, always with thankful acknowledgement of the source whence it was taken; for we are not, like our opponents, anxious to conceal the fact that we utilise the labours of the other school when they are suitable for our purpose. Several knowing ones in the old school have had the wit to perceive that the proving of medicines on the healthy could be of no earthly use to them in their allopathic treatment, and have denounced them as "contrary to nature and common sense." No doubt they perceive that if persevered in they must lead straight away to homoeopathy, as they did in the case of Professor Zlatarovich, of Vienna, Dr Schrön and some others.

The experiments carried on with unabated zeal in the so-called "physiological laboratories" so universal in the medical schools of Germany – which our zoophilist friends call vivisection – promise to be crowned with triumphant success in the "near future." For we read in the *Lancet* of the 19th of last month: "Thanks largely to the laborious investigations of the German physiologists we may now say that it looks as if, in the near future, some definite method will be discovered by means of which we may be enabled to assert whether any particular stomach which may claim the attention of the scientific physician is or is not in a healthy condition." Well, now, that is "grateful and comforting," like Mr. Epps' cocoa. In the "near future" – the "near future" seems to be the favourite period of the accomplishment of all the prophecies of medical triumphs, but as we advance it always recedes, just like a will-o'-the-wisp – well, in the "near future" the scientific physician will probably, or possibly, be able to tell us whether our stomach is or is not in a healthy condition; but in the meantime let no one rashly presume to decide whether his stomach is or is not out of order. Only let us entreat these German physiologists to hurry on their laborious investigations, so that there may be a chance of our getting to know whether our stomachs are disordered or not within a reasonable period of time, for till then, of course, we must remain in doubt about our diet, and continue to eat our dinner in fear and trembling.

The partisans of old-school physic take as many of our remedies as they like, and when they are taxed with using homoeopathic remedies, not being able to deny the charge, they loftily assert that medicine knows no "pathies," but has a perfect right to take her remedies wherever she can find them – from savages, shepherds, old women, and *even* from the homoeopathic Materia Medica; but as, no doubt, they are the people, and wisdom shall die with them, they alone know how to employ the medicines they condescend to borrow from us. The latest work on therapeutics, by Dr Mitchell Bruce, is permeated with instances of homoeopathic treatment. Thus he says: "In the intestines, copper is an astringent [according to scientific medical nomenclature, a medicine is said to be astringent when it stops diarrhoea] in small quantities, an irritant purgative in larger quantities. Small doses are given for some kinds of diarrhoea." Again: "In doses of 15 to 30 grains, *Ipecacuanha* acts as an emetic; in very small doses it will arrest vomiting." "*Rhubarb* is used in small doses as an intestinal astringent; larger doses are given as a purgative." "Many inflammations of the skin and eyelids are treated by weak solutions of *corrosive sublimate*; stronger solutions cause inflammation of the skin." "Boils, scrofulous sores, suppuration are to be treated with *sulphide of calcium*" – our *Hepar sulphuris*; "spasmodic asthma with *Arsenic, Nux vomica, Hydrocyanic acid*;" "bronchitis with *aconite, Ammonium carbonate, Antimonium tartrate, Ipecacuanha, Senega*;" "bruises with *Arnica*;" "cholera with *Camphor*;" "constipation with *Nux vomica*;" "delirium with *Belladonna, Opium*;" "diarrhoea with *copper, rhubarb, Arsenic*;" "fever with *Aconite*;" "inflammation with *Aconite, Belladonna*;" "pleurisy with *Aconite*;" and so on. In fact, all the common and well-known homoeopathic remedies and their indications are transferred to Dr Bruce's work without a word of acknowledgement as to the source whence they are derived. Probably, if hard pressed, Dr Bruce would say he took them from his friend Dr Lauder Brunton's work, who, as he has lately told us, took his from the *Comparative Therapeutics* of Dr Potter, a graduate of an American Homoeopathic College. But whencesoever directly taken we know, and every one knows, that their real source is the homoeopathic Materia Medica. It is curious to note that Dr Bruce calls his work on the title-page "*An Introduction to the Rational Treatment of Disease*," and that the "rational" treatment he introduces to us is mostly, if not entirely, homoeopathic. Now, it is well known to you that the title Hahnemann gave to the first edition of his great work was "Organon of *Rational* Medicine," so it is a significant coincidence that the author of a work which introduces a whole crowd of Hahnemann's medicines to his readers should call in an introduction to the *rational* treatment of disease, alias *rational medicine*. Dr Bruce, besides being lecturer on Materia Medica and therapeutics at the Charing Cross Hospital, is examiner in Materia Medica to the University and the College of Physicians of London. Intending candidates for the diploma of these two institutions might do well to read up a work on homoeopathic therapeutics to prepare themselves for examination by Dr Bruce.

Though our opponents largely adopt our therapeutics they do not *voluntarily* say anything to betray the fact that they have borrowed many of their remedies from us. It is only when driven into a corner, and compelled as it were to stand and deliver, that they confess to having "accepted truth *even* at the hands of homoeopathists." But they impertinently classify us with the old women and uneducated savages to whom they are indebted for some of their most accredited remedies and modes of treatment. They continue to deny us the right of brotherhood, and affect to regard us as not even belonging to the profession – pariahs, in fact, on whom any insult may be passed, and any injustice perpetrated, not only with impunity, but with applause from their allopathic colleagues. They cannot, indeed, proclaim our associations, break up our meetings by force, shoot us down with rifles if we object, and imprison our leaders, after the manner of a firm and resolute Government; but they can boycott us out of their societies and periodicals; they can intimidate our publishers, so that these tradesmen cannot publish, or even advertise, our works; and they have frequently tried their hand at evicting us from our hospital appointments, successfully in the cases of Henderson, Horner, Reith and others, but unsuccessfully in their most recent attempt of this sort at the Margaret Street Infirmary for Consumption, where two of the medical officers having become convinced of the superiority of homeopathy, the remainder of the medical staff, with one honourable exception, sought to oust them from their posts. In this attempt, as you know, they, for a wonder, signally failed, for the general meeting called to consider the matter passed a resolution in favour of liberty of opinion and practice for the medical officers. This led to the resignation of the anti-homoeopathic members of the staff. That the representatives of established medicine could remain in an institution where a resolution in favour of liberty of opinion and practice was passed, stamps their school as a sect of the narrowest description, intolerant of any opinions but those they themselves hold. But the sectarian character of the old school has quite lately received a still more striking illustration. It so happened that the surgeon elected by the governors of the Margaret Street Infirmary to take the post vacated by the former surgeon, who resigned along with the other members of the staff, was also surgeon to a newly-started hospital, called the Jubilee Hospital. The executive committee of the latter, mainly composed of the medical staff, were scandalised by the fact that their surgeon should hold a post in an institution where liberty of opinion and practice in matters medical was allowed, so they addressed a collective note to him requiring him to cease his connection with the Margaret Street Infirmary, or else resign his post in the Jubilee Hospital. On his refusing to submit to this piece of tyranny, the executive committee superseded him, and appointed another gentleman to take his post. In this instance there was no suspicion and no accusation of homoeopathic heresy against the surgeon; as a fact, he has no belief in homoeopathy. He was dismissed solely because he belonged to an infirmary where liberty of opinion and practice was accorded to the members of the medical staff, and where, consequently, homoeopathy, or any other line of treatment, might be practised by the medical officers according as they judged proper in the interests of the patients. Of course, a dismissal from a post on such a flimsy and frivolous pretext is wrong in law and equity, and the dismissed surgeon has commenced an action for wrongful dismissal against the tyrannical bigots of the executive committee. Let us hope a jury will award him a good round sum in damages, to teach the bigots that there are limits to their power to oppress those who differ from them, or, as in this case, who approve of according to others the same liberty they themselves claim.

I might enter on an enquiry as to the reasons why our colleagues of the old school still maintain their hostile attitude towards us, though they are so largely indebted to homoeopathy for the boasted progress of therapeutics both in the remedies they use and the injurious modes of treatment they have abandoned. But this enquiry would lead me too far, and would be taxing your patience too severely. I would merely mention that the reasons are manifold. There is the difficulty of bringing men to acknowledge they have been wrong in their conduct towards their homoeopathic colleagues, the reluctance to admit that methods and labours which they have been continually vaunting as the only possible means of developing scientific medicine are fallacious, the negative answer these controversialists always give to the question "Have any of the rulers or Pharisees – the big-wigs of the profession – believed on him?" – though, as a fact, we can point to many illustrious converts from the old school, including no less than five Professors of Pathology in ancient universities, such as Edinburgh, Zurich, Tübingen and Montpelier – and above all these is the well-ascertained fact that homoeopathy does not pay. It diminished the duration of diseases, it renders the frequent visits of the practitioner to watch the effects of his remedies superfluous, and it enables patients to treat themselves for most of the slighter ailments and many of the serious diseases which under the ordinary system have hitherto required the aid of the family medical attendant. The diminution of the number of the sick, and of the duration of their sicknesses implying a diminution of the fund whence the medical practitioners derive their means of living, in the face of the over-crowding of the profession – 1,200 young doctors being annually added to the profession to supply the places of 600 dead or retired practitioners – is not calculated to make the medical profession enthusiastically desirous for the triumph of homoeopathy.

Dr Richardson has lately shown in the *Asclepian* that the improvements in sanitary matters and in preventive medicine have seriously affected the incomes of the profession, and the instinct of self-preservation will lead its members to resist to the utmost any farther diminution of the sources of their incomes.

Partial compensations to the profession are occasionally found. The encouragement given by the bulk of the profession to the indiscriminate use of narcotics is one of the most objectionable of these. The doctrine that wherever pain exists it must be instantly choked off with a narcotic, has led to the manufacture of some of the most distressing maladies. Numerous asylums exist on the continent for the treatment of morphinomaniacs, whose insanity has been caused by the extravagant use of morphia, chiefly in the form of hypodermic injections, originally introduced and practised upon them by their medical advisers, but which they keep up for themselves. A Pravaz syringe or a bottle of *chloral* is looked on as indispensable to every fashionable lady's or gentleman's toilet-table – at least in Ouida's novels. Other narcotics are also extensively employed, such as *bromide of potassium, ether, chloroform, cocaine*, and lastly *hashish,* not to speak of the continual and pernicious use of alcohol in extravagant quantities. While temporarily relieving suffering, these poisonous drugs not only mask the signs by which the cause of the disease reveals itself and its remedy may be discovered, but they lay the foundation of other and often more serious diseases, which not only destroy the bodily health but injure the mind and weaken the moral sense of their victims.

Any theory or mode of treatment that promises to give the doctor more to do is eagerly accepted by the great bulk of the profession. The germ theory, which offered the practitioner many opportunities of fussing about his patients, examining their secretions with his microscope, and applying his microbicides, was very popular for a long time, but its day has gone by. In surgery, the carbolic acid antiseptic system, which brought a baronetcy to Lister, was received at first with acclamations, but is now seldom spoken of, as it has failed to effect what its promoters promised. While the delusion lasted there was a rare time for the surgeon, with his spray producers, his antiseptic bandages, plasters, lint and so forth.

That the medical profession, as a rule, are more addicted to credulity than to scepticism in regard to medical innovations which do not tend or threaten to diminish their profits, is shown by the uncritical haste with which they adopt the most fanciful theories regarding disease, and the most absurd and pernicious modes of treatment. The germ theory, with its corollary germicide remedies, the doctrine of the prime importance of subduing pain and procuring sleep, with its corollary of the indiscriminate employment of narcotics, prove this; and further evidence of this credulity is afforded by the acclamations with which the whole medical profession, as represented by their periodical organs, received the miserable delusion of Pasteur's anti-hydrophobia inoculations, the excellence and efficacy of which we have lately seen testified to by a British Committee, consisting of some of the most distinguished and highly considered men of this country, when the most cursory examination would have shewn them that so far from Pasteur's inoculations having proved successful, the rate of mortality from hydrophobia in France has been actually much higher during the year when his inoculations were in full swing than the average of a long series of years. By far the greater number of these deaths in France occurred among patients who had been subjected to Pasteur's inoculations, and there is not a shadow of a doubt that a good many of the deaths were really owing to the inoculations, which caused a new and hitherto undescribed form of rabies – rage de laboratoire, the French call it. Perhaps the recent death of a British Peer, who had been most carefully inoculated by Pasteur, will open the eyes of Pasteur's admirers to the fallacy on which the whole system is based. It was said, I think by Sydney Smith, that railway travelling would never be rendered safe until a Peer or a Bishop had been smashed; so, perhaps, now that a Peer has in his own person demonstrated the fallacy of Pasteur's inoculations, the tide of opinion will turn against them and the ludicrous pretensions of their inventor be discredited.

For the reasons before stated I do not anticipate any very speedy general adoption of homoeopathy by the profession nor any immediate general admission of the claims of Hahnemann to be considered the greatest physician whom the history of medicine can show. But the time will come when all this will happen. The flowing tide is with us, and though it seems to flow but slowly in Britain and in Europe it makes perceptible advances. This very year we have witnessed two rather significant events, one of them is the transfer of the Margaret Street Infirmary for Consumption, not exactly to a complete staff of Hahnemann's disciples, but at all events to a staff who are willing to accord perfect liberty of opinion and practice to their colleagues, and the majority of whom are open and avowed believers in the therapeutic rule we owe to Hahnemann. The other significant event is the opening of the Hahnemann Hospital in Liverpool, a magnificent gift from a public-spirited citizen and a zealous believer in Hahnemann's great reform – Mr. Henry Tate – a gentleman well known to you as a munificent supporter of this hospital.

Hahnemann has been dead forty-four years, but unlike most medical celebrities, whose names are hardly remembered a few years after their death, and whose systems have generally been discredited and discarded before they had shuffled off this mortal coil, Hahnemann's fame has gone on ever increasing, and his system gathers converts daily. New hospitals are founded in almost every civilised country for the practice of his doctrines, new periodicals are established everywhere for the propagation of his therapeutics, the whole medical world is adopting more or less completely his remedies; if you seek his monument you have only to look around you at such noble institutions as this we are assembled in, at the crowds of grateful and enthusiastic friends who owe their health and often their lives to his brilliant discovery, at the "animated busts" which smile benignantly on us from hundreds of chemists' shops, one of which nearly spoilt the holiday of his American traducer, Dr Oliver Wendell Holmes at Malvern as he tells us. No medical reformer since the days of Hippocrates has ever obtained anything like the following of Hahnemann. What remains to us of the schools founded by Galen, Paracelsus, Sydenham, Boerhaave, Van Helmont, Stahl, Cullen, Brown, Broussais? They are nothing but mere *nominum umbre*, but Hahnemann lives and flourishes in scores of colleges and universities, in hundreds of hospitals and dispensaries, in thousands of qualified and busy practitioners, and in millions of lay adherents in every civilised country in the world.

References

1 Dudgeon, RE. The Hahnemann Oration, *Monthly Homoeopathic Review*, 1887; 31: 719-741.
2 Hahnemann, S. Quin, FFH. Ed., *Fragmenta de Viribus Medicamentorum Positivis: sive in sano Corpore Humano Observatis 1805*, London, Samuel Highley, 1834.

14

THE SYCOSIS OF HAHNEMANN

Introduction

No discussion of Hahnemann is complete without a consideration of his theory of miasms. We have already seen that Hughes, for example, was a sceptic. Here is an erudite paper by Burnett (see Chapter 8), which deals with gonorrhoea and its relationship with sycosis. As far as I can discover it has not previously been reprinted as one of Burnett's 'little books'. He regards it as a continuation of his first lecture, *Ecce Medicus*. His thesis rests partially on a discussion of his interpretation of Dudgeon's view of sycosis. And he outlines a question, which we still ask, to what extent sycosis is the same as gonorrhoea.

A short series of letters and opinions about the relationship of Hughes and Burnett by Clarke completes the chapter.

On gonorrhoea in its constitutional aspects with special reference to the *sycosis* of Hahnemann[1] 1888
By James Compton Burnett

For years past I have thought it would be a very desirable task to be undertaken, to investigate afresh those diseases that give the ground work of the biopathology of the Seer of Köthen, and I have often wondered that the vigour and enterprise of some of our number of this generation have so long left this field of research comparatively untilled; that is, untilled in this generation. For, in our gropings after truth, each succeeding generation gains a little on its predecessor, by the general progress of knowledge, and by the slow movings of the human mind towards as much of certainty and of finality as seems attainable for the limited and finite.

And then, whether we believe in psora, syphilis, and sycosis, or not; that is, as they are taught by Hahnemann, a large part of the work done by the homoeopathic school during the past fifty years is more or less tinged with these doctrines; and, moreover, anything taught by so able an observer, as was Hahnemann, deserves serious investigation at our hands. And whatever may be said of the therapeutics of general medicine, positive diagnostics has distinctly advanced during the past decade, and I submit that it is desirable that our own position should be review in the light of this advance.

When I had given the *First Hahnemannian Lecture*, known as *Ecce Medicus*, I certainly thought one of my followers in the orator's chair would have tackled the Köthen phase of homoeopathy and exhibited it in the light of modern research and experience, so as to determine for us of this generation, how much of it still holds good, and what part, if any, must be considered as no longer tenable. But, thus far, the work has not been done since then, and I therefore will proceed to consider the subject in part here.

Mr. Punch is a great authority for us in this country of spleen and gravity, and, as we all know, his reiterated advice in regard to things to be done is, that if you want them done well, do them yourself.

Hahnemann, as is well known, spent his younger and more vigorous days in demolishing theories and hypotheses; indeed, he threw them all right out of his mental window and made a fresh start altogether with medicine sans pathology, sans theories, sans everything in fact, but the therapeutic law of similars, which is still for many a very filmy theory indeed. However, the law of likes is no mere theory for us; for us it is the one thing common to our body; outside of the law we practically agree about nothing, and yet, notwithstanding this almost general disagreement amongst us, our friends, the enemy, will have it that we and the medical profession at large are not *solidaire*: surely the fact that we disagree about almost everything that is of vital importance should offer them sufficient internal evidence of their and our solidarity.

But, as I said, we agree on our fundamental law, except, indeed, that some of our number of late years have had sad searchings of heart about the law also! It is a rule, they say, not a law! Or again, it is a method. So that, as a matter of fact, we do not quite agree about anything whatsoever! Therefore, we may at any rate claim still to be very professional to the full extent of the proverb, that "doctors differ."

And as to whether we should speak of the idea of similars as a law or as a rule, the contention is that it is a rule rather than a law is, I submit, quite groundless. But as some have been captivated by the reasonings of those who pose as the champions of rule as against law, it might not be amiss to point out that the whole contention for the rule is based upon the poor grammar of the disputers. I have, thus far, never known of a German or a Frenchman go in for "rule," and that for the very sufficient reason that they understand the use of the subjunctive mood, which cannot be said of all Britishers, no matter how learned they may be. In order to really understand Hahnemann on this point, it is absolutely essential that one understand Latin and German composition, more particularly in regard to the use of the subjunctive. Those who contend for "rule" had better scuttle out of their position as quietly as they can, lest someone, one of these fine days, take the trouble to pour out a vial of wholesome ridicule upon their "rule." The same remarks apply in regard to the question of the noted formula of the homoeopathic school, viz., whether should we say *similia similibus curantur*, or *similia similibus curentur*? Or course, the reply is that both are correct, they both express precisely the same thing, only one is in the indicative and the other in the subjunctive. I do not admit that it is in the imperative. In some of the old Hermetic works you will find it put *similia similibus curare*, which is, of course, precisely the same thing, only in another mood. You will also find *simile a simili curare*; hence, it is really, in more ways than one, merely a matter of mood.

However, everything in this world is comparative, and, comparatively speaking, we do agree that like cures like; and be it notion, principle, law, rule or method, we so far agree to admit that these words, *similia similibus curantur*, express something positively demonstrable in clinical life. All this falls within that phase of the development of homoeopathy anterior to the sojourn of Hahnemann at Köthen. And this part has been really almost completely exhausted, so let us go over to Köthen and hear the oracular pronouncement that all chronic disease is primarily due to three somethings – *psora, syphilis* and *sycosis*.

When a man comes out of the land of darkness of school teachings and throws over school physic (I do not mean brimstone and treacle, which was *my* school physic), and passes into the comparative glare of Hahnemannic therapeutics, he is generally considerably perturbed by the violent change of climate, *i.e.*, from darkness to light. He requires some time to acclimatise. At first he usually has an acute attack of homoeopathic enthusiasm, a veritable fever that yields neither to *Aconite* nor to *Pyrogenium*, and he makes a *tabula rasa* of everything and a good deal besides.

But when a few failures have sobered him down a wee, he goes back into himself, and finds out a few things for himself. He finds that *Belladonna* will cure the delirium of tuberculosis of the meninges, and other of its symptoms, but the patient in the end dies all the same. He gives *Baptisia, Arsenicum*, serpent poisons, acids, &c., in low fevers, but his patients are very apt to die in the end all the same. He has a patient given to picking his nose, or things in general, and after considering the merits of *Arum triphyllum, Conium, Helleborus, Lachesis, Selenium, Stramonium* and the like, and exhibiting them, he finds – the worms live on still!

In fact, he learns to discriminate and to differentiate between true initial and all-along-the-line similarity and that which is ultimate and superficial only. When a man in his homoeopathics arrives at this stage of his developmental process, he is apt to do one of three things, viz: he may, 1st, throw your homoeopathy clean overboard; or, 2nd, admit the limitedness of its sphere of application; or, lastly, he may set about procuring a pathology to fit his therapeutic doctrine. I have gone through all these stages myself now, and am beginning to understand the Köthen etiologic phase of homoeopathy. If space would allow I would seek to encompass this etiologic phase of homoeopathy in its entirety; but, as it will not permit of this, I have chosen one only of the three Hahnemannic, chronic, so-called miasms for consideration, and that *sycosis*.

I have a special reason for choosing *sycosis*. I mean the *sycosis* of Hahnemann, and not the *sycosis autorum*, viz., our knowledge on the subject has much increased of late years, for science has been shining upon it.

Now, leaving syphilis and psora quite out of consideration, I propose to enquire into the Hahnemannic doctrine of *sycosis* in the light of modern science and experience.

First of all, I would make a preliminary observation in respect of the word *miasm*, which is current in homoeopathic literature in a very peculiar sense. Hahnemann himself calls the supposed causes of chronic diseases *miasms*, and his translators carefully and conscientiously translate the word by itself!

Now, in English, *miasm* means an infection floating in the air; the effluvia or fine particles of any putrefying or noxious bodies rising and floating in the atmosphere, in fact, exhalations. Therefore it is hardly accurate to use the English word *miasm*, or its pure Greek form *miasma*, as the English equivalent of the word "miasma" as used by Hahnemann, or if you do, you must carefully define the use of the word first, for our word miasm, being derived from $\mu\iota\alpha\iota\nu\omega$, to soil, to defile, to pollute, to dirty, might etymologically stand as the translators of Hahnemann have it, but $\tau\delta\;\mu\iota\alpha\mu\alpha$ means not only a defilement, a soiling, a befouling, but also an impure exhalation, in which restricted sense only it has come into use in English. Miasm in our vernacular means impure particles or effluvia in the atmosphere, and nothing else. What Hahnemann meant when he used the Germanised miasma was not at all what we understand by miasm, but was rather what we now understand by *virus* when applied to the primary form of a disease, and *taint* when used to denote the later phases. If in speaking English in these days we talk of the syphilitic virus or taint, the gonorrhoeal virus or taint, the virus of itch, the itch-taint, we are expressing ourselves, so far as the words are concerned, accurately, and everybody knows what we mean, but when we speak of the miasms of these diseases we are really, as I must submit, using jargon, and so gratuitously mystifying ourselves. Ague is supposedly due to a miasm, syphilis to a virus. So much, therefore, for the word miasm, as wrongly used in homoeopathic literature. I say wrongly, because it tends to obscure, and in all conscience the thing is obscure enough without any verbal mystifications.

Now, let us go on to enquire what Hahnemann understood by *sycosis*. The highest English authority on the exegetics of homoeopathy is, I think all will admit, Dr Dudgeon, and he says:

"As regards the third of Hahnemann's chronic miasms *sycosis*, or the condylomatous venereal disease, the notion of its independent nature has been considerably contested, not alone by allopaths, but also by some of our own school. The disease always arises in consequence of impure coitus, and appears in the form of dry or nasty-looking, or soft and spongy excrescences in the form of a cocks-comb or cauliflower, easily bleeding, and secreting a fœtid fluid, and sometimes accompanied by a sort of blennorrhœa from the urethra. Their seat is the glans or foreskin in the male, the vulva and its appendages in the female. Their removal by the ligature or cautery, actual or potential, is, according to Hahnemann, followed by similar growths on other parts of the body or other ailments, the only one he mentions being shortening of the flexor tendons, particularly of the fingers".

"It is, Hahnemann alleges, the rarest of the three chronic miasms, and, as I before observed, it is very doubtful if it be a peculiar disease, and not rather a form of syphilis. The secondary effects Hahnemann describes as arising from it must certainly be rare, for I can state from my own experience that I know several persons who have had such venereal condylomata burnt off many years ago, and who have never had the slightest trace of those after effects Hahnemann alludes to; though at the same time I am bound to admit that think I have observed a connection of certain pseudo-rheumatic affections and inveterate gleets with the figwart disease." Thus far Dr Dudgeon.[2]

So the *only* after-effect of the figwart disease mentioned by Hahnemann is a shortening of the flexor tendons, particularly of the fingers, and yet Dr Dudgeon speaks of "those after-effects Hahnemann alludes to!"

It can thus hardly be maintained that Dr Dudgeon puts *sycosis* before us in a very clear light, though his remark in regard to gonorrhoeal rheumatism shows the accurate observer, and John Hunter had observed the same thing long ago. That people do get venereal warts admits of no doubt whatever, that they are a form of syphilis, as stated by Dudgeon, is not now generally admitted.

Hahnemann very clearly differentiated between syphilis and *sycosis*, because he found *Mercurius* helped to cure syphilis but not figwarts, and modern experience and science are seemingly on Hahnemann's side on this point. Dudgeon very properly objects to consider diseases as *sycotic* simply because they can be curatively modified by *Nitric acid* and *Thuja*. But then we cannot entirely ignore the aid obtainable from this source; for instance, a very bad chronic ulcerated sore throat that yields straightaway to full doses of the *iodide of potassium* tells a tale we all understand without any commentator. I have long been puzzled with Hahnemann's divisions of drugs, i.e., how he arrived at them; and I am beginning to suspect that he made them largely by an appreciation of the *ex juvantibus et nocentibus* teachings. And a number of his indications are, beyond any doubt, derived from the time-old *signaturæ rerum naturalium. Thuja* to wit.

Now, I complain that the great exegete of homoeopathy, Dr Dudgeon, whom we all delight to honour, devotes too little attention to the doctrine of *sycosis*; he neither establishes it nor does he demolish it. Dr Dudgeon mentions it in passing, throws doubt upon it, and then leaves it. Dudgeon's doubt as to the separate nature of the condylomatous venereal disease is based upon his observations that he had known persons in whom the condylomata were burnt off many years ago, and yet the flexor tendons of their fingers had never become shortened! I can say the same, and, no doubt, we all can, but we have equally seen plenty of people who had syphilis many years ago, and who have never had any later manifestations of the disease, but that in no way militates against the specific nature of late, later, and latest manifestations of syphilis where they do occur.

Dudgeon speaks with no great respect of those homoeopathic practitioners who have regarded ordinary warts as evidence of *sycotic* infection, because Hahnemann distinctly declares such warts as of *psoric* origin. This looks like a formidable indictment, but one which vanishes when more closely examined. It is quite true that Hahnemann puts common warts, encysted and other tumours, down to the very large account of psora, but he does not say "all" warts, only some. And herein lies *des Pudels Kern*, as I will proceed to show.

Let us now go to Hahnemann's own account of *sycosis* and see if it tallies with Dudgeon's. Turning up the *Chronische Krankheiten* we come upon the chapter devoted to the subject, and find it is just as scant and unsatisfactory as Dudgeon's exegesis of it. Hahnemann only devotes one small chapter of four pages to it, and Dudgeon's account of it is quite correct, except that he fails to point out the strange statement by Hahnemann that *sycosis* is an epidemic affection, "Nur von Zeit zu Zeit herrschend war," and ever getting more and more rare.

Common gonorrhœa, Hahnemann says, does not appear to penetrate the whole organism, but only to irritate the urinary organs locally.

His remedies for are a few globules of *Thuja* 30 and *Nitric acid* 30. His remedies for the common clap are a drop of fresh parsley juice, if there is much urging to urinate and *Copaiva balsam*; about one drop of the mother tincture when there is less inflammation, and if these do not do the trick, why you get a gleet which is *psoric*.

According to Hahnemann, therefore, there are two kinds of gonorrhœa, or clap; the one with condylomata, which is constitution infecting, and in which the urethral flux may occasionally but not often be wanting, and which constitutes his sycosis, and which must be monoposically cured by *Thuja* 30 and *acid nit.* 30, leaving each from 20 to 40 days time of action.

I would here remark, with some emphasis, that Hahnemann very distinctly differentiates between local irritation and an organismic evil in regard to the dose; when he wants to treat the organ or the part, *topico* – specifically he uses the mother tincture – or simple juice of the plant, and when he wants to treat the organism he uses the higher dilutions; and I may say that my own observations tally with this view exactly, with this difference, viz., that for the topic action the small material dose has to be often repeated. Before we go any further, let us note that Hahnemann uses the word *miasm* for the cause of the common non-condylomatous clap as well as for the other.

Let us now resume for a moment. According to Hahnemann there are two kinds of clap, the condylomatous, which is constitutional, and is to be cured monoposically by *Thuja* and *Nitric acid*; and the common clap, which is a merely local affection of the urethra, and is to be cured by the juice of *Petroselinum sativum*, monoposically also, if much urging to urinate; or a drop of the alcoholic solution of the *balsam of Copaiva* when there is less inflammatory irritation.

This is, practically, all that Hahnemann tells us about his *sycosis* and his common gonorrhœa.

We have now considered Dudgeon as exegete and Hahnemann as the originator of the doctrine of *sycosis*, but we have herewith not overmuch light, and conceptions not too clear. During the past forty years there have been very numerous authors who have written on Hahnemann's *sycosis*. Boenninghausen, Wolf, Grauvogl, Hering, H. Goullon, and many others, and it would be very interesting to follow these thinkers in their yearnings and gropings after truth, in their desire to harmonise the facts of science with their veneration of the master.

But I am afraid the task is too great, and, moreover, I prefer another plan. I suggest that we take first of all Hahnemann himself as likely to know most of his own mental offspring. I suppose the majority of us feel that we know most of our own children after the flesh, and a man may fairly, I should think, be considered an authority on his own mental offspring also.

I quite agree with the principal exegetists of Hahnemann that it does not follow that because *Thuja* and *Nitric acid* may cure a complaint that therefore said complaint is of a *sycotic* nature as Hahnemann understands it; but inasmuch as we conclude that grave ulcerations, which readily yield (at least temporarily) to the *iodide of potassium*, are in all probability of a certain specific nature, so in like manner it may fairly be conceded, at least for the sake of study and argument, that what can be cured by the two grand antisycotics may very probably be of a sycotic nature.

Let us take merely the standpoint of probability, that much may be safely conceded without any great danger to scientific truth. Therefore, I invite you to consult Hahnemann on the subject of *sycosis* under the headings of *Thuja* and *Nitric acid*.

Well, the Hahnemannian pathogenesis of *Thuja* does not help us a bit, and, oddly enough, *nitric acid* is classified by Hahnemann as what? as an antipsoric! So we see that Hahnemann classifies *nitric acid* as an antipsoric after having mentioned it as second in order for the radical cure of sycosis. Then, again, although he classifies *Nitric acid* as an antipsoric, he mentions warts (of the *psoric* kind?) and also condylomata and inguinal adenomata as curable by *Nitric acid*, while the symptomatology of this acid clearly portrays gonorrhœa (S. 375 to 389).

Hughes tells us that our only pathogenesis of nitric acid was first published in the second edition of the *Chronic Diseases*, containing 1,426 symptoms. This cannot be correct, for my edition is the first, 1828, and it contains a pathogenesis of nitric acid, with 803 symptoms.

Well, with all this we get no clear conception of Hahnemann's sycosis, as an adequate basis for the huge structure which some of his disciples have built upon it, and which is the sycosis of the homoeopathic authors, but I am not satisfied that it is Hahnemann's.

I propose now to consult Ameke's *History of Homoeopathy* on the point,[3] and on page 138 of Drysdale's translation, read "Besides this 'psora' there were other fundamental causes, viz., 'sycosis,' the phenomena connected with gonorrhœa and 'syphilis.' Though there may have been some substratum of truth in these views, Hahnemann nevertheless far transcended the limits of probability and fell into a great error." Here, then, according to Ameke, as translated by Dr Alfred Drysdale, and edited by Dr Dudgeon, we find sycosis defined as "the phenomena connected with gonorrhœa." So, according to this, sycosis and the clap disease, the *Tripperseuche* are identical. This positive statement of the identity of the gonorrhœal disease in its entirety and the sycosis of Hahnemann so surprised me, that I turned to the original and find the translator has interpolated the definite article *the*, which makes all the difference. Ameke's words are "ausser dieser Psora blieben noch als Grundursachen übrig die Sycosis, mit dem Tripper zusammen-hängende Erscheinungen, und Syphilis," and these mean "sycosis, phenomena connected with clap," not *the* phenomena.

The words of Ameke, viz., "there may have been some substratum of truth in these views" (of Hahnemann) really pretty nearly epitomise the actual attitude of the homoeopathic practitioners of the world at large. Speaking broadly, you to whom these words are addressed do *not* accept the etiologic phase of homoeopathy, and yet almost every man of you is daily, almost hourly, influenced by it in his modes of thought, of practice, and of writing and speaking. You do not accept the doctrines of psora, syphilis, and sycosis, and yet you do not quite reject them; you seem to think there is something in them after all.

Now, to keep within the bounds of my plan, viz., of sycosis, surely we ought to be able to *know* whether the doctrine of sycosis is true or false. Indeed, I think it about time sycosis were elevated from the position of a scholastic doctrine to that of positive scientific demonstration, at least clinically, or else cast out altogether; for it must be manifest that there either is, or there is not, a condylomatous venereal disease which we call sycosis.

At this stage of our inquiry we are encountered with a difficulty, for to my mind it is very questionable whether sycosis and the entire gonorrhœal disease are identical. We have seen that Hahnemann differentiates two kinds of clap, the one a local affection of the urinary organs, and the other sycosis, in which there may be no urethral pyorrhoea or blennorrhœa at all. And this quite coincides with what we no doubt have all seen over and over again, viz., condylomata, or *verrucæ accuminatæ*, in persons who have had no gonorrhœa at any time; but in all the cases which I have ever observed, impure coition had probably taken place (the hereditary ones in children always excepted), and hence these warts are certainly venereal; but are they always gonorrhœal? To say that the principal exegetes of homoeopathy and the pro-sycosis writers, such as H. Goullon and the various and numerous authors quoted by him in his admirable prize essay on *Thuja and the Lues Gonorrhoica*, accept sycosis as synonymous with the whole gonorrhœal disease, which Autenrieth and other writers before and at the time of Hahnemann fully recognised and proclaimed as due to a constitution-infecting virus, and which they termed *Tripperseuche,* or clap disease, and which they also ascribed to a miasma or virus, as did Hahnemann. To say this does not satisfy my mind that Hahnemann thought the gonorrhœal virus as the primary cause of figwarts and other constitutional ailments: I think everything must hinge upon the answer to this question. I have weighed the matter carefully and have come to the conclusion that sycosis for Hahnemann, was the *condylomatous venereal disease* indeed, and nothing else, and not the *Tripperseuche,* or clap-disease, of Autenrieth in its entirety.

If you will take the trouble to read the greater medical writers of Germany of the first four decades of this century, you will find (and I am sure Drysdale, Dudgeon, Hughes, H. Goullon, to name no others, will all agree with me) that gonorrhœa was considered by very many of them as a *Seuche,* or constitutional affection, and as the prime cause of many specifically gonorrhœal ailments or manifestations, only one of which is condyloma.

The clap-disease, *die Tripperseuche,* was a recognised prime cause of chronic disease years before our founder promulgated his sycosis, and if you admit that sycosis and clap-disease are synonymous terms, then sycosis is not the mental property of Hahnemann at all: this much is certain, either sycosis and clap-disease are not the same thing, or else if they are, there is no such a thing as sycosis to be attributed to the genius of the founder of homoeopathy.

We must not forget that Hahnemann differentiates two kinds of clap, the common variety and that of the condyloma, so he evidently did not include the whole clap disease in his sycosis.

It is seemingly no use for us to hunt about in Hahnemann's works for any real enlightenment on the subject of sycosis, as they contain none, and why? Simply because Hahnemann himself had but very little knowledge on the subject, as he practically admits on page 63, of vol. 1 of his *Chronische Krankheiten*. I should not be surprised if he had set aside sycosis for study and consideration in a future time, but apparently that time never came, that is it never came so far as we know; possibly the Paris MSS. may contain something on the subject.

We are then brought face to face with this primary question. Is the sycosis of Hahnemann identical with the gonorrhœal disease of Authenrieth? If so, then it is not the property of Hahnemann; and if not identical, what is it? syphilitic, gonorrhœal, chancroidal, or a separate and independent disease *sui generis*?

These points being settled, we could proceed to a comparison of gonorrhœa in its constitutional aspects, with the sycosis delineated in the original works of Hahnemann. For I for one cannot admit that the *sycosis autorum homoeopathicorum* is the sycosis as painted by Hahnemann himself.

Authors' comment

We must not assume a monolithic view of how our homeopathic ancestors related to each other. Homeopathy grew and progressed through the talents of all of these men, (and it was only men in this era). Burnett, Cooper, Drysdale, Dudgeon and Hughes had their own talents and strengths. Hughes had a 'purist' view of homeopathy, as all knowledge of material medica originating from proved symptoms; hence his assistance in editing the monumental encyclopedia of Timothy Field Allen with the title *pure* material medica.[4] He appeared not to tolerate Burnett's interest, for example, in Rademacher,[5] vaccinosis[6] and new nosodes,[7] all of which have long since been accepted into the canon of homeopathy. Burnett had a talent for anatomy, for which he won prizes, and German so he could read original literature. Maybe Hughes was jealous, while Dudgeon appears to try and conciliate.

General Correspondence: Hughes and Burnett[8]

> **To the Editor of the *Homoeopathic World***
> Sir: there is a passage in Dr Cooper's appreciation of Dr Hughes in your last number which calls for some remark from me. It is this: Dr Hughes "instead of welcoming with enthusiasm the most distinguished and by far the most learned of his converts into the bosom of homoeopathy, the late Dr Compton Burnett, be invariably looked askance at the man, and it is a noteworthy fact that it was Hughes himself who prevented the confirmation of Compton Burnett's appointment many years ago as co-editor of the British Journal of Homoeopathy. It is an allowable inference that the untimely ending of . . . the British Journal . . . was due to a mistake that would never have occurred had a man of Burnett's intuitive perception of human nature been installed upon the editorial staff."

I am not qualified to give an opinion as to whether Dr Burnett was "the most distinguished and by far the most learned" of Dr Hughes' converts. You, sir, being as you tell us a convert of our lamented friend, are better able to decide that point, but I don't know what authority Dr Cooper has for his statement that Dr Hughes "invariably looked askance at the man." I don't know exactly what is meant by the expression, surely nothing so bad as this:

> "His wannish eyes upon them bent askance,
> And when he saw their labours well succeed,
> He wept for rage, and threatened dire mischance."

But probably Dr Cooper means nothing more than that Dr Hughes did not like Dr Burnett, or perhaps did not feel that amount of enthusiasm at his conversion to homoeopathy, which Dr Cooper thinks the convert merited. I never heard Dr Hughes say an unkind or disparaging word about Dr Burnett; I know that he appreciated Dr Burnett's skill as a practitioner of homoeopathy; and it will be found when Dr Hughes' work on the *Principles and Practice of Homoeopathy*, of which he had not finished correcting the proof-sheets when he died, is published, that he gives Dr Burnett credit for many valuable additions to our therapeutic knowledge. What authority Dr Cooper has for his statement that Dr Hughes "prevented the confirmation of Compton Burnett's appointment many years ago as co-editor of the *British Journal of Homoeopathy*" I know not; but I know this, that there never was any question of Dr Burnett's joining the editorial staff of the *British Journal*, at least I never heard of it, and surely if there had been I would have heard of it.

What Dr Cooper means by saying that the "untimely ending" of the *British Journal* "was due to a mistake that would never have occurred had a man of Dr Burnett's intuitive perception of human nature been installed upon the editorial staff," I am quite at a loss to understand. Cessation of a medical quarterly after forty years of life can hardly be called an "untimely ending". Few British medical quarterlies have attained that age. Our reasons for ceasing the publication are stated in the last number of the *Journal*, and I am not conscious that we made any mistake in the matter. What Dr Cooper means by "Dr Burnett's intuitive perception of human nature," or how that incomprehensible quality would have saved the *Journal* from an untimely ending, I cannot comprehend.

Yours faithfully,
R. E. Dudgeon.
22, Carlton Hill, N.W., May 12, 1902

From the Editor of the *Homoeopathic World*

The story of the invitation given to Burnett to become one of the editors of the *British Journal of Homoeopathy* we heard from Burnett himself, and, as we understood it, it came about in this way. Drysdale was at one time very desirous of having Burnett on the staff of that journal, and asked him if he would be willing to join. Burnett said that he would. Later on, Drysdale told Burnett that he had been overruled by Hughes, to whom he had mentioned the proposal. Hughes would not hear of Burnett's being made one of the editors. Nothing, therefore, came of the matter. Drysdale's wish was a very natural one, for between him and Burnett there always was a very strong bond of affection and regard. When Drysdale died Burnett wrote: "A big slice of my life is buried in his grave."

Perhaps the best idea of how Hughes regarded Burnett may be obtained by quoting a passage from the obituary notice of him written by Hughes in the *Journal of the British Homoeopathic Society* for July, 1901 (p. 281):

> "His [Burnett's] practice, as shown by his books, was singularly eclectic. Now borrowing organ-remedies from Rademacher, and giving them in ten-drop doses of their tinctures; now practising isopathy with the 100th dilutions of 'Bacillinum'; now treating every chronic case with Thuja where there was suspicion of 'vaccinosis,' pure homoeopathy assumed less and less place in his therapeutics; yet he clung to our system as his home and starting-point, and was never ashamed of identification with it. Sit levis ei terra: we shall hold him in kindly memory."

The writer who penned this never took a frank view of Burnett. That Hughes could have thought it a compliment to say of Burnett that he was "never ashamed" of his association with homoeopathy proves that he never knew the man – the author of "Fifty Reasons" – at all. As well think of complimenting the Gracchi by saying they were never ashamed of their mother! The idea that homoeopathy was something to be ashamed of, or apologised for, could never by any possibility have found lodgement in Burnett's mind when once he had apprehended the principle: the idea seems never to have been wholly absent from the mind of Hughes. – Editor, *Homoeopathic World*.

References

1 Compton Burnett, JC. On gonorrhoea, in its constitutional aspects with special reference to the *sycosis* of Hahnemann, *Monthly Homoeopathic Review*, 1888, 33, 15–27.

2 Dudgeon, RE. *Lectures on the Theory and Practice of Homoeopathy*, London, Henry Turner, 1854, p. 300.
3 Ameke, W. *History of Homoeopathy, its Origins; its Conflicts, with an appendix on the present state of university medicine*, London, E Gould & Sons, 1885.
4 Allen, TF. *Encyclopaedia of Pure Materia Medicc*, 10 volumes, New York & Philadelphia, Boericke & Tafel, 1874-1879.
5 Oehmen, F., Rademacher, *Johann Gottfried, seine Ehrfahrungslehre und ihre Geschichte. Ein Beitrag zur Geschichte der Medizin des XIX Jahrhunderts*, Bonn am Rhein, Verlag von P Hanstein, 1900.
6 Burnett, J.C., *Vaccinosis and its cure by Thuja; with Remarks on Homœoprophylaxis* 2nd edition, London, Homoeopathic Publishing Co, 1897.
7 Burnett, J.C., *Five Years' Experience in the New Cure for Consumption by Its Own Virus*, London, Homoeopathic Publishing Co., 1890.
8 Dudgeon, RE. General Correspondence: Hughes and Burnett, *The Homoeopathic World* **37**: 2: June 1902.

15

THE CLARKE MEMORIAL MEETING

Introduction

The British Homoeopathic Society organised a meeting in memory of Dr John Henry Clarke on 7 January 1932.[1] It was attended by many prominent homeopaths of the day including Doctors: Le Hunte Cooper, Giles Goldsbrough, Granville Hey, Powell, P Hall-Smith, Thomas Stonham, Margaret Tyler, Charles Wheeler and H Fergie Woods. Apologies were received from Dr John Weir. The meeting was opened by the President, who introduced Dr George Burford, the principal speaker.

The proceedings

The President, Dr P Hall-Smith, said that the Society was met that day to do honour to the memory of its late colleague, Dr John Henry Clarke, who was among the foremost homoeopaths of recent times, and whose work for homoeopathy would bear comparison with that of any of those great figures who had represented the cause since the time of its founder Hahnemann.

It was unusual to devote the whole of a meeting of the Society to the memory of the life and work of one man, but such was the esteem in which Dr Clarke was held that is was unanimously decided at the last meeting of the Society to devote this meeting to his memory.

Those present would hear from those who had been most in touch with Dr Clarke and his work, and therefore best qualified to speak, something of the life of a colleague whose loss all deplored. Unfortunately, it had not fallen to his own lot to come into any close connection with Dr Clarke, as he was of a later generation, and Dr Clarke had given up his active connection with the Hospital before his advent there in 1910. However, from occasional contacts and from what he had known of Dr Clarke's work and interests, he had been impressed with one strong characteristic, namely, independence of thought and judgment, and this was an asset homoeopaths could ill afford to spare. There was always the danger in the case of any body of people attempting to carry out precepts laid down by a great founder and leader, to interpret his teachings too rigidly in accordance with the letter of the law, and they often failed to adapt them to the conditions of the day. If homoeopathy was to progress there must be that freedom and independence of thought which was always ready to discover fresh adaptations of its principles in relation to modern conditions and the spirit of the time.

There must be many of the rising generation of homoeopaths who knew very little of Dr Clarke and his work, and it was to be hoped that his independence of thought and outlook and his great industry might prove an example which would be considered well worthy of emulation. If the result of this meeting should be to extend the knowledge of what Dr Clarke had done for homoeopathy, and to inspire others to endeavour to follow in his footsteps, it would not have been held in vain.

As would be seen from the Agenda, Dr Burford was to give the inaugural address on Dr Clarke and his work, and no one was better fitted to do so.

> **About George Henry Burford**
> Dr George Henry Burford was born in Desborough, Northamptonshire, England in 1856. He practised in Aberdeen, Berlin, Vienna and London and was appointed Senior Surgeon and Physician for the Diseases of Women at the London Homoeopathic Hospital, He was President of the British Homoeopathic Society, President and Vice President of The International Homoeopathic Congress, and Secretary of the British Homoeopathic Association, Soon after the British Homoeopathic Association (BHA) was formed in 1902 its Educational Committee, in conjunction with the London Homoeopathic Hospital, formed a Missionary Sub-committee under the chairmanship of George Burford, to promote a course of instruction for non-medical missionaries[2] George Burford was also involved in the setting up of The Homoeopathic Hospital at Neuilly in France in 1914-1916.[3] Following his death in London 1937 the BHA Library was named in his honour.

Masters in Homoeopathy: the persistence of their work through time: John H Clarke[4]

by George Burford MB
Senior Gynaecological Consulting Physician to the London Homoeopathic Hospital

We meet today to affirm the continuity of the work of the great masters in homoeopathy of the past, and of their successors in the present, with that of the greater masters in homoeopathy of a yet more brilliant future. The channel through which runs this stream today contains the best work of those *Dii Majores* who but yesterday were of the present. Because the impress of their personality is still upon us, their inspiring spirit still lives, moves and has its being with us. While they were with us as contemporary original thinkers, they had not proved their survival values; now, some have already been received among the immortals in homoeopathic history. Such, within the present knowledge of many of us are Skinner, and Dudgeon, Cooper, Burnett and Hughes; the latest and possibly the greatest of these our nationals who have crossed the bar is John H Clarke. His work has already passed from the agora of contemporary judgment into the studium of survival values. For them, the tumult and the shouting have died: for us, the work of these captains and kings endures.

The pious duty of commemoration

From time immemorial, alike by tradition and instinct, great nations – and causes greater than nations, because international – these, I say, have publicly commemorated the passing of their great men – men of light and leading each in his day and generation. It is such a commemorative duty that brings us in assembly today. In this *éloge* I express the deep consciousness of all, that it is meet and right that we pay public tribute to this great homoeopath, for the dynamic he imparted to the homoeopathy, not only of his own country, but to the values of homoeopathy the world over; and not of his own century merely, but for all time. Clarke was imbued with the conviction that the profession of medicine was a liberal profession: and of the various forms of the practice of medicine, homoeopathy was the most liberal form – that its survival value was chiefest. On the occasion of the demise of Lord Kelvin – Professor of Physics, not Physic – Professor Sir Joseph Larmor said that he could not conceive that so powerful a mind, activated by the study and discovery of truth, should suddenly cease its interest in things of time and space, cut short by the limitations of this planet. I affirm the name of Clarke – in his translation to a "purer ether and sublimer air."

At an epoch in this country's history, on the death of an historical personage a great parliamentary orator rose in the House of Commons and said, "The Angel of Death has been abroad in the land: we can almost hear the beating of his wings." During your tenure of the Chair, sir, it has been your dolorous duty nearly every month to rise in your place and announce the withdrawal from this world of one and another of our colleagues – Nankivell, McLachlan, Cavendish Molson, Gerard Smith, Reed Hill – and still the list extends. At the last Society meeting the name of Clarke was inscribed on the Society's tablets as *fuit*. Form a homoeopathic point of view here was the "noblest Roman of them all"; each of them had been "faithful found," but Clarke had flown the homoeopathic flag longest and highest.

My just right to present to you for homage the record of the man who made so much homoeopathic history, is that of close personal acquaintance and friendship for half a century.

A homoeopathic novitiate and wanderjahr

Our mutual introduction was before 1880, he having recently settled in Ipswich as assistant partner with Dr W. Roche.

Here he remained for several years, working hard and reading hard. Here also he gained a *proxime accessit* to a prize offered by the London School of Homoeopathy for the twelve best clinical cases worked out on the homoeopathic plan. Here also he made his debut as a social reformer, on the lines of John Ruskin and Charles Kingsley - potent names to conjure with in those days. To him these reformers were as inspiring spirits, and he contributed a series of articles to the proletarian local press, and entitled "Men and Brethren." I fear, sir, that is farther than some of us would care to go now. When John Henry Clarke left Ipswich for London, his homoeopathic place was taken by Percy Wilde.

Clarke's first introduction to homoeopathy was made by a relative - a layman - who, finding him at a loose end, after graduation - a not infrequent episode among us - asked him boldly, "Why don't you look into homoeopathy?" He looked, and came to stay. He joined up with the famous dispensary in Liverpool, and commenced under tutelage the practice of homoeopathy. His first homoeopathic cure was of a bunch of warts, on the forehead of a boy; cured with *Thuja* in fractional doses, and effected in three weeks; the warts had lasted eighteen.

But those were spacious days for homoeopathy. In Liverpool, Compton Burnett, Hawkes, Drysdale, with his classical provings of *Kali bichromicum.* published *in M.M. Phys. and Applied*, the Haywards to whose boldness and dexterity are due the elaborated provings of *Crotalus*. (One of the allopathic journals commenced its narrative of the affair thus: "Now the serpent was more subtle than any of the beasts of the field, but he was not subtle enough for the homoeopaths of Liverpool".) This was the intensive environment in which young Clarke made his homoeopathic debut. What an inspiring experience for a homoeopath in his novitiate!

Thence to London to take up residence as House Physician at the London Homoeopathic Hospital; here the growing assurance of his homoeopathy was made doubly sure. I wish the name of every house physician who has worked for a year as resident here could find some permanent record on these walls! On the conclusion of this hospital appointment, next to Ipswich, as already recorded, for further experience and success: and ultimately the lure of London drew him to South Kensington into private practice, which with a true homoeopathic instinct he continued up to the end of his days. The period of this Wanderjahr culminated in a higher flight.

The consolidation of the homoeopathic character

By this time Clarke's star in the East had risen to some purpose, and was well on its way to the meridian. He had obtained the professional confidence of Bayes and Leadam and Dudgeon – with the latter he was always a special favourite – and others of the homoeopathic notables, sufficiently to be entrusted with their private patients. He was next elected as Assistant Physician to this Hospital; then lecturer on materia medica to the London School of Homoeopathy; and ultimately full physician in the wards where he had formerly done duty as house physician. Clarke's homoeopathic evolution up to this time had proceeded according to plan.

As full physician to the LHH came a development of private practice from general to consulting, a change of residence to Harrington Gardens and afterward to the Piccadilly area – plus chambers in Cornhill. He was now approaching the commencement of his fourth stage.

The evolution of a higher grade homoeopath

Clarke's years as physician to this hospital were useful to it – but not altogether happy to him. His colleagues were a remarkably able cohort of 3x men – S Yeldham, Galley Blackley, Byres Moir, Washington Epps, Knox Shaw, etc. And about 1890 he had made the acquaintance and received the inspiration of Dr Thomas Skinner, whose forceful personality led Clarke into the uplands of Hahnemannian homoeopathy. (Skinner, by the way, apart from his keen homoeopathy, was a notable man. He had been assistant to that equally masterful personage, Sir YJ Simpson, at the time when Simpson was experimenting with anaesthetics. Skinner was one of the fateful four who inhaled the new fluid chloroform, tumbled under the table, and came round in time to hear Simpson ejaculate, "This is better than ether.") Skinner's proselytism of Clarke was viewed with extreme disfavour by Clarke's colleagues – their aforetime close association with the new Hahnemannian heretic gradually lessened, until in the later nineties he resigned active duties at the hospital and was made consulting physicians. *Sic itur ad astra*.

The homoeopathic physician as the apostle of a minority cause

It would be well-nigh inconceivable to those who did not live it through to hear resuscitated the price Clarke had to pay for what his erstwhile compeers chose to regard as his apostasy. The natural evolution of his career of progress was blocked; the offices of dignity and honour – the Secretariat, the Vice-Presidency, the Presidency – of the various homoeopathic bodies in this country were denied to him – the boycott was complete except for his own journal, *The World*. Impossible, you say? This was a time when Dr Cooper, Sr., reading a paper at an annual congress meeting in this building, and lauding the use of nosodes, was stopped in his address, hissed, and compelled to leave the meeting – the assembly refusing to hear him further.

The discourtesy of such procedure was equalled only by its folly. There were others beside Clarke who refused to remain in bondage to tangible dosage, and who were driven into a fellowship of their own, where privately, without official publication, the finest homoeopathic work of the time in this country was reported and discussed. The members of that close confraternity were Burnett, RT Cooper, Clarke, and one or two others who thought as Clarke did. *Primus inter pares*, of course, was Burnett.

What a mass of new knowledge – what records of therapeutic victories, what ruthless deletion of the word "incurable" from the vocabulary of these masters in medicine! But the pace was too fierce to last; it killed Burnett at 61, RT Cooper at 59, and Clarke had a severe illness from which he narrowly escaped with his life. Fortunately the net result of these conferences sank so deeply into Clarke's homoeopathic mind that he envisaged the incorporation of this new knowledge into the old – and welded into the massive whole of his *Dictionary of Practical Materia Medica* the available totality of verifiable fact in the realm of the cure of disease by the methods of Hahnemann. This collocation of the *experimental* with the *clinical* sides of homoeopathy by analysis and synthesis was a vast undertaking. It was activated throughout by the clinical results of Burnett and Cooper and Clarke himself, plus the homoeopathic knowledge of the time germane to the undertaking.

I well remember Clarke presenting this newly issued work to the International Homoeopathic Congress held at Atlantic City in 1907. He introduced it to the assembly as a new endeavour to ensure the unity of homoeopaths and homoeopathy; and the embodied sentiment was *Hands across the Sea*. He received quite an ovation on that occasion.

The homoeopathic physician as man of letters

Classical literature

Carlyle, you will remember, retired for a couple of years to Ecclefechan, away from the madding crowd, for the production of *Sartor*. Clarke's detachment for the enormous work required by the *Dictionary* was of a different type, but more severe. Every day, every hour, every few minutes available were sacrificed on the inexorable altar of the *Dictionary*. Family life, recreation, social functions – one and all went by the board, for the creation of the *magnum opus*. Here is an instance; "Do you never leave the house except on professional duty?" "Yes," said he," sometimes. I like to get a change by dining *en famille* out of doors; my favourite restaurant is only a few streets away – but I always take a hansom there and back, that time and energy for the *Dictionary* work may be conserved." Samuel Johnson, the prince of British encyclopaedists, never went thus far. And the issue? A work that will endure so long as Hahnemannian homoeopathy endures.

While all this was going on, the *Homoeopathic World* was edited and published with regularity and up to 1910, when the responsibility was passed on to another distinguished colleague - to be resumed later. The *Monthly Homoeopathic Review*, the semi-official journal, would not publish his cases or his methods. Nothing daunted, he utilised the *Homoeopathic World*, then at his own editorial disposal: but like Edith Cavell in similar plight, this was not enough. Out came that series of small books whose like had made Burnett famous everywhere. Clarke had had the *Homoeopathic World* for the publication of his own methods and results, but this was not enough. Year by year he published his further original work also in handbook form. Here are the titles of some: *Radium as an Internal Remedy, Whooping Cough and Coqueluchin, Indigestion, Heart Disease*, and various others.

In such a narrow confraternity were men burning with zeal to exalt the values of homoeopathy, but excluded from the wider opportunities of evaluation and discussion available to less original minds. But there is no doubt that homoeopathy, by and large, gained enormously by this segregation and production of original observation and research, which but for this policy of exclusiveness had never seen the light.

Journalism

The *Homoeopathic World* for many years was JH Clarke's *alter ego*; by the courtesy of Messrs. Whitaker he was allowed to say in its columns just what he pleased, and this journal reflected his keen personality as the *Times* did that of Delane, or the *Review of Reviews* that of Stead.

Clarke's first principles of the editorship of a homoeopathic journal for free issue to any who chose to buy, were often enough expounded to myself and others:

I. *Homoeopathy*, first, last and all the time!
II. The criterion of the suitable and useful for publication was, "What good will it do for the cause of homoeopathy?" He ranked as nothing, or less than nothing, the quibble about professional or lay authorship, providing the facts were true.
III. He adhered closely to the theorem of Plato, his master, that "the medical art did not exist for the benefit of the medical art."

Clarke's mind was a scintillating mind easily dynamised into coruscations, if and when any cause or subject seized his imagination. He frequently and powerfully contributed to the *Zoophilist* in the palmy days of its editorship by Frances Power

Cobbe. He annotated Grauvogl's *Constitutional Medicine* and made it a handy book of reference. He refined and amplified the *Prescriber* through eight editions. Paracelsus and William Blake were both reinterpreted by the addition of Clarke's personal equation, and *nihil tetigit quod non ornavit*.

The best lecture series I heard him give were those delivered year by year in the early days of the British Homoeopathic Association when it held its meetings in the top room of a tall building in Regent Street. And the endowment of the Compton-Burnett Lectureship in memory of that great man was an abiding proof of Clarke's generous appreciation of his *confrére*.

L'envoi: Mr Chairman, Ladies & Gentlemen:
My commencement was of the nature of a dirge. My conclusion should rise to the height of a paean. Homoeopathy in this country has never lacked the enduring and wholehearted service of men and women of clear vision who were determined that sooner or later it should prevail, even when the forces of stolid reaction were dominant. These have been from time to time a remnant of independent thinkers, nothing daunted by the antagonism of *vox populi*, a remnant who kept the sacred fire of law and fact in homoeopathy burning, later to revive. John Epps, Curie, David Wilson, as well as Alfred Pope, Richard Hughes, Dyce Brown – these never kept their courage more tense than when the pressure and threat of opposition were greatest. Of such was Clarke, who in his public and private homoeopathic life was consumed by the fire of insistent necessity to leave homoeopathy better than he found it. And that inspiring spirit led him on – from Clarke, the Edinburgh graduate, whose homoeopathic history was at zero point – to Clarke upon whom, as at a loose end, homoeopathy was thrust – Clarke who drifted into rather than deliberately sought the homoeopathic life – Clarke the house physician, afterwards the country practitioner – then the suburban aspirant with views – then the hospital physician and society Fellow – to Clarke who had to endure detachment from association with his aforetime friends – into a more or less solitary career, during which his best work was done. Such is the typical history of great men, and it can be worked out in principle by every one of us: such are the men and women who make homoeopathic history for their own day and generation – and for all time. We may not pray to be delivered over to the tender mercies of such a career, but we may remember, each and all of us, that only by such blood-and-iron experience of its noblest and best is any Cause made truly great.

> "This is the happy warrior, this is he
> Whom every man at arms would wish to be."

Dr Le Hunte Cooper said he would like to say a few words in memory of his old and revered friend, Dr John Henry Clarke. It seemed to him that with so great a man one could only say "a few words," for if one spoke for a week the words would still be too few to do him justice.

Personally he owed Dr Clarke a very great debt, for when his father died in 1903, and it became necessary for him to leave the army, it was Dr Clarke's help and encouragement which enabled him to take up the reins of his father's practice, and it was Dr Clarke who vouched for his credentials to his father's patients.

A man of such attainments lived in one's memory not so much for what he *was* as for what he *did*. He was remembered for what he *was* by those who were most near and dear to him, but what he *did* would be remembered and treasured by countless thousands in generations to come long after his immediate contemporaries had passed away. His great genius lay in seizing on a fact and worrying it, like a terrier with a meaty bone, till he had got the most out of it, but unlike the terrier, he gave all thus he obtained, in assimilable and easily available form, to others; and hence arose that *monumental* work of his: *A Dictionary of Practical Materia Medica*.

Dr Clarke used jokingly to say that he wrote this to save himself time. It may have saved him time latterly, but there was no doubt he spared himself no time in its compilation He did not allow himself even an additional walk across the room, and practically denied himself all recreation in order to conserve his energies for the great task.

Dr Cooper once, and only once, heard an adverse criticism on Clarke's *Dictionary*. It was by a past member of the Society, who complained that "it contained too much." This seemed to him an unintentional compliment, for no dictionary could contain too much, provided the matter was important, and relative to the subject dealt with, and he had never found anything in the *Dictionary* which was not both. Later on he heard that the individual responsible for the above criticism prided himself on never needing, or using, more than nine remedies, which accounted for his having no use for the *Dictionary*. Whether this critic had any success in treating difficult chronic cases, he did not know, but believed he confined his attentions to those of a simple and acute nature. Under these circumstances, he might get along fairly well with a few remedies, but when it was realised that there was not a single substance on, or in, the earth which was not a potential homoeopathic remedy, and that any one of these might cure some obscure and otherwise intractable malady, the vast importance of a comprehensive work like Clarke's *Dictionary* became at once apparent.

Some men did good by stealth, and Dr Clarke was one of these. Investigations of his affairs showed that numbers of his patients came to him complaining not only of their bodily health, but of their poverty, and they did not go empty-handed away. Once this became known, was it surprising that he became surrounded by a host of harpies! It certainly was a fact that when his breath ceased, several hitherto mysterious incomes ceased at the same time. The effect of this on his own exchequer might be imagined, but imagination failed to compass the reality, which was disastrous in the extreme.

Like many other great men, Dr Clarke was often misunderstood during his lifetime, and this was largely due to his great breadth of outlook. The "low potency" men objected to his dealing with "high potencies," and those who favoured "high dilutions" considered that he ought to have dealt wholly in the rarefied atmosphere of the "higher potencies." His comprehensive brain, however, recognised the value of all potencies when appropriately used, and he was prepared to consider *anything, whatever its nature*, which could be of use in restoring health.

Before the *Dictionary*, and its satellites, the *Prescriber* and other works, were published, infinite time used to be wasted in getting the essentials of any particular drug from various divers sources, and this hampered many from adopting the system who might otherwise have done so. In putting all these vitally important facts in a handy and agreeable form, Dr Clarke immensely benefited homoeopathic science, and as time went on and the ranks gained in numbers, this work would become more and more indispensable.

What finer monument to a great man could there be than this? No one deserved ultimate peace and rest more than did Dr Clarke. His great mind could not be tied to any one particular religious dogma of faith, but he had a great comprehension of the eternal fitness of things and the beneficence of a Deity controlling human destinies. The following lines seemed to fit him peculiarly well:-

"Perplexed in faith, but pure in deeds,
At last he beat his music out,
There breathes more faith in honest doubt,
Believe me, than in half the creeds."

Dr Goldsbrough expressed his great interest in Dr Burford's and Dr Cooper's addresses. They represented a very large aspect of the man who to Dr Goldsbrough had been to a certain extent a somewhat hidden personality. There were, however, one or two facts to which he would like to refer, and which he thought even Dr Burford did not know, as they were largely personal.

Dr Goldsbrough first met Dr Clarke in the Liverpool Homoeopathic Dispensary, when studying medicine. This was in 1876, having been a homoeopath from his birth upwards, there was nothing new in going to a homoeopathic dispensary to see and hear what he could. He found Dr Roche and Dr Clarke sitting at the dispensary table and dealing with the cases there and he remembered one of these men saying, "We will now give that medicine and then give another alternately with it." Dr Goldsbrough was rather impressed at the time by this procedure. The liberality of Clarke's mind, however, led him to take the broadest possible view of homoeopathic principle and its application.

That was the first point. The second point was the following. Dr Goldsbrough came to London in 1877, twenty-one years of age, and newly qualified. (Dr Clarke was his senior by five or six years.) They both joined the London School of Homoeopathy instituted by William Bayes, of which Hughes and Dyce Brown were then lecturers.

Clarke and himself were the only two students. At the end of the session, Dr Bayes was so enthusiastic to get the best results that he offered a prize of ten guineas for the best answers to any questions that might be put on the lectures. Clarke won that prize, but Bayes then offered an additional prize of five guineas to Dr Goldsbrough, and with that prize he was able to purchase the already issued volumes of Allen's *Encyclopaedia of Materia Medica*. Clarke was then house physician of the Hospital, but after that he soon went to Ipswich. From that time until his death Dr Goldsbrough seemed to have had very little to do with Clarke, as somehow or other he was following the lines of Hughes and some others, and his mind was diverted from the broad conception of homoeopathy that Clarke maintained, so well illustrated by Dr Burford and Dr Cooper.

He did not wish to compare the two sides of the question, but there was another side to Clarke's view, which would have been originally represented by Hughes, but Hughes did not appreciate that the physiological side was obscure. Hughes did not appreciate the fact it was impossible to interpret symptoms in terms of physiology. His was a hopeless task, as it was there that the two men diverged. Clarke's work was before them, and the world would have to judge of its value. There could be no question that it would be of permanent value. One seldom heard of a drug that he had not dealt with; every drug that had ever been used up to the date of its publication could be found in the dictionary. The dictionary was an unique work; it could not be limited any way.

The *Prescriber* was also of the greatest value to many practitioners of homoeopathy. Dr Goldsbrough said that to anyone with a mind like his own, which seemed naturally bent on the source or original aspect of things, the way of Clarke was a divergence. He did not seem to trouble much about that aspect, but passed it over to what he conceived to be the clinical value of the facts.

The world would have to be judge of what Dr Clarke had done.

Mr Granville Hey said that he was called upon to address the meeting because the President of the International Homoeopathic League, Dr Pierre Schmidt, of Geneva, was unable to be present, and had therefore delegated his official duties to him, as Vice-President.

For the League's sake, and for that of his hearers, he was sorry that he was not better equipped for the task placed upon him, as he had very little first-hand information from which to speak.

Dr Clarke's international appreciation depended almost entirely upon his writings, and of these, *The Homoeopathic World*, had by far the widest international circulation, being distributed all over the world, especially in India. The *Prescriber* had also had a wide distribution, especially in India. A *Dictionary of Practical Materia Medica*, Clarke's masterpiece, and the most enduring monument to his memory, was also widely known, this also especially in India and America. It was known to a less extent in Africa and only a comparatively few volumes of the *Dictionary* had found their way on to the Continent of Europe.

Of Clarke's other writings, the two most largely called for were his books on *Indigestion* and *Colds*. There had been a great demand for these in India and not a few have been called for in America.

The publication of these volumes had made Dr JH Clarke's name more widely known probably than that of any other homoeopath, except Hahnemann, and their appreciation led to his becoming a corresponding member of many foreign societies. Dr Clarke visited the Quinquennial Homoeopathic Congress in Atlantic City in 1906; this widened his connection, and he had a most enthusiastic reception from the homoeopaths assembled there.

When the Quinquennial International Homoeopathic Congress was held in London, in 1911, the foreign members quite expected that Dr Clarke would be elected for President, but the Council who had to do with the election thought otherwise, and Clarke did not receive that honour on this occasion.

The next time the International Congress was held in London, in 1927, Dr Clarke was elected an Honorary President, which was the highest honour that international homoeopathy had conferred upon Dr John Henry Clarke. That his writings would be missed, there was no doubt, especially in India. India, being an English-speaking country, could better appreciate his writings than could the continent of Europe, and very few of his books had been translated into other tongues.

That Dr Clarke would be missed by a wider sphere than the members of the Society, there could be little doubt, because although the *Dictionary* was at the time of its publication as complete as he could make it – and all those who knew Clarke had no doubt whatever on this point – for the last two or three years he had been publishing more details of drugs as they had been worked out, both at home and abroad. These had been published in the form of inserts in *The Homoeopathic World*. It was uncertain whether these would be continued; if not, it would be a great loss.

Mention had been made of the inception of Clarke's *Dictionary*. On one occasion, when Mr. Hey and Dr Lambert were listening to Clarke giving a lecture, he explained how it came about. He told how when he wanted information on many of the homoeopathic remedies, he found it scattered widely through the writings of Farrington, Hering, Hahnemann and others, and it was necessary to spend a great amount of time hunting for it. He therefore determined to get the work over and done with in order to have an easier time of it in the future. He said that it was not energy but laziness that compelled him to compile the *Dictionary*.

In the name of the International Homoeopathic League, Mr. Hey tendered sincere sympathy with Mrs. Clarke in her loss, which would be felt world wide.

Dr Fergie Woods said there was one feature that had not been mentioned, and that was Dr Clarke's persistent opposition to vaccination and vivisection. As regards vaccination, he saw, as did all homoeopaths, the immense harm that could be done to the patient therebye, harm lasting very often a whole lifetime. As for vivisection, besides his views from the humanitarian aspect, he thought it was opposed to the spirit of essential homoeopathy, which was concerned with provings on human beings. His attitude of mind on these two points coloured Dr Clarke's work and writings, and had an important influence in his life.

Dr Hall Smith said that he had received the following notes from Sir John Weir, who was unfortunately prevented from being present.

Sir John Weir regretted his inability personally to pay his tribute to the late Dr John Henry Clarke. Much would be said about his literary efforts, with which he was in entire agreement, but he would rather like to draw attention to one phase, which had an object lesson for all.

During the last twenty-two years Dr Clarke, to many, was more or less a name. All knew and valued his books, but the personality of the man was seldom seen, as he did not attend the Society Meetings. Sir John was more fortunate, as he was invited to the Cooper Club Meetings before the War, and Dr Clarke had felt more kindly disposed towards one who used the potencies to which he had been accustomed. In 1925 he asked Dr Clarke to come back to the Society, and give the members the benefit of his experience; unfortunately, however, he was still indignant of the treatment he had received twenty years before, when he went into splendid isolation. This was very unfortunate, as his mind still retained the impressions of twenty years previously, when the attitude of the profession generally towards homoeopathy was not too kindly. In this way he failed to recognise improvement in the relationships between allopathic physicians and homoeopaths. He would have learned that they, too, had progressed, but not, of course, enough. Still, they were making honest endeavours, and who knew that, had he remained in contact with doctors, he would not have aided them in their research? All could not see alike, but each must carry on according to his own conscience, and be judged thereby, leaving others to work out their salvation as best and conscientiously as they could. It took all kinds to make progress. He undoubtedly had great literary ability, and his books were daily help to all homoeopaths, who would ever be grateful for his arduous labours on their behalf, and his books would live long after him.

If the late Dr McLachlan (of Oxford) and Dr Clarke had only remained in the Society, and not gone into the wilderness, thereby losing much of their influence, homoeopathy would have gained much: but they were sensitive souls. Homoeopaths must all pull together; be diligent in their own sphere, and pool their resources, so that they could leave the world of medicine, and especially homoeopathy, better for their existence. They should train others, so that they, too, might carry on in their day, as they were endeavouring to do at present.

Dr Wheeler said that ever since Dr Clarke died his mind had been very full of thoughts of him, and his heart of memories, and he felt he could not let this occasion go without saying something, although he had not come prepared to speak.

Dr Clarke had certainly been to him the greatest influence in homoeopathy that he had ever known. During the most important years of his homoeopathic life after his return to London, no one could have been more helpful to him, more kind or more personally generous in every possible way. Unfortunately later there arose a misunderstanding – Dr Wheeler honestly thought through no fault of his own – and he felt that for the last twenty years of Dr Clarke's life he was more a source of annoyance to him than anything else. However, he would never forget, and could never lose, the deepest respect and most complete admiration for so much of Dr Clarke's work, and the very deep affection that he had always had for him. Clarke was one of the heroes of homoeopathy, the last of the heroic age, and it had been very well said that there should be no long faces when a hero died. Clarke lived out his life fully to the end, keeping his faculties to the utmost, knowing that his work was well done; the author of more contributions to the cause of homoeopathy than any man had made, known all over the world, having achieved fame and as much success as he wanted. He had all that, and his was a heroic life to the end. There was nothing there for tears, but Dr Wheeler's sorrowing was of a different nature; it was that for the last twenty years, partly owing to the causes to which Sir John Weir had referred, those who had come into homoeopathy had found it difficult to realise fully what Dr Clarke was. The issue was confused for them by things that were now relatively of no importance. Dr Clarke's work would abide, but it would be cause for sorrow if the more recent homoeopaths were to approach it knowing only the circumstances that had been forced upon them in recent years. It was a kind of ghost that might haunt Clarke's memory if it could not be laid now once and for all.

When he called Clarke "heroic," he gave the clue to the misunderstanding. The heroic age of homoeopathy was over; he took that age to be the time when, if a homoeopathic doctor were confronted by an allopathic practitioner, they had no common ground at all. In those days there were little surgery, no rays available for diagnostic and treatment purposes; the resources of the medical profession were limited to making a diagnosis, and then the doctor, whoever he was, homoeopath or non-homoeopath, would administer a drug or drugs as the case might be. Therefore, seeing that the treatment of medicine would be the giving of medicine, the homoeopath and non-homoeopath had no common meeting ground; they took diametrically opposed views. That being so, what should be the attitude of the homoeopath? There was no possibility of compromise; the rest of the profession would never so much as listen to the argument; what was to be the attitude of homoeopaths in that time? It was by no means an easy matter to decide. No one could have foreseen the developments that would take place in the medical profession. The homoeopaths knew that they had incomparably the better method, and also that the other side did not intend to pay the slightest attention to anything they said. The problem for homoeopaths was to decide upon what alternative to take of two possible courses. Hughes said, "We can do nothing in this matter without the profession. I will therefore try and interest the profession," and to that end he set all his powers. He was a most persuasive man, and he tried to put the things in which he believed into the language, which the men to whom he spoke would understand and possibly listen. He had very great success, and if homoeopathy had any converts during those years, it was more due to Hughes than to any other man, because the inquirer found someone speaking something like his own language. There were, however, great limitations in Hughes' method, to which Dr Goldsbrough had referred.

The other way of attacking the problem was the way chosen by Clarke, and that was to leave the profession entirely alone, to answer scorn with scorn, and blows with blows, and to rely for the expansion of homoeopathy on an entirely fighting attitude, to fight and assert his views on every occasion. Not that Hughes was in the least afraid of putting his case, but Clarke would be assertive where Hughes would be persuasive. If others wished to proclaim him a fool, he was quite prepared to call them the same. He relied to some extent for the practice of homoeopathy on the unqualified physician. That, to-day, to many would sound absurd, but it was not so absurd then. It was not until the nineties that doctors were forbidden to have unqualified assistants, and until that time many unqualified men – in the sense now known – had charge over sick people. Homoeopathy had from its onset been widely practised by the unqualified. Clarke was well aware of the success achieved. What did it mean in those times? Any patient treated by anyone was treated by the administration of medicine; the other methods hardly came into consideration at all. To Clarke the advantages of being given the remedy by a mature homoeopath were far superior to being given something by someone who knew nothing about homoeopathy at all. He therefore decided that homoeopathy should be forced upon the profession by the public, he looked forward to such a demand for the homoeopathic treatment that the fact that it was needed would be forced upon the profession, who would have to accept it.

Dr Wheeler admitted that that would never have been the way that would have commended itself to him or to a great many others, but it was a tenable position. It was not the way of Clarke, having taken up a position, to do anything but go in for it whole-heartedly. As a result, Clarke's method might be summed up in the phrase, "If you see an allopathic head, hit it." It was his persistent teaching that, provided homoeopathy was practised, he did not care whether the person was qualified or not.

When Dr Wheeler was a resident at the hospital, Dr Clarke was on the staff. He was frequently accused of self-advertising, on the ground that his little books were so many advertisements. No man can publish a medical book without carrying his name a little further afield, but anyone who thought that Clarke's idea in working on these lines was an attempt to get into the limelight knew nothing about the man; he was not a limelight seeker. Some people went to the limelight because they had an instinct for it; there was a ray of limelight somewhere, and somehow they found themselves in it.

Clarke was absolutely certain about his facts, and having arrived at that conclusion, doubt was useless, and interfered with things. He was annoyed with Dr Wheeler, because for himself the fact was sufficient, and he did not worry about theoretical explanations. His relation to Blake was interesting; it was not so much the mystical side of Blake that attracted Clarke, but their minds were alike in an absence of any kind of questioning.

On the occasion of Clarke's last address to the Society, Dryden's words applied to his attitude:-

"Thrice he vanquished all his foes,
Thrice he slew the slain,"
and Dr Wheeler sorrowed think that that was so.

But all this arose out of Clarke's certainty as to the policy he had taken up, and his determination that everything was to be subordinated to it. Many of his books were written for the domestic prescriber and untrained worker. All the flouting of the profession, all the attacks on them, were expressions of his confident belief that there was nothing to be hoped from the profession unless they could be forced into taking an interest in homoeopathy by pressure from the public.

Things did not work out as he hoped and he lost touch with what was going on outside. The great sorrow was that he lived the last ten years of his life feeling far too much that his colleagues had let him down, that if they would have seen things his way, homoeopathy would have progressed. He was constantly accusing homoeopaths of "placating" the allopaths. Dr Wheeler felt sad to think that that great heroic figure should not have realized that the heroic age had passed away, and that homoeopaths would never again be confronted with the other side as Clarke was, and that he should have lived so much of those last years in isolation.

It was that which undermined the influence he might have had, because so many complained of the attitude he took, and the emphasis with which he took it.

That was the real sorrow at present, and it was with the hope of in some way making more realise why it happened, and that the way in which he took it was an element in the make-up of the man, that Dr Wheeler had spoken as he had. When one thought of the work of Clarke, he was not dead.

> For truly when a man shall end,
> He lives in memory of his friend,
> Who doth his better parts recall,
> And of his faults make funeral.

How very small and insignificant were his faults; he was a monument of homoeopathy for all time. So long as one dwelt upon his extraordinary powers, upon his courage and his devotion, he was not dead; he need not die.

Dr Hall-Smith said it had occurred to him that it might be a good plan after the finish of these personal tributes to Dr Clarke, to have a discussion for the rest of the time on Dr Clarke's actual work. There were on exhibition many volumes produced by Dr Clarke, which had been lent for inspection by Dr Whitaker of the Homoeopathic Publishing Company. Any who wished to look at these books after the meeting were welcome to do so.

Dr Tyler said: In Dr Clarke, homoeopathy had lost a great champion, and a world-wide celebrity.

A brilliant writer, he wielded a very caustic pen. But his influence for good might have been greater had he been less fierce, and made a little allowance for those whose real sin was ignorance. The old school was to be bullied and rated. Ignorance was "cussedness" to be bludgeoned into knowledge – rather than tactfully helped and taught. He was so sure on his own ground that he had no mercy on the man on the other side of the fence. Pandering to the allopaths was his name for courtesy to men who are, after all, our brethren in the healing art. He set his flytraps with vinegar.

His great work, which will secure him life after death, is of course his *Dictionary of Practical Materia Medica*. Nothing in our vast literature at all takes its place, or is likely to do so. It has done what no other work has done, or even attempted to do – collected a vast drug-lore, or drugs proved – drugs partly proved, drugs that need proving. Clarke realised that everything that can hurt is something that can heal. He has bequeathed to us, not only records of past work, but a store of work for the future. Where our great authorities stop, Clarke takes up the tale. He gives us data regarding many valuable remedies – such as *Ornithogalum*, valuable in gastric ulcer, simple or malignant, which it would be difficult to come by but for Clarke's *Dictionary*. Here, too, we find more of the essential facts concerning the nosodes than are to be found in the earlier books.

Clarke had once a keen controversy with the purists, as one may call them, in regard to the use of a remedy, which was unproved, but had been found useful in certain conditions; and he was jubilant when the remedy in question was found to produce the symptoms it was known to cure. He contested that his must always be so. Such remedies he called "born by breech presentation."

I have been told that, many years ago, Drs. Clarke, Compton Burnett and Robert Cooper, three men of genius in their different ways – used to meet frequently to compare notes.

Dr Cooper had an uncanny genius for discovering unusual remedies: some of these he got, no doubt, from old herbals; but it has been said that he used to lie down before a flowering plant by the hour, dragging from it its virtues of healing. He made extraordinary play, in cancer, with some of his flowers, and one heard him called "the man who can cure cancer." But his son can tell more about this.

Dr Burnett would give these remedies a fragmentary proving in his own person, and so wring from them the salient symptoms that enabled him to employ them to great effect in his huge practice. For instance, when *Cundurango* was being exploited as a cancer-cure, Burnett, having satisfied himself that it *had* cured some cases, poisoned himself with the drug, till he got definite, peculiar symptoms, which he published in one of the Society's journals. Among his drug-symptoms was an induration and ulceration at the corners of his mouth, torpid and longlasting. And when a case of cancer of breast came to him, with ugly, indurated, torpid cracks at the corners of the mouth, *Cundurango* generally cured. If a drug *could* cure, he wanted to know *which* cases it could cure.

The third of this brilliant trio, Dr Clarke, recorded the experiences of his friends, and fixed them, so far as they went, for posterity.

Mach's nach, aber mach's besser, was Burnett's plea, difficult to translate, but, "*get on with it, but go one better,*" about expresses what he meant. And this applies to much in Clarke's *Dictionary*. It is, what it calls itself, a *Dictionary of Practical Materia Medica*, a place where one should find anything and everything; rather than a cut-and-dried scientific work, like *Allen's Encyclopaedia*. In Clarke's work you find what is known of numbers of drugs that ask for further proving to make them really useful.

Dr Clarke once told me that all his work was to save himself work. He wanted all the knowledge he had gleaned from a hundred sources in a place where he could lay his finger upon it.

His *Dictionary* is also invaluable for the drug-pictures and clinical experiences, written in his own lucid style, that precede each remedy all through the book. These little essays (and Clarke fully appreciated their value!) provide ideal last-hour reading of a drug, before bed.

But what one does miss in the schema that follows, is the indications provided by type, in regard to the greater value of certain symptoms. Black type, for symptoms over and over again clinically verified, dates from Hahnemann, and has been carried on (Boeninnghausen gives even *four* types!) till Clarke. Clarke told me once, "I have omitted the types, because all symptoms are of equal value." One feels that this was a great mistake, and that it detracts from the value of the work, and may even be misleading. For example, the thirstlessness of *Antimonium tartaricum* is a great and important symptom in diagnosing the remedy in, say, a broncho-pneumonia. But it appears in equal type with "thirst" in Clarke, thirst being merely its inevitable reaction. And one more criticism; one occasionally finds something of supreme importance omitted as the power of *Thuja* to determine lumps in the breast. This designates *Thuja* as a probably important cancer medicine, where the economy has been permanently damaged by vaccination. Allen gives these lumps, but on looking the symptom up in Clarke one fails to find it. One can only imagine that he intended to transfer it to a more appropriate place, and accidentally omitted it. But such omissions are probably rare. Of course for actual work, or when one is writing, one needs the provings as recorded in Allen; but one could not, and would not for anything be without Clarke's *Dictionary*, which follows up and supplements the others; providing later knowledge where they stop.

Many of Dr Clarke's minor writings were telling and delightful – as one remembers them – and should be republished.

As to Clarke's *Prescriber*, my own experience is that it may act as an excellent reminder when one has learnt how to prescribe and has grasped the inwardness of homoeopathy; but that it is not very helpful to beginners.

Dr Clarke sought, by its means, to make homoeopathy easy for students and lay prescribers. In my early days I used to have it always beside me, with countless notes and emendations – how I worked at that book! But my results were not really good. Perhaps my own fault, since others do not seem to have had the same experience. But one thing Clarke did teach, that if one really masters a couple of dozen of the most useful medicines – *Sulphur, Bryonia, Lycopodium, Calcarea carbonica, Sepia, Silica,* &c. – one can spot the remedy for the majority of the cases that turn up during a day's work, and only needs to study and puzzle out the more occasional cases. But this takes one back to the purely homoeopathic standpoint, *the patient*, each time; whereas the *Prescriber* starts on *the disease*.

In memory of Dr Robert Cooper, Dr Clarke started the Cooper Club for the study of remedies. This is long since dead. But his efforts for establishing a Chair of Homoeopathy in memory of his other great friend, Dr J Compton Burnett, have indeed borne fruit, and are of enduring value.

Dr Clarke was very kind to me in my early days, and I have treasured many of his charming and encouraging letters, which took some deciphering. I remember he wrote me once, "It is a great pity that you have not got to earn your livelihood!"

Remembering and realising by a late experience, how eagerly he caught at anything that would be helpful or telling for his *Homoeopathic World*, I have felt regret and remorse that we did not help him more, of late years, by writing for him.

Well, the world is the richer for what Dr Clarke has given it of his genius and industry – severely practical always. And he is therefore one of those on whom death has no power.

Dr Stonham said he had known Dr Clarke ever since he came up to London, having met him very occasionally at the meetings of the Society, but more frequently at the Cooper Club. This Club met about once a fortnight, or month, at Clarke's house, and several members would sit round his table and a subject would be chosen and discussed. It proved to be a most useful series of meetings. Dr Clarke presided in his usual generous and affable manner, and made everything pass off agreeably. Since that time he had met Dr Clarke occasionally, and took one or two patients to him for his advice in consultation. They last met one day last year; Dr Clarke happened to be staying in Worthing and called to see Dr Stonham. At that time he was the same as ever and seemed in good health. Dr Stonham said he would always have pleasant memories of his old friend.

Dr Wheeler thought the keynote of Dr Clarke's work in homoeopathy was his catholicity. Dr Wheeler said he had never understood how the high potencies came to be so entirely superseded by the lower ones in the seventies. Clarke, in reviving their use with Skinner and others, was really doing great service had it been known, because Clarke was convinced that the high potencies were invaluable in treat chronic disease But he never lost the knowledge he had gained through using the low potencies. Clarke was one of the few homoeopaths who really practised what he said, "that there is a place for every potency, from the mother tincture to the highest, and that the physician's skill consists in knowing which to choose and when." Clarke had no hesitation. He would give remedies within extraordinary short range of one another; he would give one on top of another, and resort to different potencies.

Dr Wheeler said he would never forget one case he had the honour to watch with Dr Clarke. The case was a desperate one. The patient was a poor man, but Dr Clarke was seeing him four times a day. Dr Wheeler was called in for the chest condition and found the man had an empyema which had ruptured into the lungs and pus was being discharged through the lung. The man was in a pretty desperate condition, but even when Dr Wheeler first saw him he was astonishingly well for his condition, which gave a certain amount of hope in the prognosis. Clarke pulled that man through, and he got steadily well. That man was given six remedies in a day, every time Clarke saw him he would give him something else.

Dr Wheeler saw the case six times, and sometimes he was having low potencies, and then the 30s, and after an hour or so he would be given a low potency. Nothing could have been more satisfactory than the progress that that man made, and not long afterwards one would never have known that he had ever had empyema at all. That case was a very cogent example of what he would call Clarke's catholicity. Inside the four corners of homoeopathy he was prepared to consider and to use any procedure.

As a resident at the Hospital, however, he had not found Dr Clarke satisfactory as a chief; this was probably his reaction to the way in which he was being regarded by his colleagues. Although he was a lone fighter, he did not in the least mind standing alone, and in many ways rather preferred it. This was encouraged by the attitude of his colleagues mentioned by Dr Burford. It may have been that he was afraid his Residents might take their colour from his colleagues, but he used if possible to avoid going round with them, and would come at odd hours, so that it was only with the greatest difficulty that one could manage to arrange to go round the ward with him. He would not attempt to explain what he was doing, and he used terms that were very strange to the newcomer. On one occasion he said, "I regard that as a very psoric girl," and left his resident wondering what he meant. Most at that time he was giving fairly high potencies, 30s and 200s for chronic cases, but he would give no idea as to how long it would be before one could look for a result, so that if he did not come round again, or if the patient did not seem to be any better, Dr Wheeler might think himself forced to act upon his own responsibility, simply thinking that as nothing had happened yet that was probably as much as was expected from it. If, however, Dr Clarke saw any kind of glimmer of interest as a resident, he would follow that up. Now and again with acute cases he obtained the most striking results.

Dr Wheeler wished particularly to stress the catholicity about Clarke's work. He was always a homoeopath, but there was nothing within the four corners of homoeopathy that he would not use and turn to advantage. He was always prepared to try another potency; he really believed that there was a place for every potency, and used them.

Mr. Granville Hey wished to refer to what Dr Tyler had said about the *Prescriber*.

When he first came to the London Homoeopathic Hospital, Dr Clarke had already left the Hospital two or three years earlier, and there were no classes for teaching homoeopathy excepting an occasional lecture given at Regent House by Drs. Clarke, Stonham or Lambert, and Dr Tyler had said she did not find the *Prescriber* of value until she knew a good deal about homoeopathy, whereas it was the *Prescriber* that had led him to believe in homoeopathy. He was often alone in the hospital with no chief. He had often referred to a case of facial erysipelas that appeared in the casualty department soon after he came; on that occasion he had nothing to help him other than Clarke's *Prescriber*, and he read up there the drugs for erysipelas and used them with great success. He would have no hesitation whatever in advising any young man who wanted to try homoeopathy for himself in general practice to procure a copy of the *Prescriber* and use it every day, and if he were not convinced of the truth of homoeopathy in less than twelve months he would consider that man to be a poor observer.

Such symptoms as indigestion, distension, heaviness after food, and thirst, &c., if looked up in Clarke's *Prescriber*, would be found to have *Bryonia* running through them. It was the same with *Sepia* and many others. Mr. Hey obtained his first knowledge of *Sepia* by hunting things up in the *Prescriber*. Even today he sometimes referred to it when in a hurry.

The dominant note that had been maintained almost throughout that evening had been *de mortuis nil nisi bonum*, and he hoped he would not be considered as striking a discordant note when he said that although all found themselves in agreement with Clarke's work for homoeopathy, many were out of sympathy with his strongly-expressed anti-Semitic views; especially were these to be deprecated when expressed in a medical journal which had a circulation over all parts of the globe and among all races and all varieties of religious thought. He mentioned this to stress a point already mentioned, that Dr Clarke all too obviously demonstrated that he did not lack the courage of his opinions, no matter what they were. He never lost an opportunity of displaying his colours at the masthead, especially when those colours were those unfurled and fearlessly flown by Samuel Hahnemann.

Dr Powell thought that whatever views Dr Clarke held, anti-Semitic or other, he modified them generously, and his own personal experience of Dr Clarke was that he was friendly and helpful in all things homoeopathic. Although he was opposed to operations, he had to undergo one himself at which Dr Powell gave the anaesthetic, and subsequently he allowed Dr Powell to perform a small operation upon his wife's face. Although he had some sharp corners like the majority of us, homoeopathy would always bring him down to geniality and helpfulness. Dr Powell believed they would be as pleased to meet Clarke as he would be to meet them.

Dr Burford said that the remarks made during the evening made clear the loss sustained by the detachment and isolation on the part of leaders of homoeopathy from each other and from their colleagues in various parts of the world. Dr Clarke was a firm believer in Dr Clarke; he liked all people who followed him to do so, body, soul and spirit; then to them he became a fount of inspiration. Clarke had made his own contribution to homoeopathy, and in the course of time his detached personality would tend to become more and more dim. There was an enormous amount of homoeopathic dynamic lost to the world because so many people preferred to travel so much alone.

After a considerable amount of study of the point, Dr Burford had come to the framing of the following sentence: "Homoeopathy is what its institutions make it." It was not so much what its men individually made it, because all good men tend to incorporation with their fellows. Thus is created what is called a "school" of newness in thought. The longer he lived the more was he convinced of the truth of this particular dictum, and if it was desired to get the best possible out of homoeopathy it was necessary for each to be unified with the whole. The genius of homoeopathy was bigger than any individual.

But if Clarke had not drifted into detachment, the probability was that homoeopathy would have lost the best of his literary work. The value of Dr Clarke's books would be enduring. Dr Burford hoped that those present would take away the inspiring and spectacular lessons of this man's life. No public man was sufficient by himself; he represented a cause much bigger than himself. Homoeopathy would be altogether different if only it were a little better regimented; if they recognised their chiefs as chiefs in their day and generation.

Dr Hall-Smith, in closing the meeting, said that a great deal had been heard that evening about their esteemed and respected colleague; he hoped all would go away refreshed by what they had heard of his life.

References

1 Addresses given at the Clarke Memorial Meeting, 7 January 1932, *British Homoeopathic Journal*, 1932; 22: 115-143.
2 Price, P, *Touching the ends of the earth, The story of the Missionary School of Medicine 1903-2003*, Missionary School of Medicine, Ware, 2003.
3 Henryson Caird, R, *The Anglo French American War Hospital at Neuilly, An Account of the Work Carried on under Homoeopathic auspices during 1915-1916*, British Committee at the London Homoeopathic Hospital, London, 1916.
4 Burford GH., Masters of Homoeopathy: the Persistence of Their Work Through Time – the Dr Clarke Memorial Meeting, *British Homoeopathic Journal*, 1932; 21: 116-143.

16

THE PORCELAIN PAINTER'S SON

Introduction

As a finale here is a piece written in a completely different tempo and style. It is a fantasy from 1898 by Samuel Arthur Jones (1834-1912)[1] and presents the life of Hahnemann as hagiography.

This script requires no further commentary except an expression of my deep and continuing sadness at the loss of my dear friend and fellow bibliophile, Julian Winston who died in New Zealand in 2005. He suggests that Jones' work takes us through Hahnemann's life like a script:

> We are aware of biographical films that take literary license (Amadeus and Armisted spring to mind). Here is a book that could serve as the beginning of a wonderful script. It is the flowing pen of Jones at his best.[2]

About Samuel Arthur Jones[3]

Born in Manchester, England, Jones' family moved to the United States and he grew up in Utica, New York. He served as a surgeon in the Civil War. Jones was the dean of the homeopathic department at the University of Michigan in Ann Arbor in 1880. Described as "a live wire," he was a most outspoken proponent of homeopathy. He authored a little book published in 1880 called *The Grounds of a Homoeopath's Faith*. It is the transcript of three lectures he gave in 1879 to the students of the "regular" medical school at Ann Arbor, Michigan.

Dr James C. Wood, one of his students, said, "All who knew him dreaded his caustic pen and still more caustic tongue." Small in stature, he was known in Ann Arbor as "little pill Jones."

Upon being called a "damn liar" by a prominent physician, Jones quietly said, "You are a gentleman, sir; now we have both lied."

Jones, in an argument with an administrator of the school at Ann Arbor, wrote: "You have not enough calcium in your backbone to whiten your pate."

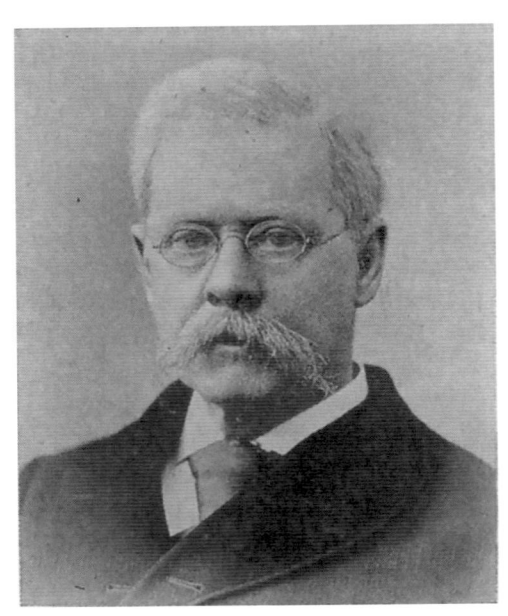

Figure 16.1 Samuel Arthur Jones (1834-1912)

Reproduced with permission of Homéopathe International & Dr Robert Séror.

His adversarial nature appeared at an early age. He enrolled at the Homoeopathic Medical College of Pennsylvania, took some courses, and then left. When he decided to return, the administration could not find his record of attendance. Expressing disgust with the school's incompetence, he enrolled in the Homoeopathic Medical College of Missouri in St. Louis, graduating in 1860. He then returned to Philadelphia, with his medical degree, attended one year at the school which had previously denied him admission, and received his MD from there in 1861.

As a hobby, Jones collected the writings of Thoreau, Hawthorne and Melville. The University of Illinois at Champaign-Urbana has a number of original editions of these works belonging to Jones.

Dr Wood tells the story: "Jones had been called into consultation the week before to see a farmer's wife, living six miles in the country, desperately ill with a colic of some sort. On this particular morning the father came in to pay him. His report was that Jones had relieved his wife almost instantly with the medicine he had prescribed and she had remained well since. Jones' fee for the consultation was thirty dollars, at least twenty-eight more than the farmer had ever paid his regular physician for the same trip. With great deliberation he extracted from his wallet three ten-dollar bills and grudgingly handed them over, saying as he did so, "Dr Jones, thirty dollars

> would hire me two good men on the farm for a month. I think your bill is robbery." Jones replied, "Well, damn it, the next time your wife gets a belly-ache, hire two good men for a month!"
>
> Jones' legacy remains with us to this day. In 1985 Jones' grand-daughter, Carol Jane Prescott, established a $75,000 fund through the National Center for Homeopathy for the "education of physicians in homoeopathy." The "Samuel A. Jones Scholarship" has provided several physicians with their homoeopathic education.

The porcelain painter's son: a fantasy[1] 1898
By Samuel Arthur Jones 1834-1912

"Is this not something more than fantasy?" Hamlet, Act I, Scene I.
Inscribed to the memory of AJT "Faithful amongst the faithless found."

Foreword
The editor is of the opinion that many a reader of *The Porcelain Painter's Son* will ask, "Is not this something more than fantasy?" In very truth it is; for the author, whom we have known long and very intimately, is, as he himself puts it, 'too near the end of the road' for idle trifling. It is a fantasy, but one that is founded upon a solid substratum of fact – serious fact to the porcelain painter's son, who lived it nearly a century agone. Fact and fancy are united to form the fabric; the web of a man's life is here, the flowers of fancy are wholly in the woof. He who has combined these in this fantasy felt to the very core of him that some salient facts of Hahnemann's life should not be allowed to pass into forgetfulness so long as it is needful that any physician shall be distinguished by the adjective 'homoeopathic,' and he is fully assured that the flowers of fancy need not disturb the most serious reader: they are allowed only that they may embellish the dusty wayside of a fellowman's life just as they do our own. It is then as a sprig of rosemary ("that's for remembrance") that his fantasy is laid on the grave of him whose life-journey it briefly outlines with only so much of over-coloring as flings a deeper shadow here and there but gives the salient points a bolder relief, while if faithfully preserves the perspective.

The author writes to us, "You will see that I found the web of fact in Hahnemann's life; the woof of fancy alone is mine. The fantasy is a 'projection' not at all difficult when a deep reverence inspires the attempt to people the dead past, to even live therein in the company of actors upon whom the prompter has long since rang down the curtain. It is not surprising that, in imagination, one should be able to enter Frau Weber's Wirtshaus and both see and hear her guests without stepping out from his own latter-day surroundings; and such is the power of sympathy that many of us can actually feel the good-hearted schoolmaster's 'katzenjammer' – we *know how it is ourselves* – so very human are we all!"

Both the author and his publishers have asked a slender service of the editor: to separate web from woof, and this for the sake of those who are not possessed of that knowledge of Hahnemann's career which the benefits that many of such readers have had from his labours would seem to make the obligation of a becoming sense of gratitude. These, it is to be feared, are not to be found only among the laity. We do not learn that Bradford's Life of Hahnemann is 'out of print,' nor are we especially concerned when a generous publisher finds himself 'out of pocket' for an endeavour to provide us homoeopathic physicians with the bread of professional life – if indeed many of us are alive, at least, to our duty!

First then as to the staple of fact, indisputable fact. It is true that Hahnemann's father was a decorator of the porcelain ware for which Meissen was famous, and a by no means contemptible artist. True it is also that he was intellectually superior to many of his class, that he was a man of original ideas, and one who did make it a special duty to give his son 'lessons in thinking.' He sowed the seed of a harvest which many of us are selfishly reaping: our ingratitude therefore being equalled only by our ignorance thereof – and both a mute reproach to any breed of parasites. The morning interview in the garden is a pure figment, but the clay-lamp and the piously-purloined oil are the simple truth. It is equally true that Herr Müller's discernment of the latent promise of the boy Hahnemann prevented the porcelain painter from apprenticing his son to his own trade. The graduation thesis, with its significant topic, is happily 'yard wide and all wool.' The delighted schoolmaster's post-graduate jubilation – well, if Herr Müller didn't have the precise experience, he did have every justification for such an one, and he certainly neglected a golden opportunity: surely Solomon's 'time' is good enough for saint and sinner!

The patrimony of only twenty thalers is the unadorned truth, as the many privations of Hahnemann's student life in Leipzig could amply testify – but the benedictions often come to us veiled, and we recognise them not until after many days. The student life in Leipzig is not at all exaggerated, and the timely friendship of the physician Von Quarin is the greenest leaf in that worthy's chaplet: "As ye did to the least of these!"

The teaching and the night translating-work – honest wage-earning – are literally true. So, alas! was the salubrity of Dessau. Gommern was indeed terribly lanigerous. It is only a fond hope that there were 'two blankets' o' winter nights, for love alone is poor fuel. The pitiful accident during the exodus from Gommern did happen, but in the happier after years the memory of it lost its old-time pang.

After the physician's 'renunciation' there was found no need for the fictions of the fancy; the harsh realities of poverty furnish material more than enough. The clothes-washing, with potatoes for soap and the physician himself officiating at the tub, are such truths as adorn – do they not? –

"The short and simple annals of the poor."

And lo! in the radiance that now invests these stern privations we cannot see the sordid for the very shine of the metal of which those trusty hearts were made.

True also to the letter is the tale of the treasured hoard of dry crusts; and to-day we moisten them with our tears.

"All else of this fantasy," writes the author, "is the truth and the triumph of the truth – *the end of which is not yet!*"

The address, which is put in as an appendix at the editor's sole instigation, was not written for publication; but this editor heard it delivered, and it is his conviction that it should be published, and precisely where it now appears. Evidently in the author's mind the two writings are closely related. In the address he openly reproves the homoeopathic school in America for lapses that are not to its credit. He plainly intimates that homoeopathy to-day is taken up as a trade rather than espoused as a cause needing advocates who are penetrated by its truths. He insinuates, at least to our understanding of the address as we heard it spoken, that the mercantile spirits rather than the scholastic prevails in both professor, practitioners and students. The supreme aim and end of the student is the diploma rather than the qualification for it; the legal right to practise, without that moral right lacking which no graduate in medicine is other than a peril to whomsoever shall entrust life to *him*.

He by implication arraigns ever homoeopathic college that teaches the practice of homoeopathy without full inculcating its principles. He evidently ascribes the murrain of unbelief that pervades and perverts American homoeopathy to this shameless dereliction.

He most earnestly believes that Hahnemann is worthy of better advocates; and he is persuaded that every college of homoeopathic name or pretense can do no worthier work for years to come than teach the matriculate at least something of *the stature, the acquirements, the labors and the teachings of him who founded the homoeopathic school.*

He has his triumvirate of worthies, Hippocrates, Sydenham, Hahnemann, and measuring these by the record of their life-work, he acknowledges with devout gratitude obligations to each that are not to be measured with words; but when one asks him why do you bear the name of a 'sect,' he makes reply: *"In common gratitude for the truth he brings that cannot be found elsewhere."*

Contents

Introductory and explanatory: A Foreword for the lay-reader.

The artisan
The village *Wirtshaus* and its guests. The Porcelain Painter. The boy who was taught to think. "Mein Herren, I must go and give my boy his lesson in thinking."

The student
The interview in the garden. "*Mein lieber Freund*, what is this I hear from little Fritz?" "I, too, am a worker in clay, and shall I not seek for the fitting ornament?" The boy's clay lamp and the stolen oil. The schoolmaster's mishap in the *Wirtshaus. Sehr gemuethlich.* The graduation thesis. The graduation night: "He can only sometimes talk, but always drink." To Leipzig.

The physician and his renunciation
The medical student. Von Quarin's friendship. Baron von Bruckenthal's librarian. The graduate of Erlangen. The world as an oyster. Dessau. The largest old school dose the Porcelain Painter's Son ever took. The good folk of Dessau are so terribly healthy. The sheep of Gommern – both species. The exodus and the accident. The perils of thinking. The renunciation. "God help me, I will practise no more?" Chemist and translator. Potato soap. The bequest of the crusts.

The philosopher and his reward
Cullen's *Treatise of The Materia Medica*. The spark and the illumination. The application of the Baconian method. The philosophy of homoeopathy. "You can learn what any medicinal substance is capable of doing in the human organism by administering it, in suitable doses and for a sufficient period of time, to persons in health." The experiment *in corpore sano* enables the demonstration *in corpore vile.* The sunset. "And he arose and followed him."

Appendix: "Under which king, Bezonian?"
"*Under which king, Bezonian?*" A shoe which may fit various feet, but pinching as all "tight fits" do.

The artisan
From its two side windows the candle light was gleaming and flickering upon the facing leaves of the ancient oak that overshadowed Frau Weber's *Wirtshaus* in the quaint and quiet village of Meissen. Now and then a falling leaf would swirl through the line of light to be lit up by a transient gleam of radiance ere it sank into the shadow of the night. Even so did those artless villagers, one by one, themselves drop away: the gladness of an upright life lighting up their wrinkled faces as they too passed on into the shadow of the night.

Though cheery from without still cheerfuller was the *Wirtshaus* within. The Frau's genial *Gut'n Aben'* made the passing stranger welcome, and the comforting porcelain stove added its friendly warmth to hers. The ashen floor, nearly as white as a wheaten loaf, and the snowy sand that glistened thereon bespoke the tidy house-wife, while the polished lids of the row of beer mugs told at once of industry, cleanliness, and a wise concern for the comfort of her guests. In the place of honor on the wainscoted wall hung an old engraving of *Unser Fritz*, as the people still delighted to call him, and directly opposite, a series of old woodcuts illustrative of *Reinicke der Fuchs*. A vigorous likeness of Luther's rugged features and one of the good-natured face of Hans Sachs completed the collection, and suggested that Frau Weber's *Wirthshaus* had patrons of an unusual order. That fact was, indeed, the crowning glory of the Frau's life, for the choicest of the village were her nightly visitants. Yes, at the Frau's tables, which were polished until they were almost mirrors, gathered a variety of groups hardly to be met out of Germany. In the *Herren Stuebchen*, the *Pastor, Burgomeister, Doktor,* and the *Amtsnotar* met evenings, and over their wine talked upon matters too high for the common ken: their select company being shared on rare occasions by some passing traveller whose bearing denoted his superior station in life. In the main room a couple of toothless *Stamgaste* sat by themselves, and smoked and drank their beer, and exchanged their respective gatherings of the village gossip, and laughed and laughed again at the thousand-times-told jokes that were far older and even drier than themselves. Not far from these the always-jolly miller, the baker and several of the small shopkeepers met each other to discuss the crops and the market. Yet another group was composed of artisans from the porcelain factory, for which Meissen was chiefly renowned.

At this particular table might be seen a man of extreme plainness of dress for even one of his class, but whose face was singularly attractive. He had a broad, high forehead, dark, flashing eyes, that were overshadowed by the heavily-barred brow, and a well-shapen head, which was fitly crowned with luxuriant brown curly hair. Whenever he spoke his companions seemed to forget their beer and were intent only on listening. They rarely made a direct reply to him, but were prompt enough to put their questions. He always spoke in an unassuming manner and with evident deliberation, as if he held himself accountable for his lightest word. He had learned, long before Schiller had written it, that *Ernst ist das Leben*, and with that conviction constantly present, he lived as one realizing that he is ever in his great Taskmaster's eye.

Though one of the poorest men in Meissen, no one was more respected. The *Pastor* had always his friendliest greeting for the painter on porcelain – for that was his handicraft, and Herr Mueller, the schoolmaster, was never happier than when in his company; for which purpose, indeed, he had some time since forsaken the grander guests in the *Herren Stuebchen* in order to be with his favorite at the artisans' table. One attempt, at least, had been made to beguile the porcelain painter from the table at which his fellow-workmen gathered to the more pretentious one that was graced by the village dignitaries, and none other than the admiring *Pastor* had sought to bring about this change. But the prompt reply to the suggestion had been: "No; he boils himself a bad soup who forgets amongst whom he was born." Despite the reproof, the more than ever admiring *Pastor* could not keep this incident to himself, and when it became known the hearts of the artisans grew closer than ever to their manful companion.

The porcelain painter's home was rich in children – the poor man's wealth, whatever else the Fates deny. These were sent to the village school as soon as they were old enough, although the teacher's stipend was a serious drain upon the meager earnings of the father; but he and his good wife were adepts in those self-denials of the poor that give a heavenly luster to the lowliest lives.

On little lad, some twelve years of age, was the constant companion of the porcelain painter in such hours of leisure as his toilsome life allowed. Sunday after Sunday and on all holidays hand in hand they took their walks; and the father made Nature the book from which he taught his child. From flower, and leaf, and bird, and beast he had gotten his fresh and faithful designs for the pictures he painted on the porcelain vessels; and from long communion with nature he had learned something of the rare art of seeing. This he fain would teach his boy, leading his fresh young mind the while from the wonders of the created thing to the grandeur and glory of the Creator.

On these delightful days the sports of his schoolmates lost their zest for the porcelain painter's son. Nothing could then beguile him from his father's side; no schoolboy games could charm him into forgetfulness of the pleasant rambles when they strolled afar and ate their frugal noonday meal by the side of some rippling brook or in some nook filled with the hidden music of the forest's birds. The boy's grave thoughtfulness, his curious questions, and even the depth of his insight, filled the father's heart with thankfulness; and, lo! poverty forgot its every pang in a child's companionship the father tasted the delights of Paradise.

As was the custom in those days, and indeed is yet in *Vaterland*, each evening the father sought the *Wirthshaus* and there rested from his day's toil in the delightful calm which shuns the gilded palace for that humbler place – the like of which labour finds not on this earth. It was the nightly unbending of the bow that had been tightly strung all day, that would be re-strung day after day until the tired hand had lost its cunning and the eye grew dim and the worn out toiler became the pensioner of God. At these evening gatherings his companions observed that, invariably, at a certain early hour the porcelain painter emptied his *stein* and bade them *Gut' Nacht*. It mattered not how interesting the conversation or how rapt his listeners – as the finger of the clock pointed to the precise minute, he uprose and took his departure.

Such was the force of the porcelain painter's personality that none of his companions had ever dreamed of calling him to account for these abrupt leave-takings, which left them a silence that they still preferred to the platitudes of common talk – although that silence was as the ceasing of pleasing music. But one memorable night the talk had soared beyond its usual wont, and their pipes had gone out, and their beer had grown flat – and still they listened. The clock finger pointed to the well-known minute; the porcelain painter arose, his face shining with the light of the high truths they had been considering, and with his familiar smile, he had spoken his hearty *Gut' Nacht,* when Hans Lindermann, the very oldest of his companions, grasped him by the arm, exclaiming: "*O mein lieber Freund,* why do you leave us in the sky, from which we cannot get down unless we tumble, like Satan from Heaven!"

The porcelain painter smiled gravely and with a parting bow said: "*Meine Herren,* I must go and give my boy his lesson in thinking."

The student

The porcelain painter was an early riser, one who spent the sluggard's hour in the care of his little garden, which was one of the thriftiest in Meissen. He was tilling the cabbages that were to furnish the winter's *Sauerkraut,* when the schoolmaster approached, uttering a cheery *Gut' Morgen.* The salutation was returned ere the two were face to face, and before the hand-grasp was over the schoolmaster began, with the eager manner of one who had business near to his heart – "*Mein lieber Freund,* what is this I hear from little Fritz?"

"Ach, I am afraid you and the house-mother are teaching the boy to be rebellious," replied the father, laying aside his tool with the air of one who is preparing to make good his words.

"I teach your boy to be rebellious?" repeated the schoolmaster with deliberation in his every word as if he doubted his ears.

"Have you not counselled him to stick to his books; did you not tell him his fingers were never made to mould clay or wield a painter's brush? Tell me that, Herr Mueller." The enquiry was made with an earnestness that had in it a tinge of severity as from one who was being trifled with.

Said the schoolmaster: "Of a truth, I have." The words were spoken firmly and with the deep feeling that betokened a profound conviction of the probity of his counsel.

"It was not kind. You know my family is growing; more mouths to fill and broader backs to cover, and only the same two hands. And I have brought up Fritz to follow me in my ways of thinking; and I have always wished to see him as good a workman as ever moulded clay or painted porcelain. And I need his help to carry the load that is getting heavier every year. You, Herr Mueller, are putting yourself between the boy and his duty to me; and he is so fond of you that had you advised him properly, he would long since have been an entered apprentice. Is that right; is that friendly?"

The schoolmaster was deeply moved. "*O mein lieber Freund*, what if I did put myself between the boy and his earthly father, if I was then showing him his duty to his Father in Heaven?"

"Not so fast, Herr Schullehrer. You forget your lesson: what means it when that heavenly Father says, 'Honor thy father and thy mother?'" There was fire in his words and the flash of his dark eyes showed rising anger.

The schoolmaster's matutinal visit was made by pre-arrangement with the porcelain painter's wife; she was his ardent ally in abetting what her husband called his son's "rebellion." She had watched for the pedagogue's coming, and with a woman's wit had waited for the fitting moment to join the group in the garden, and this her husband's rising voice had indicated. As she drew near, the schoolmaster gave her his morning salutation with grave dignity, adding, "You have come happily, for my best friend is blaming me wrongly."

"Answer my question; do not hide in the bush, Herr Schulmeister," said the father sharply and sternly.

"House-father," interposed the wife. He turned her quickly: "Stop! Christina; *I am at school now*, and I have asked my teacher a question which he forgets to answer; you know not what it is."

She held her peace and the schoolmaster made reply. "What said the Christ when he left his father and mother in Jerusalem and they were obliged to turn back and seek him: 'I go about my Father's business.' I have studied your son as you do the piece of porcelain you are about to ornament. Has it been said that you ever put an improper design upon anything you have painted? You are an artist as well as an artisan, and you consider the fitness of the vessel for its ornament. *I, too, am a worker in clay,* and shall I not seek for the fitting ornament? My work is for the temple of the living God, and to Him must I make answer for any neglect of my duty. That you could teach your son the cunning of your hands is undoubted; but that he was not made to mould or paint porcelain my heart believes and my head *knows*. He has the divine gift for learning languages, and the tasks that are as mountains to his schoolmates are only ant-hills which he gets over with a single stride; and do you think I do not know what all this means. A precious stone of singular size and beauty is polished for the Emperor's cabinet, and a mind of rare promise must be cultivated for the glory of God."

"Amen!" said the mother, her eyes brimming with tears, as from under her apron she reached out her hand to her husband, holding in it a rude fashioned from unbaked clay: "O House-father, strive not against the will of the Lord! See this." She placed the little lamp in his hand. "When you forbade the boy to go on with his books, he made this lamp that he might secretly study with the oil I stole for him. Had he taken a house-lamp you would have missed it and found him out. You can put out the boy's lamp, but, O house-father, there is a light in the boy that only God who gave it can put out."

There was silence, and the porcelain painter stood holding the lamp in his hand, and the birds sang in the cherrytree, and the laughter of little children came ringing from the house.

"Perhaps you are wiser than I," said the father, speaking slowly and in a subdued tone, "but the little ones, whose laughter you hear, must be clothed and fed, and I not only cannot spare the help of my son: I *need the very money that must be paid for his teaching.*"

"That is already provided for," said the teacher eagerly, "nor is it charity, for even now he can assist me for as much as his teaching would cost, and soon he can earn something beside. You see, my friend, the God who endowed him is also shaping his way."

Slowly the father said: "I will think of this," and he parted with the rejoicing teacher after a hearty shake of the hand.

As the husband and wife entered their dwelling the schoolmaster was closing the little gate behind him, and a passer by could have heard him thinking aloud "I shall see that boy in the pulpit before I die!"

That night the schoolmaster went to Frau Weber's *Wirthshaus* with unusual eagerness. He knew the porcelain painter's promptitude, and he felt sure that his decision would have been made long before sunset. He went there with joyful expectation, for he saw that the father's heart had been deeply stirred at that morning's interview in the garden.

Alas, for the frailty of poor human nature! After the porcelain painter had left the *Wirthshaus*, it was soon to be seen that the schoolmaster was going beyond his allowance; *stein* followed *stein*, until he suddenly jumped to his feet and declared that every soul in the *Wirthshaus* must join him in singing "*Eine feste Burg ist unser Gott.*" The hymn was sang to humor him, and in the second stanza the schoolmaster's voice soared far above the rest.

"Mit unsrer Macht isn't Nichts gethan, Wir sird gar bald verloren:Es streit't fur uns der rechte Mann Den Gott selbst hate erkoren."

A little later, when the last belated guest had departed, Frau Weber's manservant was helping the *gemuethlich* schoolmaster to a friendly bed in the *Wirthshaus*.

There was but one other transgression of this nature during all the remainder of the schoolmaster's life, and that occurred on the evening of the day wherein his favorite pupil was graduated in the *Fuersten Schule* of Meissen.

Nearly the whole village turned out to hear the porcelain painter's son read his graduation thesis, *On the Wonderful Construction of the Human Hand.*

How the artless villagers did stare at one another and at the young man who had grown up under their very eyes, and yet could tell them so much about their own hands of which they had never dreamed. They had indeed found fingers and thumbs exceedingly convenient and useful, but until that day they had not really known what a hand is. The student's thesis pleased the exoteric hearers, who never think of reading between the lines; while the esoteric few fancied they discerned in it a delicate tribute to the well-known skill of the porcelain painter's hands.

Of this few was Doctor Poerner, and his delight surpassed all description. On one point, however, all were agreed, namely, that the porcelain painter had most assuredly given his son "lessons in thinking," had taught him to look beyond the mere surface show and to discern occult qualities that are so plainly discovered when once genius had pointed them out.

It was on the night of the graduation that the *Pastor, Burgomeister*, and *Amstnotar*, led by the exuberant Doctor Poerner, left the *Herren Stuebchen* and, gathering around the artisan's table, drank the porcelain painter's health, especially thanking him for the bringing up of a son who would "one day do honor to Meissen." Wineglasses clinked, beer mugs resounded on the oaken table, and a chorus of *Hochs!* Went through the roof of the *Wirthshaus* in a manner that might startle the stars.

When the toast had been duly honored, the porcelain painter arose. His face had a strange seriousness, and his voice sounded as if it came to him from afar. "*Meine Herren*: the praise is not mine. I would have made a horn spoon of that from which he," and he fixed his eyes upon the schoolmaster, "has produced a sword handle for the King." And then he impressively related the long-past interview with the schoolmaster in the garden. "Never," he continued, "can I forget his words: I, too, am a *worker in clay*, and shall I not seek the fitting ornament? My work is for the temple of the living God, and to Him must I give answer for any neglect of my duty.'"

Then upspoke the wealthy Burgomeister, addressing himself to the astonished schoolmaster: "Her Mueller, you are an honor to Meissen. Blessed is he that magnifieth his calling. Frau Weber, all these guests will drink with me the health of our faithful Schulemeister, and in your best wine."

The health was drank with fervor, and the overwhelmed schoolmaster attempted to make reply but his tongue clave to the roof of his mouth, and he could only stammer in helpless confusion.

"More wine!" shouted the blacksmith. "He can only sometimes talk, but always drink."

The Burgomeister clapped his hands at this sally and gave order for unlimited wine.

"Wein auf bier das rath ich dir."

So runs the rhyme; but, alas! the overjoyed Schulemeister was again put to bed in the *Wirthshaus*.

When the autumn came the porcelain painter's son started for Leipsic to prepare himself for the medical profession. He had twenty thalers in his pocket his whole and only patrimony; but he had in his heart principles that would bloom perennially, and on his head a father's blessing; and with him went a mother's prayers. Nor had Dr. Poerner forgotten him. The world is before him, and it is "a mad world, my masters."

The physician and his renunciation
"I can myself testify that while I was at Leipzig I honestly tried to follow my father's injunction neither to play a merely passive part in the matter of learning. Neither did I neglect exercise and fresh air, in order to preserve that strength of body by which alone mental exertion can be sustained." This is a glimpse from a retrospect taken when the seamy side of life was safely passed; but the testimony is too modestly stated. With his whole fortune of twenty thalers in his pocket, and that pitiful pittance much lessened before he had reached his destination, he who was to attend lectures and provide clothing, food and lodgings for himself must either find a Fortunatus' purse or make one.

But his graduation thesis had so pleased Doctor Poerner, Counsellor of Mines at Meissen, that he had written to the Faculty at Leipzig, telling them of the promise that lay unfolded in the poor student, and everyone of the professors remitted his fee. This was a precious lift, and the student proved his worthiness by the most unremitting attendance upon their lectures. He also taught languages, and made translations for the booksellers: Leipzig being even then the chief book mart in Germany. His zeal and industry were such that he often worked throughout the night. Without robust health and one of the best of constitutions he could never have withstood such wearing toil.

After two years of study at Leipzig he went to Vienna for the sake of that hospital experience which was not then to be had at the former place. There his exemplary conduct won for him the esteem and friendship of the Physician in Ordinary to the Emperor; and of whom the grateful student wrote, in happier days that were still far off, "Freiherr von Quarin singled me out, loved me and taught me as if I were his sole pupil in Vienna, and even more than that; and all without expecting any pecuniary from me." We are not obliged to take only the grateful student's word for this – Professor Bischoff also has written: "Freiherr von Quarin bestowed on him his special friendship." It is also well known that this favourite student was the only one whom von Quarin took with him on his visits to his private patients. And later on, when his slender earnings were insufficient to enable him to continue his studies for the obtaining of his diploma, it was still von Quarin whose good word secured for the porcelain painter's son the position of resident physician at Hermannstadt, under the patronage of Baron von Bruckenthal, of whose extensive library he also took charge. "No, your Excellency; not yet a graduate, but fully competent for the professional responsibilities of the physician; and your Excellency will also find him a scholar, a fine linguist, and one not a stranger to the value and uses of a library"

Twenty-one months' service in this field enabled him to earn sufficient to go to Erlangen and take his degree.

Now the world is before him; as a duly qualified physician he can choose his abiding place. Softly! the world is the oyster of only him who can open it.

The heart of the porcelain painter's son hungered for Saxony, as he says only a Cur Saxon can, and he settled himself for practice in the little town of Hettstadt, but only to find, after a nine months' sojourn, that it had little need for a physician. He then removed to Dessau, where he found some patronage and, what was better, a wife. The largest "old school" dose he ever took was a druggist's daughter; and in his circumstances it must have been that two blankets are better than one which determined the bold step for the impecunious physician. Alas! the wife and the supplementary blanket were about all that he got in stony Dessau; and wives must be fed and blankets wear out, and the good folk of Dessau are so terribly healthy!

At the end of the first year of his marriage he was appointed District Physician at Gommern, in which position he will receive the Government's stipendium as an official. Bravo! the oyster is opening! Courage, and patch the thin blankets! The young wife shared his delight to the full, and to Gommern the couple went. Never before had there been a physician in that place; he had a fresh field and all to himself. Surely, his prospects were rosier than even the blushing dawn of his double-blanketed wedding-day!

Three years this couple existed in Gommern, but how they only know, for the State stipend was but a pittance, and not even the apothecary father-in-law could coin the gold in stony Gommern to help them: the daughter and her blanket being all that he could bestow.

Lack practice? Bless you! he never lacked practice; he was busy enough to satisfy even so earnest a man as he. He was gathering precious experience every day; he was putting drugs to the test, and in after years he naively admitted that his patients would have come off better had he given them nothing – and that is more than true of much of the therapeutics of the lecture room and the laboratory to-day. Strange as it may seem, breeding bacteria is a costly pastime for even a philosopher; naming them affords harmless occupation for bookmakers, and such breeding and christening is called "science." Now there is both the science and the art of Medicine; let the philosophers have their fill of science, but in God's name! let the sick have the art. They do not need your "cultures;" they are asking, and largely in vain, for "destructions," and *that* not of *themselves!*

They physician, let it be known, has to deal with four species of patients; the rich and the poor. But that is only two varieties! Aye, but the poor are subdivisible: there are "the Lord's poor, the devil's poor, and the poor devils." Before leaving Gommern the famishing physician approached one of the first class in this category, a well-to-do farmer, and asked him frankly why he had never patronised him. The reply is worth preserving: "Herr Doktor, we people have lived in Gommern four hundred years without one of your kind, and we cannot play foolish now for your sake. If you could do anything for a sick sheep, we might find use for you."

The disgusted District Physician sought a place where sheep were not supreme. He hired a *Fuhrwerk*, packed into it his household goods, wife and children – for, somehow, children come whether practice pays or not – and shaking off the dust of his feet as a testimony against all swine, departed from Gommern.

O implacable Misfortune, thou who delightest in doubling the misery of those on whom once Fate has frowned, why art thou so relentless, why dost thou shower they fiery darts as well upon the just as the unjust, on gray-haired sire and helpless babe alike? Doth the old, old *Weltschmerz* need aught from thee!

Whilst journeying from Gommern a bad place in the highway caused the *Fuhrwerk* to overturn and tumble down a steep declivity until it rested in a brook swollen by the rain that had undermined the road. An infant son was so severely injured that he shortly after died; an older daughter broke her arm, and as if this were not enough, his household effects were sadly damaged by the water. Some peasants helped the unfortunates to the nearest village; and when the fractured arm was healed the father's slender purse grinned gauntly in his face.

It is a sordid picture but it is the truth. In the mysterious orderings of Providence this discipline was needful for the developing of even so upright a man as the porcelain painter's son. But, although he had not been able to emerge from the poverty in which he was born, he still had a robust body, a brave heart, and the patience and the indomitable courage that are akin to these – and these must sustain him when there comes to him the still darker dispensation.

If my reader has been led to regard this man as merely an unsuccessful practitioner he must rid himself of that most erroneous conception. He was, instead, that most successful of all practitioners – a thinking one! In the unremunerative years that he had lived he not only faithfully followed up his father's "lessons in thinking," but he had also carefully husbanded, rigidly scrutinised and unflatteringly questioned every day of his professional life; and all this was to bear precious fruit, although as yet not even the bud could be seen. In the several insignificant villages wherein he had valiantly struggled for a bare subsistence, he had nevertheless written some books that were not unheeded in their day, and are noteworthy even to-day. His contributions to chemistry had won for him the encomiums of Berzelius, and Hufeland ranked the struggling physician among the very first of his profession in Germany. Jean Paul, *der Einzige*, termed him that "double-headed prodigy of leaning and philosophy," – and yet this learning and philosophy were destined to bring him to the very brink of despair. O ye who would go smoothly through life, swim with the tide, spread your sail to catch the "trade winds;" ask no troublesome questions; let others do the deep-thinking, and the challenging of the old beliefs: then shall you never behold the bottom of your meal tub grinning at your greenness.

The porcelain painter's son had already asked too many questions, and still each day brought a new one, deeper-reaching and more perplexing. In Gommern, in sheep-loving Gommern, he had owned to himself that the sick would really have done better had they taken no medicine whatever: yet he was fully abreast with the so-called science of his day. Hufeland's famous *Journal* had no contributor whose papers were more warmly welcomed. But his questions led him deeper and deeper, while day after day his doubts grew stronger and stronger, and in vain did he say to himself: "It is not I who am at fault; it is the art of Medicine that is wrong." Daily this unwelcome conviction deepened, until at last he asked himself: "If I think that the sick will fare better without our hap-hazard medicines – and in my heart I do so think – why do I practise? Am I honest in so doing? I know that I can prescribe as skillfully as the best of those who now give medicine; but if I am convinced that the *sick will do better with no medicine at all* – God help me! I will practise no more!"

From the hour of his renunciation he turned to Chemistry, and he has left an enviable name in the history of that science; he also worked night and day as a translator for his old friends the booksellers. But with all his toil, and he could, indeed, *toil*, the publisher's pittance was small, and even German frugality was taxed beyond its possibilities. O genius of Poverty, help this struggling pair with every honest device that Necessity can conceive; help the good house-mother's needle to out-do the cunning of Penelope so that she may indeed.

"Gar auld claes luik amaist as weel as new."

Alas! one may cheat the back, but the belly is inexorable; and the cry of a famishing child – merciful God, is *that* ever heard in Heaven!

One day his faithful wife's face betrayed her; she was in the depth of a quandary; her husband saw this, and questioned her.

"Well, House-father, our clothes, although they are poor, must not also be dirty: I want to wash them and I have no soap."

He turned to look at her, dropping his pen, and he could be see that the rosy cheeks, that won him in those early days at Dessau, were worn and faded. He sprang from his table and kissed her. "No soap? Well, I must teach you a trick; and as I must also show you how it is done, I will wash the clothes, and without soap."

His little son, Fritz, looked on with a pair of wondering eyes, and soon called his sister from her play to see the grave House-father bare-armed at the washtub.

Despite the remonstrance of the wife and her expostulation that for him to do her work would disgrace her as a reputable Hausfrau, he performed the feat of washing the clothes without soap – using potatoes because they were so much cheaper.

The thin, worn cheeks were not forgotten, and until the coming of better days one of the most learned physicians of Germany assisted in doing the family washing.

And now, brave heart, be stronger still, for there is yet a cup of bitterness that shall search thee still more sorely.

They were living, oh, how frugally, on the small earnings of the father's pen; their only bread the black, barley loaf of the peasant, and that there might be no words of complaint about the equitable sharing of it, the father dealt it out by weight, each receiving the portion due. One day a little daughter, who had long been dropping, fell seriously ill. The poor sufferer could not eat, but she piously treasured up her daily portion of black bread against the time of her recovery, when the accumulated hoard would enable her to enjoy, oh, such a bountiful meal; and her eye lit up as she saw her hoard increasing.

Perhaps it was in a dream that the Messenger told his errand, for the child knew her doom; so one day she called her favourite sister to her and solemnly bequeathed to her the dry black crusts, telling her that she herself should never recover to eat them.

Bear up, brave heart; the uttermost bitterness of thy renunciation is reached; the night is dark; there shines no star, but be steadfast to duty: lose not sight of that. Bear up:

"God's in His heaven;
All's right with the world."

The philosopher and his reward

In Medicine, the fame of William Cullen was second only to that of Hermann Boerhaave, and when the porcelain painter's son was wearing the thorn-crown of his renunciation the Scottish professor was the brightest luminary in the firmament of the medical world. One day, fresh from the Edinburgh press, there came his famous *Treatise of The Materia Medica*, and the enterprising German publisher put it at once into the hands of his hack for translation.

Now, despite the privations that had followed his renunciation of the practice of Medicine, the porcelain painter's son had kept up his habit of thinking, and whilst he was translating the Scottish physician's text there came to him a ray of light in the darkness. It was, indeed, the dawning of a brighter day for Medicine than any of which he had ever dared to dream.

How that strange *thought* haunted him; he could not dismiss it, and yet it was distracting his attention from the text he was to translate. He had not half finished his daily sting, and his children's voices remind him that they must be fed; but work he could not, that one *thought* had laid a spell on him. With a sigh he laid aside his pen and went forth into the fields, but nature had lost her charm for him, because that importunate *thought* followed him like his own shadow.

This *thought* came to him in the shape of a question, and this question challenged him to experiment. He experiment! He play the leisurely philosopher when he had barely time enough to provide a slender living for his family! But he found no peace; experiment he must and experiment he did. O Spirit of the long-dead porcelain painter, be near to him whom thou didst teach to think; guard him from error, clarify his sight, direct his steps, for he has reached the parting of the ways and the issues thereof are those of life and of death!

The *thought* that had so disturbed the porcelain painter's son had in it both a question and a conjecture; and his first experiment had answered the question by confirming the significant conjecture. For him this was not enough. He had all the sanity of Genius, and he knew that the value of a single instance must be proven to be not an exceptional quantity but an invariable; it must be the constant result of law, not the chance product of accident. How he was tempted to neglect the daily task that brought him bread in his eagerness to follow the clue that would lead him – whither? He did not know, nor did it then enter into his fondest imaginations to conceive; but he remembered those heroic student days of strenuous endeavour in Leipsic, and he lived a double life of translating and experimenting.

O Joy! after each successive experiment there came again, and again, and again, ever the same, the unvarying result. He continued piling experiment upon experiment; getting from each new experiment the positive confirmation of the first, Heaven-inspired conjecture, until it seemed as if his list of positive affirmations had been lengthened unto superfluity. Then he turned from his experiments to formulate the *thought* that had disturbed him when he was labouring over the pages of Cullen's *Materia Medica*, and the formula took on this shape:

> *Any substance that relieves diseased conditions will produce similar conditions when taken in suitable quantities and for a sufficient period of time by those in health; and it is this property in drugs that makes them medicines.*

He was ready to distrust his own formula, for was he not the first of woman born to frame it? But was it not buttressed by hundreds of careful experiments, and had he not invariably received the self-same reply whenever he had interrogated Nature with the Heaven-sent clue in his hand?

He had also the modesty of genius, and he asked himself if it could be possible that he alone of all the race had discerned the new truth; whereupon he began to ransack the records of medicine from the earliest period. Thanks to Herr Mueller, the faithful schoolmaster of Meissen, who had long before seen that the porcelain painter's son had "the divine gift of tongues," and had made a struggle that this gift might not be despised and rejected: thanks to his insight, for his pupil was now enabled by his linguistic attainments to make an exhaustive search throughout the whole realm of medical literature. On reading the records he soon found that Jewish, Arabian, Greek and Roman physicians had reported cure after cure which had been accomplished by the use of the very same drugs that had produced in him the likeness of those recorded diseases when he had experimented on himself, his family and his friends with the self-same drugs. Better even than this, he found that Hippocrates, "the divine old man of Cos," had sanctioned a method of practice based upon the very formula which he himself had reached by the strictest Baconian investigation. He found, too, that Haller had recommended experiments with drugs upon the healthy body, "in corpore sano," in order to determine the *actual effects* of these agents. But Haller had also taught that it was then necessary to experiment again with the same drugs upon the sick, "in corpore vile," in order to learn what the same drugs would do in disease. As a drug cannot possibly act the same in a healthy body and in one that is diseased, because the conditions under which the experiment is made with it are not the same or even similar, of what use, then, is the Hallerian *experiment upon the healthy body?* Suppose that Haller had learned by experiment with a hitherto unknown drug upon a healthy man that it acted by making him vomit; what value had that for a system of therapeutics whose armamentarium was already rich in emetics? But suppose that an experiment upon a healthy man with the new emetic showed the physician *in just what kind of an attack of vomiting, occurring in a sick man,* that very drug would relieve the sufferer "quickly, safely, and pleasantly?" Then, indeed, is there sense in and need for the experiment *upon the healthy man.* In fact, in this very feature alone and only is there any philosophical justification for the experiment upon the healthy: why else should a person in health be put to such discomfort? The pseudo-science that declares otherwise is a delusion and a sham, or in the words of one of its own disgusted disciples, such a system of therapeutics is "the withered branch of medicine."

The porcelain painter's son found, to his own surprise, that he had of a certainty gone beyond all the previous generations of men in the realms of rational therapeutics. He had stripped the art of its perplexing uncertainties because he had based the proper exercise of it upon a law of nature. He had learned the alphabet of Nature, and with it he could read her therapeutic method. And he, first of all men, said to the world:

> *You can learn what any medicinal substance is capable of doing in the human organism by administering it, in suitable doses and for a sufficient period of time, to persons in health.*
>
> *It will then evince its properties by producing symptoms, or "signs," of distress that were not felt before taking it; and it is this property of causing symptoms that makes it a remedy for them when they occur as disease.*

Why? Because that very drug will dissipate such symptoms in the sick as it is capable of causing in the well.

How do we know this? First, by experiments with this drug upon the healthy alone – which experiments will show what symptoms that drug is capable of occasioning – and, secondly, by administering that very drug to the sick presenting similar symptoms, which it will abolish in every case of curable disease.

This last procedure is not "an experiment upon the body in disease:" it is, instead, a demonstration of Nature's law that LIKE IS TO BE TREATED BY LIKE.

If this is pronounced only theory by some caviler, it still has this somewhat unusual merit amongst theories, as theories go, namely – it can be tested by precise experiment and thereby exposed, if false. It differs from all other therapeutic systems in that it challenges such a refutation from foe and friend alike. "This doctrine appeals not only chiefly, but *solely*, to the verdict of experience – 'repeat the experiments,' it cries aloud, 'repeat them carefully and accurately, and you will find the doctrine confirmed at every step' – and it does what no medical doctrine ever did or could do, it *insists* upon being 'judged by the result.'"

The boy who was *taught to think* is a Pontifex who could not, indeed, bridge the universal grave, but he has erected a *Pons asinorum* impassable forever to pseudo-science.

With this new light upon his path the porcelain painter's son resumed the practice of Medicine. His guide to the treatment of any disease being first to get all the symptoms, or "signs," of it by every possible method of examination known to the science of Medicine; his further process thereupon to find what drug produced a similar set of "signs," – then, upon administering that drug, *in justa dosi*, recovery followed in accordance with Nature's law of cure.

As he had discovered what symptoms each drug would produce by its action, *singly*, upon the human organism in health – for, if he mixed drugs in such an experiment, how could he learn what symptoms each ingredient produced? – it follows that he gave each drug *singly* in the disease whose total symptoms most closely resembled the total of effects it produced in the healthy experimenter. This, too, is not the device of a theorist; it springs directly from the very therapeutic law which selects a given drug from all other drugs for a given congeries of symptoms, on account of the nearness of similitude.

Having discovered the therapeutic law by experiment, and being confined by it to a single remedy in prescribing, it still remained for experiment to determine if the quantity of the dose is a matter of indifference. On resuming the practice of medicine under the guidance of the newly-discovered therapeutic law the porcelain painter's son at first administered such doses, in quantity, as were given by his fellow physicians of the method of practice that he had renounced; but he thereupon found that as a drug selected from the similarity of its action to that of the morbific cause of the disease for which it was being given, aggravated, or intensified, the very symptoms for which it had been given, it was, then, a matter of necessity that the quantity, or, as he termed it, the potency of the dose should be diminished. This reduction he soon began to make; and the same experience that obliged him to make the first reduction in the quantity, or potency of the dose, remained to denote the limit to which that reduction of the dose should be carried. In this, likewise, he was influenced by theory. This step was also the outcome of experience; so that both the single remedy and the diminished dose of direct derivatives from the law of similars and essentials for the practice of Medicine under this law.

So far the man who had learned to think had followed the Baconian path, and thus far his conclusions are impregnable. He could have burned every line that he had written in exposition of his discovery and still prove the truth of this therapeutic law *by the literature of the very school that he had abjured*; and if its doubting disciples denied the records of their own teachers, he could still challenge them to disprove the newly-discovered therapeutic law *by such experiments as had led him to its discovery*. Such a refutal can never be accomplished, because before the creation of man the fiat of the Eternal had gone forth framing the laws that were to govern the universe, and so long as the universe is governed by law the therapeutic truth that *magis venenum magis remedium est* must remain as fixed as gravity itself. To find the *remedy* in the *poison* is possible only under and by the guidance of the law of similars it matters neither how loudly the heathen rage nor how long the people imagine a vain thing.

The porcelain painter's son was granted not only a far-off Pisgah vision of the Promised Land; he was also permitted to labour therein and to partake in all honour of the fruit of his long toil. Those years of storm and stress, so sore in the time of fiery trial, so grievous to the flesh, had in them the blessing that was "for the healing of the nations."

Ripe in years, richly rewarded with earthly goods, loved by the afflicted and revered by the world's wisest and best, he found his exceeding great reward. And while he sat in the vineyard, in the cool of the evening, there came to him the messenger of the Master of the Vineyard: and he arose and followed him.

Appendix: "Under which king, Bezonian?"

"Bezonian. From *bisogno*: a new levied soldier, such as comes needy to the wars." – Florio.

A lecture delivered by request of the faculty in the amphitheatre of the first Homoeopathic Hospital at Ann Arbor, Michigan, on the evening of 13th April.

The request of the faculty that I would lift up my voice once more in this familiar place was accepted promptly, as Dr. Dewey can testify; and this not that I am particularly fond of hearing my own mouth. I have heard that so long (and so have my friends) that it is getting monotonous. My friends are too polite to tell me so; but I know it "just the same." Moreover, there is the quiet evening at home, the weary feet in the easy old slippers; the faithful pipe (almost the only friend that never "goes back" on us), the favourite books, whose charm grows stronger and dearer from the knowing that each reading is bringing one nearer and nearer to the last: all these combine to keep a spavined and wind-broken ex-professor away from places like this. Nevertheless, at the call, I at once agreed to come. Why? That is just exactly what I am going to try and tell you.

I am obliged to be somewhat autobiographic, for I am going to deal with history of which I am a small part. That is why you must pardon so much of the "I" as will of necessity enter into this talk.

Only once before have I spoken in this very room. The occasion was the inauguration of the first Homoeopathic Hospital. To me, that was an impressive occasion; to-night it is even a solemn one. Then I looked into friendly faces that have long since gone as we must all go. Well do I remember just where they sat, those faithful old members of the *Homoeopathic Hospital Association*. Believe me, you who are here tonight, I speak as one talking to the sacred dead. I may fall into error, for that is human, but not for all that I have will I knowingly utter one word which from its insincerity could disturb them where they are *now*. This is not the place for rancor; it is not the time for reproach: the utmost that can be allowed is reproof for wrong-doing, mis-doing, *not* doing - this and the friendly warning of the first and oldest worker in this field.

In the twenty-three years that this college has existed there have been many changes. This is stale news as regards the college; but it is not the college alone that I have in mind. I mean the outside changes that affect not only colleges but all in them and the great majority out of them. Civilisation, as we delight to call it, has its mumps, and its measles - diseases incident to certain periods. Civilisation is prone to delirium: what else was the Salem Witchcraft? Civilisation has also its intervals of serene lucidity, and of storm and stress through which and by which the race levels a new lift and leaves the fabled anthropoid ancestor farther and farther in the slimy depths of that Christless hypothesis. These are the changes I mean; and how strikingly and startlingly History reveals them! At times we need a long perspective to discern them, and this History affords. Contrast the England of Cromwell with that which Charles the Second directed: the one a conventicle resounding with psalm and prayer; the other a brothel of ribaldry and all unspeakable abominations. What an oscillation from one extreme to the other, from the supernal splendours of Milton's divine Epic to the unutterable lecherous leprosy of Wycherley's comedies.

Writers ascribe these mysterious transitions to an occult *Zeit-geist*, Time-spirit, Spirit of the Age. Its influence it is that inaugurates now a "truce of God" and now a saturnalia as lurid and infernal as the French Revolution. In the dark days when "the heathen rage and the people imagine a vain thing" the faint of heart despair: as if the Eternal had fallen short of His purpose, as if OMNIPOTENCE were baffled!

It is "through the shadow of the globe we sweep into the younger day." The astronomical fact is also the eternal fact behind and beyond all sublunary things. We may not question the Eternal's plan, we dare not interrogate His purpose. Duty remains; duty in sunshine, duty in storm; duty in the darkest night – and to each comes the fateful challenge: *"Under which king?"*

The now-prevailing *Zeit-geist* is a questioning spirit, a doubting spirit, a mocking spirit, and it delights to masquerade disguised as Science. Science is "knowing" and the Spirit of the Age assumes the name though it does *not* know – it only itches *to* know. Its field of enquiry is the Natural, it does not recognise the Supernatural. It does not believe there is anything above and beyond sense. It does not *know* that there is not; and yet it is science and science is "knowing." It is a pretender in "knowing." It is a pretender in all that pertains to the supernatural; it is also a pompous pretence and braggart in much that pertains to the Natural as distinguished from the Supernatural. Such is the Spirit of the Age in which we live; a questioning spirit, a doubting spirit, a mocking spirit, an irreverent spirit. To it nothing is sacred, not even the truth; for it is a falsity itself in that it assumes to know that which it does not *know*. Chemistry, for its purpose, is called a precise science; yet chemistry is playing the juggler with hypothetical "atoms." Optics is an experimental and yet is also called a precise science; yet optics is spinning cobwebs from hypothetical "undulations" in an equally hypothetical "ether." Mathematics itself, the most precise of all sciences, at last reaches a sphere wherein its conclusions are lame and impotent contradictions. "Thus far shalt thou go and no farther" is the edict pronounced to the intellect, and that by no mortal Canute.

For the science that recognises the pride-purging limitations, the science which led Newton to compare himself with a child that has picked up a single pebble on the shore of a limitless ocean – the "knowing" that it *knows* so little – for this I have only reverence. But the science that is not clothed upon with humility is an arrogant mockery, a specious pretence. It is not the science for which men revere the Newtons and the Faradays: at its best it is knowledge without wisdom and therefore without humility. It is a foolish suckling that cries for the moon. Pseudo-science is making night hideous with that very cry.

Man and the monkey have one trait in common: both are imitators. We do not, indeed, know that the monkeys are stuck up on this account; but many men are certainly proud of their proficiency in this line. Hence the popularity of the "fad." What is a fad but the device of one monkey imitated by others? Suppose "science" is made a fad: will it be obliged to offer a premium for science-aping Simians?

It does not so appear. Many men are nothing if they are not "scientific" and worse than nothing when they are. Because some other men are scientific they would be considered so.

Understand me now beyond all chance of mis-conception: I am not referring to the science represented by a Newton and a Faraday, the Science that has the meekness of humility, the *Knowing* that *feels* the Illimitable. I mean the science that falsely assumes the name, the arrogant science; and the special imitators to whom I refer – the tailless monkeys – are those whose assumptions are doubly false, because they affect this miserable "science" without even that knowledge of it which might, perhaps, palliate so pitiful an affectation. These are what might be called the pseudo-pseudo-scientific; these display all the arrogance of its assumptions without possessing what little of real "knowing" it may have. These are dreaded by all real scientists because like the bull in the china-shop, they can only make havoc with the stock in trade – they can only "smash things." Emerson has said: "The grossest ignorance does not disgust like this ignorant knowingness."

What if any number of such "scientists" should point the pop-gums of their "science" against the only system of Therapeutics that has law for its basis, law for its application, law for the experiment upon the healthy in the laboratory, law for the demonstration upon the diseased in the hospital. Suppose the noise of these innumerable little popguns were such, so incessant, so importunate, so indefatigably clamorous, that it distracted the student's attention from everything else. Suppose it dinned the ears of the practitioner at each bedside until he forgot everything else. Suppose it bewitched learned editors as the pied piper of Hamlin's tune did the other vermin. Suppose it usurped the ears of the teachers in the colleges until they, the gowned apostles of the faith, began to shoot their own little popguns and add to the clamor. Were not all this an enviable state of affairs! Thanks to the doubting, unbelieving, mocking, irreverent *Zeit-geist* and the "pure cussedness" of human-nature, such is the state of *things* to-day. The so-called "homoeopathic" medical student is insensible of the infinite riches of his inheritance as a student *of homoeopathy*; the homoeopathic practitioner is irresolute, his feet are not fixed on the bed rock that underlies his therapeutic system, but his hands are dirty with coal tar products that are a reproach to therapeutics as a science, and he himself is blown hither and thither by every varying wind of doctrine; the editors – well, homoeopathy to-day has some editors, she has also *editors* "to burn" – the boneless sardines of the sanctum; the professors – well, I want to return in safety to my family to-night, so "mum is the word!"

Professors, editors, practitioners, student I rejoice that such is the state of things, for it is the extremest oscillation of the pendulum to the sinister end of the arc, and not all the powers of darkness (editors included) can avert or pervert the directly opposite swing. That is the divine compensation for all these dark ministrations. The truth must ever be tried by fire; blow on Beelzebub, heat the crucible until the metals melt; dross shall be utterly consumed, the refiner shall see his own face clearly in the thrice-refined residuum of sterling truth. I may not behold the completion of this purification with these old eyes of mine; but the Refiner has never yet failed of His purpose, never can fail. On that you may depend forever!

The Time-spirit, flippant, mocking, doubting denying and irreverent; these I say are its characteristics. Consider the unabashed mendacity of the newspaper: who believes the modern newspaper? Consider the depravity of the modern theatre, given up to the froth and filth of the debased drama. Consider the cloud that overshadows our courts, the highest as well as the lowest. Consider the mad struggle for wealth and the paralyzing power of riches. Consider the present purchasing-power of gold – it is the Juggernaut that is crushing the death what little of truth and manliness there is left. Singleness of purpose, serious earnestness, sweet humility – all these are "Caviare to the general."

"There is no money in them," says the Time-spirit: and it does not openly say it but it means, "There is nothing else in them." The Time-spirit hath taken an inventory of all things, and marked them with their price: only the fool refuseth a good offer!

The flippancy, the mockery of all worthiness, the unbelief, the denials and the irreverence of today are the dry rot of the end of the century. And what is the outcome of all this? In the *nominally* homoeopathic school certain men have called in question Hahnemann's teachings, when the difference between them and him is such that they could not untie his shoestrings without a step-ladder. Men who are stultified by their record; testifying to the efficiency of potencies in one decade, denying it in the very next. If their first testimony is not reliable it challenges the competence of the testifier; if the first testimony is untrue what credentials have we for the veracity of the second. These are the pseudo-pseudo-scientists whom learned editors should put into the pillory, with the record of their infamy posted above their heads. But journals and medical societies have the rather encouraged and disseminated the spawnings of such 'critical' cretins.

Remember that the right to critical doubt, the right to call in question, the right to challenge is vested in knowledge alone. The ignorant, the unqualified, the neophyte should be dumb; the adept, proven and approved, should not. All else is mere babblement, idle vanity, a mockery and a sham.

When the 'scientific' homoeopath – the most perilous of wild fowl – assails Hahnemann's teachings in the windy medical journal or on the floor of the windier medical society, how many homoeopathic students are qualified to judge the critic and the criticism? Indeed, I may ask, how many homoeopathic physicians? How may of either have ever read the *Organon*; how many have given it the serious and intelligent investigation that it both deserves and invites alike from friend and foe? If one is grossly ignorant of the *Organon*[i] – that declaration of, exposition of and defence of the principles and practice of homoeopathy – by what shadow of right does such an one assume the title 'homoeopathic' physician? Does a dabster in the practice, as an art, pretend to a knowledge of the principles, as a science? Has not homoeopathy too many of such pretenders – 'doctors' that cannot for the life of them deliver the goods they advertise? Can the truth, the absolute truth, the simple truth be presented, defended and triumphantly demonstrated by such advocates?

"The mill cannot grind with the water that has passed," and I should bitterly reproach myself for my failure to include the study of the *Organon* in the early curriculum of this college, were it not for the turmoil and torment of its first five years. I appeal to any old-time student who may be present whether in those early years I did not have both my hands and my heart full.

Aside form the intrinsic value which we its special acceptors find in it or ascribe to it, the *Organon* has indubitably these merits, and has them merely as a contribution to medical literature, namely, scholarship that evinces wide research, and experimental investigation – much of which latter in is fields entirely new. Especially do I now refer to Hahnemann's *dynamisation theory*. The *Organon* is the production of a scholar and philosopher: of a man whom Jean Paul Richter pronounced "a double-headed prodigy of learning and philosophy."

I have, indeed, known some professors of the peck-measure species who called this estimation into question. They were 'all right:' what else could be expected from a peck measure? This is a free country, and every professor has the right to demonstrate his own capacity, but he shouldn't forget that in the process he is also making evident the extent of his own *in*capacity. A common jackass appreciates the difference between a peck and a bushel: some professors are not up to that discernment! Do not conclude that I am referring to professors of the non-homoeopathic variety only. No; I have heard a "homoeopathic" peck-measure derogate Hahnemann in this very room; have heard more than one of such 'do up' Hahnemann – but he did it only with his mouth. And on those very seats sat the students of homoeopathy, and the professor talked and talked at them,

> "And still they gazed and still the wonder grew
> That one small head could carry all he knew."

(The college was nearly dead in those days, and I suppose that is what brought such 'blow flies' here.)

The *Organon* has this peculiarity among medical books: it does not solicit unconditional acceptation: it does, however, challenge you to repeat the experiments upon which it is based, and to show by the results that it is a delusion and

---

i. *The Organon*, as an exposition of the homoeopathic doctrine, of necessity includes the Introduction to Hahnemann's *Chronic Diseases*.

a falsity. Read Hahnemann's introduction to the pathogenesis of *Ipecacuanha* – then ransack the literature of Medicine and find me such another challenge as that. You cannot; nor has the man been born that can.

The history of homoeopathy shows that the *Organon* did not meet with unconditional acceptation; there were those who would not swear by the words of the master.

That pioneer quarterly, the *British Journal of Homoeopathy*, bore on its title-page the significant motto: "In certis unitas, in dubiis libertas, in omnibus charitas." It is a modification of the original, which reads, "In *necessariis* unitas." The modification is too dogmatic: Unity in matters that are certain is quite different from Unity in matters that are necessary. Hahnemann's theory of dynamisation did not establish the 'certainty' of that theory, but the teachings of the *Organon* indubitably declare the 'necessity' for dynamisation. When Hahnemann challenged the world to put to the test the therapeutic system that he advocated, he said "Imitate exactly." This makes the 'potency' as we term it, a 'necessity.' This all his adherents have not allowed; but can you 'imitate exactly' without it?

It will be a fortunate day for you under-graduates when the hard knocks of experience shall have taught you that the 'potency' is indeed an essential factor. I learned this late, but I have learned it! For long years I was a 'kicker.' In my first pocket-case every liquid was a mother tincture and not a single trituration had I above the third decimal. Surely, it was a kind Providence that saved me from becoming the undertaker's delight! To tell you the truth, for confession is good for the soul, I once got an arsenical poisoning nicely started – and I wasn't making a proving on a patient, either. Oh, but I was stiff-necked bull of Bashan in those days: you see, I knew a great deal more then than I do now. A few years after that exploit with a low potency of arsenic, I was instigated by a fellow physician to turn my microscope upon the triturations of the metals. I did so, and just as fully expected to blow up the dynamisation theory as the man who touched the button did the unsuspecting Maine. I will only add that the end of that line of research led me to make some dilutions myself and to carry them as high as the thirtieth. I did this so as to know that I had the thirtieth. I began to test them clinically:

It is my firm conviction that the man who expects to *blow up*, not the theory of dynamisation, but the fact that dilutions are potential therapeutic agencies, has most assuredly "bit off more than he can chaw." The phrase isn't elegant, but the *fact* is. My faith in the potencies is not a suit of old clothes inherited from a professional god-father. It was made to order; it was made to fit; I earned it and I have paid for it; I, too, can give account for the faith that is in me. This is not egotism; I have earned the right to declare that I think I am qualified to take the stand as a witness; and for that you will find me *semper paratus*.

I do not care to specify how many years it is since the homoeopathic 'scientists' began to "get in their work" on the theory of dynamisation. They have since been blown so high that if they are "docked for the time they were up in the sky" it will bankrupt the breed. They appealed unto Caesar, and "science" is the Caesar of that appeal. To annihilate one theory they attack it with another. They took Hahnemann's dynamisation theory and Dalton's atomic theory, tied these by their tales and hung them over the clothes line to fight it out after the manner of the Kilkenny cats. Of the cat they bet on there is only the *tale* left – it is, indeed, "a thing of beauty," but it is not "a joy forever," as they would have the simple imagine.

The night would fail me to tell you of the funny things these 'scientists' did with their microscopes and of the impossible things they tried to do. I give them the 'benefit of the clergy' – and they need it.

Dalton's atomic theory needs what are called molecules. It assumes them. Hahnemann assumed his *dynamis*. As what is sauce for the goose is sauce for the gander, we will let these assumptions offset one another, and call the two theorists, Dalton and Hahnemann, "even." But, says the *homoeopathic* 'scientist,' the molecule is recognised by its behaviour under certain conditions. That is exactly true of the *dynamis*, declares the *Organon*. At the end of this round Hahnemann and Dalton are "even" again. (If it goes on in this way it is going to be a drawn battle). But long before these homoeopathic 'scientists' were clout-stainers, the *Organon* declared that a certain degree of subdivision set free a *dynamis*, or spirit in every material substance, which thereupon displayed properties not observed in the undivided substance.

That is the dynamisation theory in a nutshell. Now it had been better if Hahnemann had remembered Newton's *"Hypotheses non fingo."* Alas! it is the itch of trying to explain the unexplainable that trips us all. That trituration and succussion "set free an imprisoned spirit" is an hypothesis framed to explain a fact. The fact is impregnable; the hypothesis is a flimsy figment. You can demonstrate the fact; the explanation of the fact is a bird that you can never catch by sprinkling the sale of hypothesis on its tail.

Be it remembered, there were no hypothetical molecules dreamed of when the dynamisation theory was framed; otherwise Hahnemann might have said: liberated drug-molecules display therapeutic properties not observed in the crude substance. What then? Simply this: the latest discoveries in molecular physics would bear him out and would bring forward a Crookes' tube to make the visible demonstration of the fact. The clinical application of the homoeopathic 'potency' is the Crookes' tube that substantiates the fact in the Hahnemannian theory of dynamisation.

I said the appeal was unto Caesar, and science the Caesar of that appeal. It is to be hoped that 'scientists' of the homoeopathic species will go to school and learn the alphabet of science: then they may be able to read the hand-writing on the wall. It is quintessential irony itself that a graduate from the medical college over the way – the orthodox church around the corner – has recently written in a devastating little book that the latest discoveries in molecular bear out every one of Hahnemann's teachings that pertains to that branch of science. I have yet to read any refutal of his declaration. I commend his book to the attention of those professors who annually annihilate Homoeopathic with their – mouth. Really, I do not believe the jawbone of an ass is what it is "cracked up to be!"

Turning for a moment to the science that is not 'homoeopathic,' to the science that "has the name blown in the bottle, none genuine without it," we find in it some singularly suggestive thought for the homoeopathic physician. At present this science is deeply enamoured of what it is pleased to call "cultures." In other words, its bottled bacteria, microbes, bacilli – things that are made even more formidable by the names given them in scientific baptism. Let some of these sesquipedalian indescribables conclude to hold a 'family reunion' in the neighborhood of the appendix vermiformis, and lo! the scientist who has "caught on" has his exceeding great reward; for the inevitable "operation" fetches anything from five dollars to five thousand. "Thousands of dollars for a skilled operator," writes a New York surgeon recently, and the tender pathos with which he mentions 'our beautiful surgery' is infinitely touching. Some of these uncoscientifics say these festive picnickers are the *causes* of disease; others just as severely scientific declare that they are the *consequences* of disease; and still other scientists find that these identical critters with unpronounceable names are *present in both health and disease*. You who are students here pay your money and take your choice; but you may be conditioned at your examination if your fancy doesn't happen to coincide with the 'partikiler vanity' of the professor of bacteriology in your immediate vicinity. It is dangerous to 'monkey' with the scientific buz-saw, isn't it?

But having bereft the colon of its appendix (and pocketed the fee), the performance is not yet over. Science is as insatiable as the worm that never dies. The word reminds me that it is the patient that has to do the dying, not the surgeon.

He that cuts and gets his pay
Remains to cut another day.

That is when 'tuberculosis' sets in. The 'operation' was a splendid success, thanks to 'our beautiful surgery,' and the 'tuberculosis' is also a success. If you doubt it, just ask the sleek undertaker. And this is 'Science,' – God save the mark!

The latest pronouncement of this charnel-house science is that tuberculosis is omnipresent – it has a railroad pass and the freedom of the city; for its bacillus may play its pranks any- and everywhere.

Now you pitiful 'homoeopathic' physicians who are hankering for the flesh-pots of such 'science,' please remove the caked boracic acid from your ears and listen. I propose, as you are so fond of names, that we exchange. Just for a few minutes – I don't mean a 'swap for keeps.'

I am fully satisfied with an older name than 'tuberculosis.' Instead, then of 'tuberculosis' read *'psora.'* Science says that tuberculosis is omnipresent: it can play havoc anywhere. Hahnemann had long before said as much of *psora*. All that science to-day explains by its last rag doll, 'tuberculosis,' Hahnemann had far earlier 'explained' by his *'psora.'* One calls it a bacillus, the other a dyscrasia: what does it matter to the *pathological fact* underlying both names?

"'Tis strange there should such difference be
'Twixt Tweedledum and Tweedledee."

And while the 'schools' are splitting hairs about names, names, names the smitten are languishing and dying. O Science and pseudo-science stop your 'cultures.' Death will see that germs do not become extinct. Turn from them, and in the name of God and Humanity, provide us with saving destructives. Such songs as you are singing have no music in them for the aching hearts of the widow and the fatherless.

Having mentioned the pathological fact underlying the names *'psora'* and 'tuberculosis,' allow me to give what I believe an evidence of the existence of such a fact, call it what you will. The last visitation of the epidemic called *la Grippe* came to us in the early winter of 1889, and with some modifications has continued ever since. The genius of the epidemic has not changed, the qualifying adjectives have; but these do not perplex or deceive the philosophical observer. The homoeopathic physician who found the simillimum in 1889, and it is a single remedy, did his work 'pleasantly, quickly and safely' with it; he could, as a rule, dismiss his patient on the fourth day. Now the pathology of the epidemic disease explains the cardiac sequelae, the derangement of the heart's rhythm, the choreic ventricular action, and that "heart failure" which is such a convenient name for that shot-rubbish – a physician's ignorance.

Now in many of the cases, the majority, in fact, treated by me in 1889 the heart to-day is doing as well as it ever did, while in others the heart has never been right since. Why? I am not going to offer a dogmatic theory – for I hold all theory cheaply – but remembering what Hahnemann has written of *psora* (of the pathological fact), I incline to the belief that the cases treated by the undoubted simillimum for the *genius epidemicus*, yet having these deranged hearts in spite of it, are instances of the psoric diathesis, or dyscrasia. There is certainly in these cases something that frustrates the complete curative action of the simillimum for the grippe pure and simple. A philosopher calls it *'psora,'* a modern microscopist calls it 'tuberculosis:' be it whatever it may, the thing for you to remember is that, changing the names or throwing them both away, the science of to-day corroborates the hard pathological fact which is independent of any name.

This is all that true science can ever do for and to homoeopathy: corroborate whatsoever of truth it hath in it. There is not a single truth entrusted to the mind of man that need fear aught from science, for Science is ever and always the servant of Truth.

Considering the peculiar environment of this college, have not some of you, teachers as well as students, at times forgotten this? O ye of little faith!

Teachers and students, remember your inheritance; be proud of it; be true to its demands; forget not its deservings. Devote all that in you is to the comprehension and *apprehension* of it; make all knowledge, the fullness of knowledge, tributary to it – for such all truth is.

Like the prince in the story, Science is walking the earth with the lost glass slipper in its hand seeking the rightful wearer thereof. Many false claimants are "trying it on" and vainly. In the fullness of time Cinderella shall be known; contempt and contumely may be heaped upon her by the proud and haughty ones now in high places; but it is she only whom the prince will espouse.

Now go from hence and witness the blandishments of 'science;' behold the glamour of her laboratories, hearken to the tales of wonder told therein. Hold fast all that is good. Then read your Organon, master it, apply its truths at the bedside. Let the years bring to you the ripe fruit of all this. Do not be impatient. Remember that

"Knowledge comes, but wisdom lingers."

Perhaps when you are gleaning the precious aftermath in thankfulness, you may give a passing thought to the memory of the worn-out workman who came to you by night, bringing the challenge: *"Under which king?"*

References

1 Jones, SA. *The porcelain painter's son: a fantasy,* Philadelphia, Boericke & Tafel, 1898.
2 Winston, J. *The Heritage of Homoeopathic Literature,* Tawa, Wellington, Great Auk Publishing, 2001, p. 161.
3 Winston, J. *The Faces of Homoeopathy,* Tawa, Wellington, Great Auk Publishing, 1999, p. 15.

INDEX

Aconite 7, 123, 161, 261
Ægidi, Dr Julius 91-96
American Institute of Homeopathy 10, 88
Ammonium carbonicum 62
Anacardium 62
Anhalt-Köthen, Duke of 8, 9, 119, 180, 212, 235
Antimonium tartaricum 217
anti-psoric remedies 62
Apis 163
apothecaries 8, 212
Arnica 25-29
Arsenicum 261
Arum triphyllum 261

Bacon, Francis: *Novum Organum* 6, 143, 146, 147, 181
Ball, John: *Modern Practice of Physic* 5
Baptisia 261
Belladonna 7, 133, 16, 261
Berkley, Helen 9
Boenninghausen, Dr C von. 79, 82, 87, 92, 93, 95, 96, 97, 291
Boenninghausen, Madame 79
Borax 62
Bradford, Dr Thomas Lindsley 13, 55
British Homoeopathic Association 274, 280
British Homoeopathic Journal 140, 166-167, 268-270, 323
British Homoeopathic Society 139, 199, 273, 274
Bruce, Dr Mitchell 253
Bruckenthal, Baron von 5, 302
Brunonian system 247-248
Brunton, Dr Lauder 248-249, 251
Bryonia 163, 217, 291, 294
Büklerin, Henrietta 5

Büchner, Dr 30
Burford, Dr George Henry 274
　　Address to JH Clarke Memorial Meeting 274-280
Burnett, Dr James Compton 13, 268-270, 290
　　First Hahnemannian lecture - *Ecce Medicus* The life and work of Hahnemann 101-138, 202, 260
　　obituary 99-101
　　paper: On gonorrhoea with reference to the sycosis of Hahnemann 259-268
Bute, Dr George H. 57

Calcarics 163, 291
Camphor 8
Chlorine 62
cholera 8
chronic disease 261, 267
Cinchona 6, 13, 116, 122, 129
clap disease, *see* gonorrhoea
Clematis 62
Clarke, Dr John Henry 1, 221-223
　　Clarke Memorial Meeting - report 273-295
　　Clinical Repertory 221
　　Constitutional Medicine 221
　　Dictionary of Practical Materia Medica 221, 289-291
　　The Prescriber 280, 282-284, 291, 293-294
Cleave, Egbert
　　Biographical Cyclopaedia 3, 110
　　Biography of Hahnemann 3-10
Columbus 6
Cooper, Dr Robert 268-269, 273, 290, 291

Conium 261
Cullen, Dr William 70, 106-107, 112-115, 126-128, 146, 173, 187, 202-203, 216-7, 302

D'Hervilly-Gohier, Marie Melanie 9-10, 55, 79
Dublin 67, 69, 87
Dudgeon, Dr Robert Ellis 1, 135
  Biography of Hahnemann 106
  books on the human eye 167
  correspondence with the Editor *Homoeopathic World* 268-270
  obituary 165-168
  pocket sphygmograph 168
  The Hahnemann Oration 241-258
  The Third Hahnemannian Lecture – Hahnemann the founder of scientific therapeutics 169-195
Dunham, Dr Carroll 1, 87-89
  Essay – Memorial 89-95

Ecce Medicus, see Hahnemannian Lectures
Epsom salts 33

Falconer, William: *Waters of Bath* 5
Fleischmann, Dr 8
Frankenberg, Minister von 30
Freud, Dr Sigmund 57

Gardner, Dr WT 247-248
Gelsemium 163
Georgenthal 14
gonorrhoea 259-268
Gotha 30

Haehl, R 79
Hahnemann, Christian Gottfried 1, 4
Hahnemann, Johanna Christian, née Spiess 4
Hahnemann, Dr Christian Friedrich Samuel
  books
    Æsculap auf der Wagschaale 135
    Instruction for Surgeons in the Treatment of Venereal Disease 109
    La falsification des medicamens dévoillée 132
    Lesser Writings 201, 204

Materia Medica Pura 7, 8, 59, 68, 135, 175, 182, 212, 214
Medicine of Experience 1805 13, 135, 143, 175, 208
Organon of rational medicine/Organon of rational art of healing 2, 8, 13, 58, 68, 89, 135, 142-163, 169, 175, 181, 208
Pharmaceutical Lexicon 132
The Chronic Diseases, their specific nature and homoeopathic treatment 55, 58-65, 182
concepts
  individualisation 82
  life force 41-53
  miasm 60, 262
  minimum dose 7, 39
  provings 6, 83-84
  psora, psoric 60, 62, 259, 261, 262, 264, 266
    anti-psoric remedies 62
  similars 6, 68-69, 116, 122-123, 173, 177, 185, 195, 261
  sycosis 63, 259-268
  syphilis 63, 68, 259, 261-264, 266, 268
essays and papers
  Are the obstacles in practical medicine insurmountable? 143
  Helleborism of the Ancients 234
  Homoeopathic reminiscences 80-85
  Investigations on the nature of gall and gallstones 109
  On antiseptics 109
  On arsenical poisoning 109-110, 201
  On the human hand 107
  On the means of avoiding salination & other ill effects of mercury 109
  On a new principle for ascertaining the curative powers of drugs 131, 132, 143, 204
  On the positive effects of medicine 8, 173
  On the preparation of Glauber's salt 109
  The advantages of using coal as a means of warming 109

The genius of the homoeopathic
    healing art 41–53
followers – dates/timelines 1–2
life
    biography by Egbert Cleave 3–10
    boyhood 103–105
    defence of thesis 211–212
    life and works by Dr JC Burnett
        103–140
    life of Hahnemann written as
        hagiography by Dr SA Jones
        299–327
    old age & death 10, 212
    parents 3–4
    philosophy of life 31, 313–317
    professional life 108–110, 309–313
    reminiscences 80–85
    schooling 4, 104–105, 200, 225, 304
    student life 4, 5, 105–10, 302,
        305–309
    works and results by Dr Alfred Pope
        199–219
letters
    to Dr Stapf 7
    to newspaper and journal 36–37,
        201–202, 204
    to patient 2, 13–35, 241
locations
    Altona by Hamburg 36
    Brunswick 25, 30, 129
    Dessau 5, 134, 300
    Dresden 5
    Erlangen 5, 200
    Gommern 5, 200
    Hamburg 31, 33, 34, 36, 133
    Hermanstadt 5
    Hetstadt 5
    Konigslütter 25, 26, 27, 29, 129, 131,
        132, 133, 137, 208
    Köthen 2, 8, 9, 71, 80, 101, 130, 132,
        137, 181–184, 180, 181
    Leipzig 4, 6, 7,8, 107, 110, 136, 137,
        176, 179, 209, 300
    Meissen 3, 4, 10, 11, 70, 107, 302
    Paris 2, 9, 10, 55, 80
    Pyrmont 23, 129
    Torgau 8, 35
    Vienna 5, 8, 200

Walschleben 129
Wolfenbüttel 129
portrait by Hesse 3
prescribing
    diet 13, 14, 21, 30, 34, 84
    electricity 16, 18, 19, 20, 21, 22, 30
    exercise 14, 16, 21, 23, 28, 29, 35
    Iceland moss 35
    moral advice 31
    remedies, see under individual names
        of remedies
    silk 29
    water, clyster of 33
    whalebone 29
translations 5, 106, 134, 207
Hahnemannian lectures
    The First Hahnemannian Lecture – Ecce
        Medicus 101–138, 202, 260
    The Second Hahnemannian Lecture – The
        Organon 142–163
    The Third Hahnemannian Lecture –
        Hahnemann the founder of
        scientific therapeutics 168–195
    The Fifth Hahnemannian Lecture –
        Hahnemann's works and results
        199–219
Hahnemann, Melanie, see D'Hervilly-
    Gohier
Haller, Albrecht von 14, 113, 122–123, 134,
    154, 173, 175, 187, 204, 315
Helleborus 261
Hempel, Dr Charles Julius 41, 58, 92, 165
Hering, Dr Constantine 1, 40, 55–58
    Direction of cure, law of 57–58
    Preface to Hahnemann's *Chronic
        Diseases* 58–65
    Preface to first American Edition of *The
        Organon* 72–76
    *Guide to the Progressive Development of
        Homoeopathy* 63
Hesse, Alexandre Jean-Baptiste: portrait of
    Hahnemann 3–4
Homoeopathic Medical College of
    Pennsylvania (HMCP) 40, 55, 96
Hufeland's *Journal* 6, 71, 132, 134, 143, 201,
    204, 208
Hughes, Dr Richard 1, 268–270
    obituary 139–141

The Second Hanemannian Lecture – *The Organon* 142–163
Hyoscyamus 13, 25, 26, 69, 123

Institut für Geschichte der Medizin, Stuttgart 3
International Hahnemannian Association 39
Iodine 62

Jenner, Dr Edward 7
Jones, Dr Samuel Arthur 1, 3, 297–299
  The porcelain painter's son – A fantasy 299–327

Kali bichromicum 163
Kayser, Secretary 18, 26

Lachesis 163, 261
Leipzig Society of Economical Science 5
Lippe, Dr Adolphus 1, 39–41, 55
London Homoeopathic Hospital 101, 274
London School of Homoeopathy 101–102, 140, 168, 199, 241, 276, 277, 283
Lutze, Arthur 87, 89–96
Lycopodium 291

Maclaggan, Dr 217–218
Magendie 7, 217
Mathiolus 7
Mercurius solubilis 5, 109
mercury 68, 109
Miller, Magister 4

Nessler 22
New York Homoeopathic Medical College 88
Nitrate of potash 69
Nitric acid 68–69, 263–266
North American Academy of the Homoeopathic Healing Art 57
Nugent, C: *Essay on Hydrophobia* 5
Nux vomica 163

Opium 13, 33, 34, 69, 122
Ornithogalum 289

Peruvian bark, see *Cinchona*
Petroselinum sativum 265

Phosphorus 62, 217
Pope, Dr Alfred Crosby 1
  obituary 197–199
  The Fifth Hahnemannian Lecture – Hahnemann's works and results 199–219
Pulsatilla 163
Pyrogenium 261

Quarin, Professor (Dr) von 5, 106, 302
Quintessence of Toads 171
Quintessence of Men's Bones 171

Reichsanzeiger 29, 36
Reinicke 22, 23
Rhus tox 163
Richter, Jean Paul 7

Salmon, William 171
Sandford, Sir Daniel 174
scarlet fever 7
Schröder, Secretary 18
Schuchardt, Bernhard 13, 18, 36
Selenium 261, 291
Sepia 291, 294
Silica 62, 163
similia similibus curentur, see Hahnemann concepts – similars
Society of Homeopaths 79
Solanum dulcamara 116
Stahl, Dr 123, 146, 173, 187
Stapf, Dr 7, 182
Steadman's *Physiological Essays* 5
Stickler, Dr 33
Stoerk, Baron Anton von 122–123, 204, 229
Stramonium 123, 261
Stratten, Samuel 67
  Preface to British Edition of *Organon* 68–72
Sulphur 62, 69, 163, 291
Sympathetic ointment 172

Tafel, L 165
thaler 36
Thuja 264–265, 267, 270
timelines 1–2
Tübingen 13

UK Faculty of Homeopathy 79

Veratrum album 7

Wagner, Dr 200
Wander, Mr 33
Williams, Dr CJB 246